# Cultures of Oral Health

Oral health is integral to wellbeing and quality of life. This important edited volume brings together leading scholars to address global oral health and the multiple ways in which theory, practice and discourse have shaped it in the modern period.

Structured around key themes, the book chapters draw on interdisciplinary perspectives in order to consider the role of the dental profession, the commercial sector, charities, the state, the media and patients in shaping oral health in the past and present. Collectively, the chapters consider the extent to which each of the studied groups and actors have sought to own and control the mouth. By adopting multiple perspectives, the book highlights the importance of cross-disciplinary work across the sciences, social sciences and humanities and provides a road map for a new interdisciplinary field focused on oral health and society.

Drawing on perspectives from dentistry, sociology, history and the wider humanities, this book will interest students and researchers of dentistry, public health, sociology of health and illness, the medical humanities and history.

**Claire L. Jones** is Senior Lecturer in the History of Medicine at the University of Kent, UK.

**Barry J. Gibson** is Professor in Medical Sociology in the University of Sheffield's School of Clinical Dentistry, UK.

# Routledge Studies in the Sociology of Health and Illness

# Cultures of Oral Health
Discourses, Practices, and Theory

**Edited by Claire L. Jones and
Barry J. Gibson**

Routledge
Taylor & Francis Group
LONDON AND NEW YORK

First published 2023
by Routledge
2 Park Square, Milton Park, Abingdon, Oxon OX14 4RN

and by Routledge
605 Third Avenue, New York, NY 10158

*Routledge is an imprint of the Taylor & Francis Group, an informa business*

*British Library Cataloguing-in-Publication Data*
A catalogue record for this book is available from the British Library

*Library of Congress Cataloguing-in-Publication Data*
A catalog record has been requested for this book

ISBN: 978-0-367-49851-1 (hbk)
ISBN: 978-1-032-28907-6 (pbk)
ISBN: 978-1-003-04767-4 (ebk)

DOI: 10.4324/9781003047674

Typeset in Goudy
by MPS Limited, Dehradun

# Contents

# Figures

# Tables

# Contributors

**Catherine Carstairs** is a professor at the University of Guelph, where her work focuses on the history of public health. She is the co-author with Bethany Philpott and Sara Wilmshurst of *Be Wise! Be Healthy!: Morality and Citizenship in Canadian Public Health Campaigns* (2018) and *Jailed for Possession: Illegal Drug Use, Regulation and Power in Canada, 1920–1961* (2006). Her new book *The Smile Gap: A History of Oral Health and Social Inequality* is scheduled to be published by McGill-Queen's University Press in 2022.

**Blánaid Daly** is professor of Special Care Dentistry (SCD), School of Dental Science, Trinity College Dublin (TCD) and consultant at the Dublin Dental University Hospital (DDUH). For the past 30 years, she has combined her academic interest in DPH with the clinical specialty of SCD, returning to TCD in 2016 as professor. In 2020, she was appointed to the Lancet Commission on Global Oral Health Inequalities and was joint winner of the Aubrey Sheiham award for distinguished research in dental public health, from the International Association of Dental Research (IADR). Her overarching research interest theme is the reduction of oral health inequalities for people living with disability and vulnerable groups.

**Alison Dougall** is consultant for medically compromised patients at Dublin Dental Hospital and director of the three-year specialist clinical training and doctorate programmes in Special Care Dentistry at Trinity College Dublin. She has led dental care services for the past 15 years at the National Coagulation Centre and was awarded Healthcare Leader in Ireland in 2017 for her work in developing oral healthcare pathways for adults with bleeding disorders in Ireland. Alison is the current president of the International Association for Disability and Oral Health, and in 2021, she was awarded the prestigious John Tomes Prize by the Royal College of Surgeons in England to recognise her significant contribution to the advancement of global health care.

**Abdulrahman Ghoneim** obtained his bachelor of dental surgery from Egypt before moving to Canada where he obtained his master's in dental public health from the University of Toronto. He is also a fellow of the Royal College of Dentists of Canada and is currently pursuing a doctorate degree from the University of Toronto.

**Barry J. Gibson** is a professor of medical sociology at the School of Clinical Dentistry, University of Sheffield. His work focuses on using oral health and dentistry as a case to answer wider questions about health in society. His work has focused on questions related to accounts of illness, drug use and oral health as well as how such accounts of illness are organised. He uses a range of theoretical and methodological traditions in his work, including systems theory, grounded theory and narrative research methods. He is published widely in oral health and dentistry as well as medical sociology.

**Michael Glogauer** is a clinician scientist with a focus on inflammation, microbiome and oral cancer. He is a professor at the Faculty of Dentistry, University of Toronto, where his research over the past 25 years has focused on the mechanistic contributions and interplay between neutrophils and microbiome in oral and systemic health. He is the head of Dentistry for the University Health Network and chief of Dental Oncology at Princess Margaret Cancer Centre.

**Alexander C. L. Holden** is an executive at a dental hospital, senior clinical specialist and academic with extensive experience working within the public health and higher education sectors. Alexander holds specialist registration with the Dental Board of Australia in Public Health (Community) Dentistry and is internationally recognised for his work on oral health systems, dental ethics and healthcare professionalism. He is the head of Specialist Services at Sydney Dental Hospital and Oral Health Services and holds an appointment as a clinical associate professor with the University of Sydney School of Dentistry where he is the head of Subject Area for Professional Practice.

**Claire L. Jones** is a historian and senior lecturer in the history of medicine at the University of Kent. Her research focuses on the history of commoditized medicine and health and examines the relationship between the medical professions, the market and consumers, emphasising themes of ethics, technology, professionalisation and commercialisation. She has published widely on these topics and her current focus is the history of oral health inequalities and the role of the market in shaping them.

**Jennifer Kettle** is a sociologist, and research associate in the Academic Unit of Oral Health, Dentistry and Society in the School of Clinical Dentistry at the University of Sheffield. She has worked on a number of projects and clinical trials related to people's experiences of aspects of dental care and oral health. This includes Significance of the Mouth in Older Age, an interdisciplinary project funded by GlaxoSmithKline investigating older people's experiences of their mouths, teeth and oral health over the life course. She is interested in the sociology of health and illness, family and other interpersonal relationships, and everyday life.

**Rizwana Lala** is a dentist and dual registered clinical public health specialist – dental public health (General Dental Council) and public health (UK Public Health Register). She works as a consultant in public health and is an honorary clinical teacher in dental public health. She undertakes interdisciplinary sociologically informed public health research that bridges the research–practice gap. Her principal academic interests centre on patriarchy and coloniality in healthcare and public health practice. Her writing on dentistry, healthcare and public health has also featured in local and national magazines.

**Herenia P. Lawrence** is an associate professor in the discipline of dental public health in the Faculty of Dentistry at the University of Toronto. Dr Lawrence's research explores population-based and preventive clinical and behavioural interventions that seek to improve the oral health of marginalised populations and reduce oral health inequalities in Canada. She has received a number of grants from the Canadian Institutes of Health Research (CIHR) and published widely on Early Childhood Caries (ECC) preventive interventions. She is a vocal advocate for the oral health of Indigenous Peoples and increased access to dental care for newcomers to Canada.

**Patricia Neville** is a sociologist and senior lecturer in social science at Bristol Dental School. She advocates for a social science perspective to dental/oral health research and dental education. Her current research interests are in equality and inclusion issues in dentistry, digital technology and social media in dentistry, dental/healthcare professionalism and a sociology of oral health. These research interests build on her previous/ongoing work in the sociology of gender, health and education.

**Carlos Quiñonez** is a dental public health specialist and Vice Dean and Director of Dentistry at the Schulich School of Medicine and Dentistry, Western University. His research centres on the politics and economics of dentistry, with a specific focus on health and social equity. He is regularly called upon by government and non-governmental agencies to provide advice on issues of dental care policy.

**Sarah E. Raskin** is assistant professor at the L. Douglas Wilder School of Government and Public Affairs and member of the iCubed Oral Health Equity interdisciplinary research core at Virginia Commonwealth University. Cross-trained in medical anthropology, health services research, and public health, Sarah conducts mixed methods community engaged research on dental safety net policy and practice in the United States. Sarah is a board member with the Association for the Anthropology of Policy, and a co-chair of the Future of Public Oral Health Workforce

Implementation Team with the Virginia Health Catalyst. Sarah's research has been funded by the National Science Foundation, Agency for Healthcare Research and Quality, and Patient-Centered Outcomes Research Institute.

**Jonatan Samuelsson** completed his PhD in 2022 in the history of science and ideas in the Dept. of Historical, Philosophical and Religious Studies, Umeå University. His doctoral thesis focused the late twentieth-century dental amalgam controversy in Sweden. Among his teaching and research interests are twentieth-century history of science, medicine and media.

**Sasha Scambler** is a sociologist and reader in medical sociology in the Dental Faculty at King's College London. Her current research focuses on experiences of living with long-term conditions and disability, and the application of social theory to inequality in all its various forms. She has published widely in these areas and is currently working on applying Bourdieu's conceptual framework to health and healthcare. She is an editor of the journal *Sociology of Health and Illness* and a contributing editor of the British Sociological Association (BSA) affiliated 'cost of living blog'.

**David Scott** is a medical ethnographer, writer and film-maker. He was previously employed as a dental surgeon for NHS Scotland, then an epidemiologist for Health Protection Scotland, before taking up a fellowship granted by the National Institute for Health Research at the University of Bristol. In 2019, he returned to the University of Dundee with a fellowship from the Healthcare Improvement Studies Institute and became a visiting scholar at the University of Cambridge. His current work explores how reflexive and ethnographic film-making can be used to visualise, and intervene in, the practice of medicine.

**Helen Strong,** Helen's academic interests lie within the history of child health and welfare in the nineteenth and twentieth centuries, and the history of dental health. She recently worked as research officer at the University of Kent's School of History under Dr Claire Jones on the 'Oral Health Inequalities, Oral Hygiene Cultures in England, 1870–1970' project. Helen has also lectured at the University of Greenwich on the BA Childhood and Youth Studies and BA Education Studies programmes. She is currently writing up her PhD thesis.

**Ryan Sweet** is lecturer in humanities and director of the Humanities Foundation Year at Swansea University. Most of his research to date has centred on the cultural and literary histories of prosthetic body parts. He has published several essays on this topic, including (most recently) a contribution to Clark Lawlor and Andrew Mangham's *Literature and Medicine in the Nineteenth Century*. Thanks to generous funding from the Wellcome Trust, his first book, *Prosthetic Body Parts in Nineteenth-Century Literature and Culture*, was published in 2022.

**Lorna Warren** is senior lecturer in social policy at the University of Sheffield. Lorna's research is centred on the topics of ageing and care and she has published widely in these areas. She has held grants under four major research programmes, local (DWP/ Sheffield City Council), UK (ESRC) and European (EC). In her most recent research, Lorna has collaborated with colleagues from dentistry to look at the significance of the mouth in old age. Lorna draws from a mix of anthropological, social policy, sociological, social gerontological and feminist perspectives and approaches, which she has also applied in her interdisciplinary studies.

**Bonnie Yu** is a dental public health specialist and fellow of the Royal College of Dentists of Canada. She is an analyst at the Royal College of Dental Surgeons of Ontario, the provincial regulatory body for the profession, and an instructor at the Faculty of Dentistry, University of Toronto.

# Acknowledgements

This edited volume is supported by the Academy of Medical Sciences/Wellcome Trust through a 'Springboard – Health of the Public 2040' grant 2017–20 [HOP001 \ 1031]. The editors would like to thank the publisher and the authors of respective chapters for all of their valuable contributions to this collection.

# 1 Oral health: an interdisciplinary or multidisciplinary approach?

*Claire L. Jones and Barry J. Gibson*

'Dental crisis is a social justice issue' begins an online article by Healthwatch England, a national watchdog, from May 2021 (Healthwatch England, 2021a). Research by the watchdog suggests that 80 per cent of patients are unable to obtain timely oral care, which has been exacerbated by the lockdowns under the Covid-19 pandemic. Some patients have been asked to wait three years for an appointment, while one patient was in so much pain that he extracted his own teeth (BBC News, 2021). Some patients have been charged £400 for the removal of one tooth and one individual reported being asked to pay over £7,000 for dentures privately (Healthwatch England, 2021b). People aged over 55 from ethnic minority groups and those on low incomes have been particularly hard hit by this dental crisis and are reportedly six times more likely to avoid treatments due to costs than their White counterparts. Such findings are reflected globally, particularly in low- and middle-income countries, with children living in poverty, socially marginalised groups, and older people being the most affected by oral diseases and least able to access oral health care (Watt et al., 2019). Such reports, and the ongoing research in dental public health, not only reveal low standards of dental health provision at a national and global level but also demonstrate that social inequalities in oral health, and in health more broadly, are currently being widened by systems in urgent need of reform (Anderson et al., 2021).

As the aforementioned discussion demonstrates, oral health is a social justice issue (Otto, 2017). Good oral health is a key marker of social advantage, while poor oral health suggests the opposite. Oral health is not only a central aspect of overall health that is integral to wellbeing and quality of life for individuals of all ages but reflects the nature and priorities of the political state of which it forms a part. It is not only part of health and biomedicine but also a key subject for science, a disciplinary activity, a profession, government policy and big business, all of which have preventing and treating oral disease as their primary purpose. But oral health also has a history (or histories) that impinges on its present and future; it has a social object – the mouth – that is worked on, manipulated and changed. Across time and cultures, the mouth has been viewed as a passageway to death in the Hellmouth of the fifteenth and sixteenth centuries and of the soul to heaven,

DOI: 10.4324/9781003047674-1

and as a way of rebirth in the myth of Ngakola in Africa and the Christian Mythology of Jonah, the word of wisdom (i-ching) or God (Gibson, 2008). The mouth is a portal, an interface, an erogenous zone (Otto, 2017, p. 3). Inevitably, how societies perceive the mouth has political and social consequences that, in turn, affects state, medical and societal responses to oral health and disease. Yet, despite the fact that oral health touches upon so many aspects of the lived experience, there is no volume of research that brings together these diverse aspects in one place. This edited volume seeks to address that lacuna by bringing together some of the world's leading scholars to address oral health and the multiple ways in which theory, practice and discourse have shaped it in the modern period.

What the reader will find here is a series of encounters centred on oral health between the disciplines of anthropology, history, sociology, English and dentistry. And yet, the book seeks to go beyond studies that see oral health and the mouth, its object of enquiry, as topics of 'disciplinary work' (Nettleton, 1992). The mouth is, of course, a subject of disciplines, of which dentistry is seen as the most important. But dentistry is not the sole determinant of the mouth as an object; it is not simply something that 'dentists do', as the General Dental Council in the UK seemingly assumes, and neither is dental knowledge solely aligned to the auspices of medical science. In fact, there was no such profession as dentistry before the modern period (although the exact dates of its foundation are debated) and our understanding of the mouth as an object of this profession has been historically constructed. The case studies in this book, particularly those with a historical focus, go some way in demonstrating the fragile and contingent status of the profession. Dentistry's establishment was messy and contested and the intensity of its objectification of the mouth changed over time, aligning with different political ambitions, disease categories, technological developments and interventions from businesses and philanthropy.

The limitations of dentistry in shaping oral health in the past, present and future are highlighted by the fact that oral diseases (dental caries and periodontal disease being the two most common), among the most prevalent diseases globally, are largely preventable. It is now agreed that dentistry alone will more than likely never be able to successfully tackle these diseases. Instead, the profession has become increasingly focused on what it can 'fix' through aesthetic treatments, largely driven by consumerism. In 2019, private dentistry in the UK was worth £3.6 billion, while NHS dentistry was worth £3.5 billion (Lala, this volume). But despite dentistry's rhetoric that the profession is wholly distinct from the trade, consumerism has long formed part of the realities of dental practice and dentists have long worked with companies or conducted private practice for their own financial self-interest. Without substantial structural changes, financial incentives will continue to shape the profession and the oral care it is willing and able to provide. However, consideration and application of the findings of new research (like that contained within this volume) provide the potential to improve provision and make oral health more equitable.

As we argue in this book then, the forces that brought into focus the mouth as an object in the form that it is today are broader and more diffuse than the discipline of dentistry acknowledges. These forces are disciplinary and the mouth was (and is) subject to disciplinary surveillance, manipulation, control and resistance, but they are also creative, commercial, consumerist, legal, historical, ethical and social. We seek to articulate in various forms how the mouth came to be established through a series of social projects that have crisscrossed the past several centuries, from soldier activity in the trenches of World War One (Strong, this volume) and commercial activity in interwar America (Carstairs, Holden, this volume), through to the activities of employers in the early decades of the twentieth century (Jones, this volume) and the surgeons who operate on the heart today (Scott, this volume). Establishing 'oral care as a life course project' reveals how it is through the interactions with this broader 'social world' of oral care and dentistry (that contains a history of multiple oral care projects and regimes) that people realise the goal of keeping their teeth into later life (Gibson et al., 2019; Kettle et al., 2019; Warren et al., 2020). Our understanding of oral health, and thus our ability to improve it, is therefore lacking without uncovering the complexity of actors, organisations, institutions, bodies of knowledge and technologies that shaped it.

## Oral health disciplines or disciplining oral health?

When we speak of the interdisciplinary logic of oral health, we echo the words of Barry and Born (2013) that what we have come to know as the mouth today has taken this form because of the array of institutions, actors, technologies and practices that have been directed at it through time. Barry and Born's edited collection on interdisciplinarity provides a comprehensive outline of the many different kinds of interdisciplinary work that currently exists and the wide-ranging interdisciplinary relationships between the social and natural sciences and between the arts and sciences. Is then, our book interdisciplinary? The book's orientation around a central theme with the involvement of multiple disciplines seemingly suggests so. But what does it mean to be involved in interdisciplinary work in the humanities and social sciences on the subject of oral health? Interdisciplinary work is not straightforward. In the growing debate about its nature and purpose, certain disciplines have been vicariously described as parasitic, trespassers or poachers, taking approaches and ideas from other territories (Osborne, 2013), while others have been described as interlopers (Barry and Born, 2013). Interdisciplinary collaborations have also been seen cynically as a way to generate funding and described as little more than arid rhetoric, with the literature on interdisciplinarity called bloodless, sterile, profoundly uninteresting and conservative (Fitzgerald and Callard, 2014; Callard and Fitzgerald, 2015). Yet, the space of 'interdisciplinarity' is of course, like the mouth, a historical and sociological artefact and as such is an object that offers numerous opportunities as well as constraints (Callard and Fitzgerald, 2015). Interdisciplinarity can therefore also be useful, and like Barry and Born (2013), we see it as a way of generating new questions and reflecting on existing problems associated with oral health and dentistry.

In order to generate new questions and to reflect on existing problems, we need to identify where our project lies in relation to current work on oral health. From Barry and Born's identification of two alternative forms of relationship between disciplines within interdisciplinary work (the 'subordination-service mode' and the 'agnostic-antagonistic mode'), we can determine that most existing research on oral health to date falls within the 'subordination-service mode'. In the 'subordination-service mode', the social and behavioural sciences have commonly been called upon to help supply a social perspective or to explain errors in measurement in research within oral health and dentistry, or to provide 'higher order skills' as a way of enhancing dental education and dentists' personal and professional development. For example, the theoretical background and methods from the sociology of childhood have been used to help improve the 'voice of the child' in dental research (Marshman et al., 2007, 2015). Likewise, researchers have drawn on the theory of social practices in relation to the management of carious teeth in children during a large-scale clinical trial. Here, sociologists have helped to examine what it means to be 'doing dentistry' during the clinical trial (Marshman et al., 2020).

In the same vein, the social sciences have contributed to making dentistry more accountable beyond the profession and enabled dentists to see things from the user's perspective. For example, Exley et al. (2009, 2012) examined decision-making processes associated with the costs of having dental implant treatment and highlighted that private healthcare involves assessing not only the provider but also the product. As such, patient decisions to engage in private health care are 'distributed' beyond the single event where treatment is said to happen. This was *not* found to be the case with patients in relation to implant treatment where patients seemed to be poorly informed; these patients could very well have been exploited because of their trust in their providers. This research directly challenges the wholesale embracing of implant technology by the dental establishment without proper consumer protection. Moreover, in ground breaking work, Horton and Barker (2009, 2010) highlighted the critical role that oral health care workers play in 'racialised' politics in North America. Using the tools of critical anthropology, the authors demonstrate how dental health care workers are not simply promoting oral health when they work with Mexican American farm workers but are also promoting a 'racialised' politics that talks of Mexican Americans as containing the 'stain of backwardness', which has been a threat to the success of oral health in North America over the past century. In doing so, those involved in dental public health are furthering concerns about the pollution of the American population writ large and are thus furthering the goals of the 'neoliberal' state to promote self-governance.

Whilst Exley indicated in 2009 that there was a 'lack of a' sociology of oral health, it might now be said that this project is well underway. This is certainly less true when it comes to the arts and humanities. Oral health and dentistry have drawn less on the arts and humanities than the social sciences, particularly in the UK, presumably because their insights are considered more abstract and diffuse and accordingly, their contributions are poorly understood. More commonly, the arts and humanities (along with the social sciences) have played a subordinate role to medicine more broadly and indeed, their potential service to medical practice and pedagogy is a key reason for the foundation of the medical humanities field several decades ago and the teaching of medical humanities electives in medical schools and colleges across the world (e.g., see: Arnott et al., 2001). Nonetheless, the arts and humanities are beginning to be seen as useful to dentistry, particularly in dental education (Smyth Zahra et al., 2018; Smyth Zahra and Park, 2020). Its advocates argue that the similarities between the professions of medicine and dentistry mean that the same insights gained from the arts and humanities in medicine can also apply to dentistry. For example, the arts and humanities' provision of 'a grounding in humanistic values, principles, and skills' can promote a more person-centred, holistic and reflexive approach to dental care, as opposed to a paternalist, reductionist model of healthcare (Howley et al., 2020). Such approaches, enriched by the arts and humanities and grounded in ethics, are also predicted to reduce or remove the high levels of workplace stress that dentists commonly report once in practice (Smyth Zahra and Park, 2020), although research on whether this is the case has yet to be conducted. Moreover, art museum-based pedagogy is thought to build clinically relevant skills and promote learners' professional identity formation through activities including visual thinking strategies and group poems (Chisolm et al., 2020).

The aforementioned examples demonstrate that an interdisciplinary programme of research centred on oral health is in development and that this programme is seeking to enable oral health care to become more responsive (and indeed more responsible) for its impact on the society around it, particularly in the areas of inclusion, consumer protection and professionalism. This is important for dentistry because without such critical reflection, the profession may very well lose its protected status in society. The various disciplinary perspectives included in this book support this position by promoting a greater degree of reflexivity than would have been possible without their input, particularly on the current zeitgeist in dental public health around the social determinants of oral health. While the work of Watt (2007) can be seen as a key point of contact *within dentistry* of the necessity of understanding the central importance of the social determinants of health to oral health policy, work beyond dentistry is necessary too. Indeed, the recent statement of the Behavioral, Epidemiological and Health Services Research (BEHSR) Group of the International Association for Dental Research that to 'achieve optimal oral health globally, there is consensus that action is needed to advance and *further integrate behavioral and social sciences* as applied to oral health, healthcare, and training' (BEHSR, 2020) suggests that work to date has not gone far enough. But we suggest that the BEHSR Group's recent call for a greater degree of insight into middle range theory (i.e., theory that seeks to explain key intermediate mechanisms for social inequalities) can best be served with a widening of the current range of disciplines that can be brought to bear on the subject of oral health in global society (BEHSR, 2020). The social sciences, together with the humanities, can inform such work by demonstrating how and why certain social determinants came to be significant and what integrated upstream and community-based approaches have succeeded or failed in the past. The social sciences and humanities can, and arguably should, be more useful to dentistry and oral health through their focus on temporality, continuity and change, and context.

Yet, as we also want to make clear, there are a number of potential issues with the 'subordination-service mode' and its implications for inter-disciplinary work centred on oral health. In particular, all involved must re-cognise that the balance of power in such relationships is not equal. Oral health and dentistry are more highly valued than the social sciences and the arts and humanities, not only within an instrumentalist society but also within institutional structures and with regard to financial resources. Again, this kind of power dynamic has been constructed historically and the chapters by Lala and Jones (in this volume) highlight different ways in which dentistry came to acquire its status in society. These kinds of cultural and financial power im-balances might also go some way to explaining why the flow of knowledge is generally unidirectional from the social sciences and humanities to the sci-ences (Scott-Fordsmand, 2020)[1]. Such power relationships then could lead to the utilitarian exploitation of the social sciences and the arts and humanities, where these disciplines come to simply contextualise or illustrate scientific research and are seen to be of little inherent value in and of themselves (Callard and Fitzgerald, 2015). We would like to emphasise here that we see the social sciences and arts and humanities as having immense cultural and financial value beyond the realm of the sciences and this is the case now more than ever, as academic departments in the humanities in universities across the world are closed or are threatened by closure (Fazackerley, 2021). Not only are the social sciences and the arts and humanities vital for the health and breadth of our civic culture, and our evolving sense of self-understanding in all its nuance and complexity, but as the Royal Historical Society recently stated, an undergraduate degree in history teaches all the skills that employers want, including independence critical thinking and advanced writing, and this is reflected in the graduate employment market (RHS, 2021). As Sweet in the volume reminds us, the focus of literary studies is a reflection of what society views as important at a given time. Moreover, the British Academy's recent report 'Qualified for the Future' (2020) shows that employment levels are identical for STEM and AHSS degrees. Claims that the arts and huma-nities are less valuable in this respect smack of hubris. On a practical level, when encountering this kind of power dynamics, enthusiastic and perhaps idealistic interdisciplinary workers can become disillusioned with the project, although we are fortunate that this has not been the case with this book!

In contrast to the 'subordination-service mode', Barry and Born's (2013) 'agnostic-antagonistic mode' rarely applies to oral health. This mode refers to an agnostic or antagonistic relationship between disciplines, where a self-conscious dialogue takes place that reflects on the limits of these disciplines or the status of the underlying knowledge produced. By making an explicit commitment to contest or 'transcend the given epistemological and/or ontological assumptions' of these disciplines, this kind of research can lead to radical shifts in knowledge that otherwise cannot be grasped by one discipline or through some form of 'spurious unity' of the disciplines. It could also be described as 'transdisciplinarity'. The work of sociologist Sarah Nettleton (1988, 1989, 1991, 1992) provides an important starting point for an antagonistic relationship with dentistry through exposure of how moralistic, sexist and yet productive dental discourse constructed stereotypes of mothers as 'natural', 'ignorant', 'responsible' and 'caring' (Nettleton, 1991). Following Foucault, Nettleton (1992, 1994) went on to establish how the disciplinary power of dentistry was mobilised through micro-techniques of power involving examinations (the dental check-up), measurement and comparison (the use of epidemiology). The creation of the mouth as a dental object resulted in its subjection to mechanisms of power. Several of the chapters in this volume (e.g., Strong, Jones and Scott) pick up the themes of power from Nettleton in order to demonstrate the embedding of examinations or measurement in the army, in factories and in cardiac surgery. In a different way, the work of Barry (Gibson et al., 2004a), one of the editors and contributors to this volume, has provided an 'agnostic' glance between disciplines by examining the 'identity work' that drug users have to do when seeking to stop taking drugs. While there was no 'antagonistic' analysis of underlying ontological or epistemological commitments in Gibson's work, sociology examined the identity work drug users have to use to eventually stop drug use, noting that oral care may act as a precursor to 'becoming clean'. The data was collected by a dentist and analysed by a sociologist and two dentists who were 'in discourse'. This work was subsequently published across disciplines in sociology (Gibson et al., 2004a, 2004b) and dentistry (Robinson, Acquah, and Gibson 2005).

We can also see examples of the 'agnostic' social science and humanities within the critical medical humanities, a field founded as a dissatisfied response to the 'first wave' of medical humanities of the early 2000s in which the arts and humanities operated in the 'subordination-service mode' to medicine and medical education. The critical medical humanities aims for a more equal relationship between the disciplines and is focused on 'subject matter that somehow both straddles the disciplines and falls between them' (Evans and Macnaughton, 2004). Research projects in 'critical medical humanities', such as the Life of Breath (2015–2020), for example, which brought together medicine, philosophy, anthropology, history, arts and literature in order 'to find new ways of answering questions about breathing and breathlessness and their relationship to both illness and wellbeing', demonstrate a genuine attempt by researchers to depart from their disciplines and instead to 'build a perspective that is unique to the discipline called "medical humanities"' (Evans and Macnaughton, 2004). Similarly, the work of Fitzgerald and Callard sought to go beyond the unequal power balance in relations between neuroscience and social science through 'experimental entanglement' by setting aside the epistemological and ontological commitments from both disciplines and refusing preliminary decisions about the shape or outcome of their interactions (2014).

But the rare use of the 'agnostic-antagonistic mode' in dentistry suggests the strength of the 'subordination-service mode' and indicates that it is seen as the work of those in other disciplines, namely social scientists that have long been located in dental schools across the world, to challenge existing assumptions within dentistry and to conduct much of the reflexive discipline-traversing work required for developing truly discipline breaking work. More generously, the lack of attention paid to transcending the given epistemological or ontological assumptions of oral health at least suggests that those who are keen to do so are underfunded or so globally disparate that it has hitherto been impossible to achieve this kind of critical work to date. The potential for work focused on oral health that transcends the disciplines then is vast and under realised.

In this volume, we do not claim to 'supersede [the] prior epistemological and/ or ontological commitments' of our respective disciplines, but neither do we believe our unity is a spurious one. As we stated at the beginning of this introduction, our project seeks to go beyond viewing the mouth as solely an object of 'disciplinary work' and by doing so, begins to uncover the range of actors, institutions, bodies of knowledge and technologies that have shaped it and continue to shape it. But as the chapters in this volume and the themes under which they are organised demonstrate, our shared interest in oral health and commitment to cross-disciplinary conversations are combined with a commitment to our own disciplinary methods and frameworks. Endorsing the proposal by Fitzgerald and Callard, the book interacts between disciplines on the understanding of their pre-existing separateness (2014, p. 3). For example, a scholar of English literature, an historian, a dentist and an ethnographer share perspectives from their own disciplines under the theme of 'cultural representations of the mouth and teeth', while the perspectives of two historians and an anthropologist are brought to bear under the theme 'State, Surveillance and Social Justice'. There are certainly nods here to other disciplines. Jones, for example, draws on recent research in oral health and conceptual frameworks from sociology to demonstrate the beginnings of the major effort needed to socially construct the worker's mouth as an object of surveillance and manipulation by the state, the dental professions and industry, while Holden analyses historical evidence (advertising) with sociological theory to provide insights for a dental audience. Instead, we seek initial connections and begin the process of an engaged interdisciplinary commitment that goes beyond the simple 'subordination-service mode' that have been most typical hitherto in oral health and dentistry.

With its firm disciplinary commitments then, some may claim that this book is not 'interdisciplinary' at all and is in fact best described as a 'multi'- or 'cross'- disciplinary project. Certainly, the book offers a multidisciplinary conversation around the theme of oral health. And yet, the wide remit provided by

Barry and Born (2013) suggests that it is perfectly accurate to describe our work as interdisciplinary. Indeed, the authors in the volume seek to contribute to their own disciplines through their chapters in much the same way that anthropologists, in Barry and Born's (2013) example of 'creative parasitism', seek to make contributions to their own discipline from locations such as businesses, laboratories and clinics. In this respect, interdisciplinarity does not pose any kind of 'threat' to other disciplines but through the work, the disciplinarian is able to make valuable contributions to their own discipline, while providing insights to interested parties in other disciplines. While our case studies usefully expand knowledge within the disciplines, the chapters by dentists also navigate the historian and sociologist towards a chronological end point for the importance of the social determinants of health and those by scholars in non-dental disciplines have the potential for feeding directly into policy making, dental education and practice. Moreover, as this book demonstrates, the different disciplines brought together have more in common than first appears with their epistemological concerns with power, knowledge, professionalisation, ethics and commodification. Indeed, together, the authors address, sometimes implicitly, a fundamental question: 'who owns the mouth?' Is it the profession, the patient, the market or the state?

In what follows, we lay out the structure of the book under four main headings: Professionalism, Ethics and Inequalities; Cultural Representations of the Mouth and Teeth; The Patient's Perspective; and State, Surveillance and Social Justice. This structure around four key themes usefully expands the work of Whitehead and Woods (2016), which sees the critical medical humanities field as structured around the three 'Es' – ethics (medical ethics and bioethics); education (medical, but also increasingly health); and experience (particularly qualities of illness experience). It should also be briefly noted that the case study nature of this book means that it inevitably provides an incomplete picture of oral health. Indeed, with its focus on Britain, Europe and North America, the book is Western-centric with little discussion of ethnic diversity. Such exclusions say more about the constraints on the size of the volume than they do about the need for such studies. More in-depth and diverse studies are certainly urgently needed, not least that focus on other parts of the world, particularly middle- and low-incomes countries where oral health inequalities are at their most stark. But nonetheless, the chapters in this book provide significant insights into aspects of the past and present of oral health and as a whole, the book, part research output and part manifesto, provides a crucial first published intervention in bringing into focus the significance of oral and the mouth across numerous disciplines. It aims to be a platform on which other scholars and practitioners can build.

## Professionalism, ethics and inequalities

We view ethics, particularly professional ethics, as a key theme in emergent interdisciplinary work in oral health and it is by paying attention to ethics that inequalities within the profession are revealed. In this first section of the book, chapters by Bonnie Yu et al., Rizwana Lala and Patricia Neville provide contrasting contemporary perspectives of the profession of dentistry by analysing various threats to its integrity (or esteem). Yu et al., with backgrounds in oral and dental public health, assess the degree to which the concepts of moral inclusion and moral community can be measured and what this says about dentists' wider concerns about the health of the public. The authors seek to examine how these concepts might be used to examine dentists' willingness to be involved in health advocacy, acting beyond the remit of their daily practice to actively promote the kind of structural changes associated with the social determinants of oral health as espoused by Watt (2007). Lala, a dentist, draws on institutional ethnography and applies the cultural and symbolic capital of Bourdieu to her examination of the ways in which dental power within cosmetic dentistry can undermine patient autonomy. Through its definition of the perfect smile as symmetrical, gleaming white and modelled on European facial features, Lala's chapter demonstrates that the profession excludes those with facial disfigurements, those who are non-European or those who cannot afford cosmetic treatments. Patricia Neville, a sociologist, highlights the historical development of dentistry as a male-dominated profession in order to demonstrate gender inequality present in the profession today. In contrast to the 'gender myth', which is the widespread image of the profession (both in and outside of it) as inclusive, meritocratic and family friendly, Neville draws on feminist and sociological literature to demonstrate that the prevalence of sexism and sexual harassment within the profession, the position of women in relation to power, status and control and the specific job types or roles in which women find themselves indicate that the profession has a long way to go before gender equality is achieved.

Together, the three chapters question and challenge the professional status quo, its regulatory frameworks and everyday practices, arguing that the dental profession could and should be inclusive to patients and practitioners alike and should not be commercially exploitive. Their critiques of current professional circumstances are important because firstly, they remind us that dentistry is only a profession by virtue of the monopoly that it holds over the training and regulation of its members. This monopoly is a relatively recent phenomenon. Indeed, while some form of dentistry (usually tooth removal) has long been practised by anyone with a strong pair of pliers, it was typically seen as trade where payment was exchanged for a required service (Kunzle, 1989). The emergence of something resembling a profession, as an organised community that shared a body of knowledge (medical science), a regulating body (typically national dental associations and councils), an agreed standard of education (typically university degree) and shared ethical values and practices, did not come into being until at least the nineteenth century and then it was fiercely contested by those deemed outside of the new professional boundaries. Lala highlights the Dentists Act of 1984 as a way of regulating members of the profession, but this act built on the earlier acts of 1956, 1921 and 1878.

These acts dictated the kinds of practitioners to be excluded and included in this new profession. In Britain, for example, on the passing of the Dentists Act 1878, only 37 per cent of those practising at the time were qualified; this increased to 80 per cent by the time of Dentists Act of 1921 (Dussault, 1981, p. 72).

The Dentists Acts did not explicitly exclude women from the profession, but of course, entering dental school and qualifying as a dentist was not easy for women and wider social structures favoured male dominance. The first female dentists – Lucy Hobbs Taylor graduated from Ohio Dental College in the United States in 1866, while Lilian Lindsay became the first licensed female dentist in Britain in 1895 and went on to become president of the British Dental Association in 1946 – remained a minority until at least the late twentieth century. For much of the twentieth century, women formed part of the related but subordinate professions of dental dressers (the first of which were trained to do simple dental work in Derbyshire in 1916 by Sidney Barwise) and dental hygienists (the first of which were employed to teach dental hygiene in New York in the 1910s). In both cases, women were initially employed to fill shortages left by male dentists, but their dominance in subordinate professions is also suggestive of the kind of vertical and horizontal gender segregation outlined by Neville as existing in today's profession. In contrast to the claim of most functionalist histories then (e.g., Gelbier, 2005), the three chapters remind us that the consolidation of dentistry into a profession was not solely a bene-volent response to growing levels of oral disease in the population but was also a self-interested venture that sought to raise the status and maintain control of the occupational group. As Nettleton (1992, p. 31) has argued, it was dentistry that created the mouth as an object of dental care.

Second, the three chapters highlight the limitations of the profession's reg-ulatory frameworks, particularly with regard to its commercial relationships. The boundaries between commerce and professionalism have never been clearly defined and as historians and sociologists have long argued, much professional practice evades such formalised codes of conduct (see, for example, Jones, 2015). What is deemed acceptable practice is implicitly sanctioned by those who conduct it (see Scott in this volume on the profession's assessment of dental fitness). Despite the rhetorical power of professional codes of conduct and the medical authority they carry, dentistry in practice has remained a trade by virtue of the financial transactions between practitioner and patient or appropriate intermediary. Even the establishment of free at the point-of-use provision, such as under the National Health Service in the UK from 1948, has done little to erode the commercial element of the profession and as Lala and Yu et al. de-monstrate, public and private provision sit alongside each other in the market for oral health care where dentists have often been more free to choose their patients than patients have been to choose their dentist.

Moreover, their ambiguity aside, regulations have not always been enforced. Since their inception, dental regulators have repeatedly failed to take action against dentists who have been deemed too commercial. As Lala demonstrates, the General Dental Council has failed to take action against cosmetic dentists who use the title of 'Dr' in promoting their practice despite such use being forbidden under the 1984 Dentists Act. The controversial use of titles among those practising dentistry is not new, however, and neither is the reluctance of professional governing bodies to reprimand those who use them. Even after the passing of 1878 Dentists Act that sought to provide ethical standards, the dental and medical press was littered with complaints about those practising dentistry (qualified and unqualified) overtly using titles like 'dentist' and 'dental surgeon' in printed advertising and on name plates outside of their premises (Anon 3 June 1893; 30 November 1895; 25 August 1906). In 1893, the *British Medical Journal* (Anon) condemned such advertising commenting that 'the person who thus thrusts himself upon the public must be void of anything like professional feeling ... those who resort to such proceedings do much to injure the status of the dental branch of the profession'.

And yet, professional practice and regulation could be quite different. The chapters here remind us that while the profession has historically been unequal, it could also be enhanced in the future. Changes to regulation in medicine have followed when the profession has fallen into public disrepute as in the examples of Alder Hey and Bristol Royal Infirmary in the 1980s and 1990s, which led to the Human Tissue Act of 2004. Dentistry does not need to wait for professional crises to reform (although it is arguably in one at the time of writing). As Yu et al. point out, knowing and understanding that the profession lacks inclusivity can inform policy makers, dental educators, associations and regulators on policy strategies to address existing inequity. A new Dentists Act, for example, could for the first time include provision for public dental service and explicit clauses about advertising. More specifically on gender inequality, Neville provides four concrete and multifaceted recommendations for professional reform. Her recommendations are more concerned with changing cultures of practices rather than high-level policy or professional regulations. While cultures are often difficult to change, the adoption of these recommendations by dental schools and dental employers across the world could be the first step in changing them.

## Cultural representations of the mouth and teeth

In order to secure its monopoly over oral health, dentistry had to convince both its practitioners and the wider public of its authority. The ways in which this authority was communicated is addressed by the chapters in this section. The four chapters here explicitly address how the profession and its object have been represented in various forms and through numerous types of media since the nineteenth century. In turn, the chapters demonstrate the wider meaning of these representations in the past and present.

Both Ryan Sweet, a literary scholar, and David Scott, a medical ethnographer, focus on metaphors of the mouth and teeth. By drawing on literary critic and philosopher Bakhtin's emphasis on the symbolic importance as the mouth as grotesque, Sweet outlines how fictional writers, H. Rider Haggard and

Rudyard Kipling, represented false teeth in their writings. In doing so, Sweet provides a new approach to reading teeth in literature. By demonstrating that dentures can be read as metonym, metaphor and comic prop, Sweet's new approach provides a sense of the significance of these objects in the late-nineteenth- and early-twentieth-century literary imagination. Representations of dentures in these writings, Sweet argues, reveal contemporary attitudes to health, aesthetic standards, technology, social institutions and nationhood, but also demonstrate the power of the mouth as a symbol of cultural conformity, difference, physical fitness and selfhood. Of particular importance is the wider context of the writings. The authors were writing around the time when greater state intervention into public health followed the 1904 Report of the Inter-Departmental Committee on Physical Deterioration, which found the level of dental fitness among British army recruits for the Boer War to be alarmingly poor. Five thousand recruits were found unfit, 2,000 of whom were evacuated for dental reasons (Dussault, 1981, p. 131). The writings of Rider Haggard and Kipling then reflect cultural anxieties not only about the nation's oral health but also regarding the dwindling condition of Britain's imperial forces. Dentures, both those included in the texts and those the authors themselves wore, were a metaphor of an empire that presented itself as well formed and intact but behind the veneer was weakened and unhealthy. Similarly, Scott draws on the 1904 Report as one of the first dentally sanctioned documents that uses the term 'dental fitness' to refer to the oral health of army recruits. It was in this document that 'dental fitness' became a metaphor for military fitness (which Strong also picks up in her chapter in this volume). Through his brief history of the use of the term 'dental fitness', which emerged from dentists' acceptance of focal infection theory from the late nineteenth century, Scott demonstrates how the dental profession began to give the metaphor uncodified meaning and incorporate it into cardiac surgery, where patients are currently required to demonstrate that they are 'dentally fit' before undergoing an operation.

The portrayal of professional authority and its potential for raising the status of oral health was also beneficial for companies that supplied oral hygiene products. We can see the continuation of the use of the military metaphor in the interwar advertisements for Lavoris mouthwash in Alexander Holden's chapter, in which the image of the dentist both metaphorically and literally aimed to command the same authority as a military officer. Holden, a dentist, draws on discourse analysis from the social sciences to demonstrate how and why dentists were used to promote Lavoris' mouthwash in one of the firm's interwar advertising campaigns included in the *Saturday Evening Post*, one of America's largest-circulating newspapers. Holden demonstrates that the typical use of a particular representation of a dentist – as male, white-coated and bespectacled – was a powerful symbol of dental authority to the newspaper's growing market of consumers of oral hygiene products. These consumers were middle class, white and male. While the Lavoris campaign focused on professional image in order to target men, the chapter by Carstairs, a historian, demonstrates that the incorporation of contemporary dental science, particularly focal sepsis and oral hygiene, into advertisements of toothpaste and tooth-brushes featured in *Good Housekeeping* and *Ladies Home Journal* aimed to appeal to the journals' readership of middle-class, white women. Women, Carstairs argues, were particularly susceptible to company messages about toothpaste being an important beauty aid and as a tool to combat bad breath. Firms appealed to these women through the language of dental decay prevention and by featuring aspirational images of young attractive woman.

Of course, the rhetorical use of medical science and the authority of the professional as a symbol of authority in the promotion of products were not new to the interwar period but features were common to advertisements from the nineteenth and early twentieth centuries. For example, the *British Medical Journal* debated whether it was ethical for advertisements promoting tooth-powders to include epithets such as 'recommended by Mr A. B. LDS', as was common practice ('Dental Advertising' 1906). Moreover, as historians of medicine have shown, advertisements for all kinds of medical products, ranging from surgical instruments aimed at surgeons and disinfectants aimed at the housewife, drew on the authority of the medical profession and the language of contemporary science (sanitary science in the case of disinfectants) (Jones, 2015; Tomes, 1990, 1998). Others have demonstrated the growing significance of the white coat in portraying the authority of science in mid-twentieth century popular imagery more widely, including American comic books (Basalla, 1976; Hansen, 2004). Yet, Holden and Carstairs amply demonstrate that the interwar period was particularly significant for the use of dental tropes in advertisements for oral hygiene products. Indeed, it was in this period that not only did print media's widespread adoption of colour and photographic imaginary make advertisements more appealing to their ever-expanding readerships, but the inclusion of dental tropes aided the success of advertisers in shaping and growing markets of middle-class consumers who saw their consumption of oral hygiene products as part of their personal responsibility as healthy and modern citizens in a new post-World War world. In 1920, markets for oral hygiene products were relatively small, but by the 1940s, toothpastes in particular were one of the most heavily advertised products across the Western world with most middle-class households adopting the 'practices of hygienic modernity' (Carstairs, this volume). Approximately half of the dwellings in North America had a room with tub or shower and hot and cold running water in the 1940s, thus giving dwellers the ability to use oral hygiene products. It took until 1970 until well over 90 per cent of dwellings had fully functioning bathrooms for oral hygiene products and practices to be widely adopted across the social classes (Ward, 2019, p. 159). Nonetheless, the use of professional tropes in the promotion of oral hygiene products in the interwar period highlighted that dentistry had entered the middle-class home.

For better or worse then, the symbolic authority of dentistry and its products within popular culture that gained prominence in the nineteenth-century literary imagination, the interwar period and continued in to the post-war period also remains in the present, with the use of the professional to promote cosmetic dentistry (as Lala in this volume demonstrates) and in the promotion of oral hygiene products in a range of media beyond print, including television and social media (Holden this volume). But in their provision of contrasting accounts of representations of oral health, the teeth and the mouth, these four chapters highlight not only the efficacy of dental authority and dental metaphors but also their limitations. Sweet's chapter, in particular, suggests that not all representations of dental authority were taken seriously as demonstrated by the comedic and tragic potential of dentures. Moreover, the dentist as white and male is an image that the profession is trying to leave behind as it diversifies. Like the chapters in section one, the chapters by Scott and Holden provide further challenges to the professional status quo, and point to potential futures for the profession. Scott argues that without acknowledgement of the social and historical construction of the term 'dental fitness' and more explicit clinical guidelines on the dangers of leaving teeth that do not meet a specified criteria of the term in situ, surgeons will continue to remove what are otherwise healthy teeth unnecessarily before cardiac surgery. Holden provides current dentists with an opportunity to reflect upon the concept of fragile professionalism. The profession was fragile in interwar America but Holden argues that it is also fragile now, as non-dentists provide a growing share of oral health services and as patients increasingly rely on businesses for their oral health care.

## The patient's perspective

Chapters by Holden and Carstairs in the previous section demonstrate how the purveyors of oral hygiene products in the interwar period targeted the white, affluent, middle-class consumer. Such patient-consumers were not only able to afford dental services and products, but were influenced by the authority of dentists portrayed in print media marketing and elsewhere. The same is true today, with middle-class patient-consumers more willing and able to access dental health services and products than other types of patient-consumer. But as the chapters in this section demonstrate, there were, and indeed still are, other important patient-consumers of oral health care. The three chapters in this section then provide contrasting perspectives of the dental patient-consumer.

Helen Strong's chapter provides a much-needed account of the oral health of the British soldier during World War One, particularly those suffering from the painful condition of trench mouth. Like the chapters by Scott and Sweet, Strong picks up on the 1904 Report as a significant turning point in the state's recognition of the poor oral health of the British population, but she also demonstrates its limitations; despite the Report's significance for prompting recognition of poor oral health, the provision of dentistry within the army and the condition of the teeth of soldiers remained poor until at least the 1920s with the establishment of the Army Dental Corps. Paralleling Scott's analysis of 'dental fitness', Strong points out that part of the reason for the lack of dental care for soldiers during the war was because there no definitive 'dental standard'. Just as cardiac surgeons today are required to rely on their own interpretation of what constitutes 'dental fitness', army medical officers during the war were required to rely on their own interpretations of what constituted 'adequate dentition'. The need for troops meant standards were low and soldiers suffered. But Strong's focus on World War One soldiers also has wider significance for broadening our understanding of oral health among the British population at the time; she reminds us that soldiers' poor oral health resulted from a complex set of underlying inequalities that were present at home. While it should be noted that tooth decay was widespread across all social classes in this period, the issue was more acute among the poor. Soldiers typically came from a poor social and economic background and along with those in their class were unlikely to be able to afford the services of qualified dentists, leaving them only access to variable and non-standardised dental treatment by chemists, itinerants and non-registered dentists. The rare adoption of oral hygiene practices among soldiers, along with the wider working classes, and the high sugar content of much of their foods meant they were prone to dental caries and other oral diseases and as we have already seen, the lack of indoor bathrooms in working-class homes until the late twentieth century was a major impediment in the adoption of these practices.

But as the chapters by sociologists Alison Dougall et al. and Barry Gibson et al. demonstrate, class is not the sole social determinant by which we can analyse dental patients. By focusing on people with haemophilia, Dougall et al. demonstrate the poorer oral health status and reduced oral health related quality of life of this patient group compared to the general population. They highlight how people with haemophilia have poorer access to dental services and experience more fear and stigma during oral health care than their non-haemophilic counterparts. Extensive or prolonged bleeding from the mouth due to poor oral health, as a consequence of a dental intervention, or through trauma to the mouth, is cited as both a perceived and experienced problem for people with haemophilia. Drawing on the work of Nettleton (1992), the authors argue that while haemophilia is a well-managed condition, the peculiarities of the mouth makes the oral health of those with the condition distinct. The mouth becomes the focal point of the leaky body and 'remains largely separated out from the body, both in haemophilia care and in the attitudes and experiences of people with haemophilia towards their bodies'.

Shifting to focus on the experience of older persons, Gibson et al. demonstrate how dental perspectives among this patient group have evolved over the life course. Like Dougall et al., Gibson et al. focus on the uniqueness of the mouth and its separatedness from the body. In doing so, their chapter demonstrates the embodied enterprise of older people holding onto and maintaining their teeth. The authors highlight the importance of 'having work done' among their participants in order to restore the function of the teeth; they demonstrate that this is a life-long project as different forms of work fail and as the mouth and teeth change over time or as Gibson et al. put it as the 'body-mouth schema' becomes unstable leading to the loss of the pre-reflective harmony between her body and everyday life. Like those in the chapter by Dougall et al., the participants here express feelings of vulnerability over having their mouth in-terfered with, but at the same time, also express a sense of achievement as they keep undergoing work in order to maintain the 'body work' first undertaken by the dentist.

Yet, while each of the three chapters in this section focus on different patient-consumer groups, they also have much in common. Methodologically, their reliance on patients' own testimony in form of oral history (Strong) and in-terviews (Dougall et al. and Gibson et al.) provide us with glimpses into the lived experience of oral health. This focus on the patient's perspective is re-flective of the long-established emphasis in social and medical history since the late twentieth century on 'history from below' (e.g., Thompson, 1966). Indeed, while the cultural revolution of the 1960s ushered in the study of 'real life' and 'ordinary people' in mainstream academic history as a critical response to in-stitutionalism, Roy Porter's plea in 1985 to look beyond doctors in order to take the patient's perspective seriously has had a profound impact on medical history (1985). Likewise, there has been a shift from the reliance on medical narratives to patient experiences within the critical medical humanities since its inception in the 2000s (Whitehead and Woods, 2016). The authors' concern with 'life histories' (Strong), 'life courses' (Gibson et al.) and the 'lived experience' (Dougall et al.) thus not only demonstrate a keen interest in the patient's perspective of oral health within sociology and history but also highlight how patient experiences can radically differ to those prescribed by the profession. For example, Strong demonstrates how soldiers had trouble eating with their dentures and lost them deliberately so as not to wear them, while Gibson et al. demonstrates how older people adapted their partial dentures to suit their lives.

Moreover, the lived experiences offered here provide important insights into the emotional lives of patients and the feelings their oral health invoke, an aspect often neglected in professional perspectives. As Dougall et al. and Gibson et al. demonstrate, people with haemophilia and old people experience pain, fear, vulnerability, worry, as well as satisfaction and even joy with regard to their mouth and teeth. Among the most important emotions attached to oral health within these chapters is the feeling of being stigmatised and the navigation of oral health as a way to feel as 'normal' as possible or to 'pass' as someone without oral health problems, both in terms of appearance and function. As Gibson et al. emphasise, the goal of having work done among older people is to restore function, while Dougall et al. suggest that people with haemophilia avoid oral health practices so as not to prompt a bleed and are thus living in bodies that are not able to engage in 'body idiom' and conform to cultural expectations. As a result, people with haemophilia are forced to undertake information manage-ment to combat the negative perceptions or stigma surrounding their label. Strong not only outlines how soldiers coped with the pain of their gums and teeth in the trenches but also demonstrates how they were able to convince Army medical officers that they 'passed' as dentally fit. Like the chapters here, dentistry itself currently strives for a patient-centred approach, although the extent to which this is achieved in practice is variable.

Equally important as the experience of the dental patient as expressed in their own words is the ways in which the patient, or more precisely the patient's mouth and teeth, have been transformed into an object of study by the dental profession. As Porter argued, historians need to pay attention to the patient both as narrator and as subject (Porter, 1985). Indeed, it is important that we recognise that 'the patient' (e.g., as opposed to 'the sick') is a medical construct and only called such as a result of the medical (or dental) gaze. These three chapters bring into focus the transformation of the patient, or more precisely the patient's mouth, into a dental object. Within sociology and the history of medicine, the transformation of the patient into an object of study has been a topic of interest since Nicholas Jewson's charting of the 'disappearance of the sick man' in the 1970s (Jewson, 1976). In his influential article, Jewson charts medicine's decreasing reliance on patient testimony for diagnosis and treatment from the eighteenth century. Patient testimony (bedside medicine) was replaced by clinical tests (hospital medicine) during the nineteenth century and by laboratory tests (laboratory medicine) in the twentieth century. Although in practice bedside medicine continued long into the twentieth century, signs and symptoms from the patient's body that had to be read and interpreted by a professional gradually replaced the patient's experience as expressed by their own words. As we outlined earlier, Nettleton has provided a good overview of how the late nineteenth and early twentieth century professionalisation of dentistry brought the patient under its gaze, but her story remains vastly incomplete. Indeed, it is striking that the experiences of World War One army recruits from Strong's chapter contrast with Nettleton's narrative; these soldiers were largely left to deal with their own oral health and only became formally subjected to dental intervention during the 1920s once a professional organisation within the armed forces was established to specifically deal with oral health. Thus, as the patients' perspectives here demonstrate, the transformation of the patient to an object of the dental profession was thus more piecemeal than in medicine and occurred later among some groups. After the 1920s, dentistry extended its gaze through private practice and in publicly funded health services. The chapters of Dougall et al and Gibson et al bring the dental gaze up to the present by demonstrating how dentistry today is a fundamentally 'embodied' enterprise. By doing so, these authors highlight how the patient's body is a social entity but also a material one.

## State, surveillance and social justice

The mouth as an object of manipulation also comes into focus in the chapters in the final section of the book. As the other sections demonstrate, dentistry and commerce have long surveyed and moulded the mouth as their object of study, but as the four chapters here demonstrate, they have been aided in these actions by the state and third-sector organisations. Indeed, the state and dental charities have long sat alongside the profession of dentistry and the commercial sector as important providers of oral health care, often filling the gaps in provision among populations or patient groups identified by but not adequately provided for by dentistry or the market. Working-class children were among the first identified key target group for state-sponsored dental surveillance and intervention in late nineteenth century North America and Western Europe in the form of school dental clinics and educational initiatives (Welshman, 1998). Children were soon followed as targets of state-sponsored dentistry by match factory workers (Jones, this volume), soldiers (Strong, this volume) and throughout the twentieth century, the entire population as dentistry became fully embedded in public health services and systems (in 1939 in Sweden, as Samuelsson outlines).

Power and power relations are at the heart of the chapters in this section, as they are in all sections. As we have already noted, the increasing encroachment of the dental profession and commerce into the oral health of populations was not solely a benevolent response to growing levels of dental disease with intentions to cure it but also represented the attempted monopolisation of these groups over oral health and by extension, the mouths of the population. The chapters in this section demonstrate that similar attempts at domination occurred in dental public health and the charitable sector. In her chapter, Claire L. Jones, a historian, demonstrates how dental public health became a key concern of successive local and national governments in Britain between the 1890s and the 1930s and was provided in conjunction with manufacturers in major industries, who began to see the mouth as a significant separate entity to the rest of the body. However, the provision of oral health care by these manufacturers and state institutions was not solely about the prevention and cure of phosphorous necrosis (in the case of match factory workers) or maintaining a happy workforce (in the case of Cadbury's) but was also a way of making the nation's workforce more productive and politically compliant. Such attempts were aided by the interwar professionalisation of industrial dentistry, as a sub-discipline of dentistry, and by wider public health campaigns.

Shifting the book's focus to Sweden after World War Two, Jonatan Samuelsson's case study of fluoridation in Norrköping between 1952 and 1962 demonstrates how the state, businesses and dentists came to debate Community Water Fluoridation as a part of public health provision. In 1950s Sweden, these groups viewed Community Water Fluoridation as preferable to providing fluoride to the nation via toothpastes, mouth washes or foodstuffs because it was cheap, continuous and could improve oral health without mass manipulation of their behaviours. Shifting to the United States in the present, medical anthropologist Sarah E. Raskin draws on ethnography to outline how dental charitable volunteerism in the form of short-term dental volunteer events have become a dominant mode of providing oral health care to those who cannot afford or access private dental services – in particular those on low-incomes, the Medicaid-insured, rural-residing and non-English speaking – since the federal austerity measures obliterated state-level budgets for community dental services in the late 1990s. She argues that, in the moral economy of normative temporary dental volunteerism, the student dentist volunteers (who are socialised as 'ethical clinician-citizens'. Rivkin-Fish 2011, p. 187) wield at least symbolic power over those who get treatment and those who do not. They create what it means to be a 'deserving' patient and categorise patients so that first timers who win the denture lottery are met with ambivalence and those abusing opioids or who have poor home hygiene are not prioritised. In so doing, these students endorse and perpetuate the inequitable social structures in oral health, consisting of market based periodic and irregular treatment opportunities, that the events aim to subvert. This has clear implications for the actions of the dental profession once these students are in practice and evidence suggests that their empathy and sense of social obligation towards these patient groups declines after volunteering, thus evoking the conclusions of the first chapter of this book by Yu et al. regarding the desirability of a morally inclusive profession.

But as the chapters here also demonstrate, state-sponsored oral health services and their charitable equivalents have long had their limitations; state provision was far from straightforward, was frequently contested and piecemeal and was, and indeed still is, also largely dependent on the political priorities of those in charge. Moreover, even when provided, provision did not always achieve the desired objective of controlling the mouth. Jones' chapter, for example, highlights how some industrial workers and working-class targets of the state and manufacturers rejected interventions into their mouth by refusing to adopt oral hygiene practices and even walking out of their factories. Indeed, Jones' chapter, along with Strong's in this volume, again reminds us that professional domination over the oral health of the British working-class population was only partial by the outbreak of World War Two. In contrast, Samuelsson's chapter shows us how the contested science of fluoridation during the Norrköping Fluoridation Trial and opposition among the anti-fluoridation movement led to the eventual abandonment of the trial without any fluoridated water passing the lips of the population targeted. Debates over the trial paralleled those over fluoridation in the United States, Canada and Britain, but also formed part of debates beyond fluoridation in Sweden over whether it was in the remit of the state to medicalise its citizens, as public health in Sweden had long sought to achieve, or whether ensuring good health was the responsibility and choice of individual citizens. Raskin outlines how not all those who attend short-term dental volunteer events are seen or treated by the volunteer dentists.

Together then, the chapters highlight that government reticence in the provision of oral care traverses time and national borders but the contingent nature of these case studies also suggest that situations can also change. Reticence can be overcome with the necessary political will, although it remains to be seen whether all population groups can be, or indeed should be, controlled and manipulated by state-sanctioned dentistry. In the growing global political climate of individualism, we suspect not. Indeed, the tensions between government public health programmes and the rights and personal freedoms of individuals have been starkly highlighted during the Covid-19 pandemic. But as Samuelsson suggests with regard to Community Water Fluoridation, more international comparisons of the past and present might help us further understand the different trajectories of oral health and its inequalities around the world today and how we can best tackle them.

## Note

1 We say 'generally' because there have been genuine moves in certain humanities disciplines to incorporate knowledge and methodologies from the sciences, particularly with regard to the anthropocene and antibiotic resistance. See, for example, Thomas, 2014, Isenberg, 2014, Landecker, 2016.

## Reference List

Anderson, M., Pitchforth, E., Asaria, M., Brayne, C., Casadei, B., Charlesworth, A. et al. (2021) 'LSE–Lancet commission on the future of the NHS: re-laying the foundations for an equitable and efficient health and care service after COVID-19', *The Lancet*, 397(10288), pp. 1915–1978.

Anon. (3 June 1893) 'Dental advertising', *British Medical Journal*, 1(1692), pp. 1203.

Anon. (25 August 1906) 'Dental advertising', *British Medical Journal*, 2(2382), pp. 457–458.

Anon. (30 November 1895) 'Dental irregularities', *British Medical Journal*, 2(1822), pp. 1399–1400.

Arnott, R., Bolton, B., Evans, M., Finlay, I., Macnaughton, J., Meakin, R. and Reid, W. (2001) 'Proposal for an academic association of the medical humanities', *Journal Medical Ethics: Medical Humanities*, 27, pp. 104–105.

Barry, A. and Born, G. (2013) *Interdisciplinarity: reconfigurations of the social and natural sciences*. New York: Routledge.

Basalla, G. (1976) 'Pop science: the depiction of science in popular culture'. In: Holton, G. and Blanpied, W. A. (eds.) *Science and Its Public: The Changed Relationship*. Boston: Reidel, pp. 261–278.

The Behavioral Epidemiological and Health Services Research Group (2020) *Behavioral and Social Oral Sciences Summit: Consensus Statement on Future Directions for the Behavioral and Social Sciences in Oral Health*. [Viewed 5 October 2021]. Available from: https://www.bsohsummit2020.com/

British Academy. (2020) *Qualified for the future: quantifying demand for arts, humanities and social science skills* [online] [Viewed 5 October 2021]. Available from: https://www.thebritishacademy.ac.uk/documents/1888/Qualified-for-the-Future-Quantifying-demand-for-arts-humanities-social-science-skills.pdf

BBC News. (2021) Dentistry: NHS patients 'asked to pay for private care'. [Viewed 5 October 2021]. Available from: https://www.bbc.co.uk/news/uk-55978595

Callard, F. and Fitzgerald, D. (2015) *Rethinking interdisciplinarity across the social sciences and neurosciences*. Basingstoke: Palgrave Macmillan.

Chisolm, M. S. et al. (2020) 'Transformative learning in the art museum: a methods review', *Family Medicine*, 52(10), pp. 736–740.

Dussault, G. (1981) *The professionalisation of dentistry in Britain: a study of occupational strategies (1900–1957)*. PhD Thesis, University of London. [Viewed 5 October 2021]. Available from: https://ethos.bl.uk/OrderDetails.do?did=2&uin=uk.bl.ethos.704484

Evans, H. M. and Macnaughton, J. (2004) 'Should medical humanities be a multidisciplinary or an interdisciplinary study?', *Medical Humanities*, 30(1), pp. 1–4.

Exley, C. (2009) 'Bridging a gap: the (lack of a) sociology of oral health and healthcare', *Sociology of Health & Illness*, 31(7), pp. 1093–1108.

Exley, C. et al. (2009) 'Paying for treatments? Influences on negotiating clinical need and decision-making for dental implant treatment', *BMC Health Services Research*, 9(1), pp. 1–8. [Viewed 5 October 2021]. Available from: https://bmchealthservres.biomedcentral.com/track/pdf/10.1186/1472-6963-9-7.pdf

Exley, C. et al. (2012) 'Beyond price: individuals' accounts of deciding to pay for private healthcare treatment in the UK', *BMC Health Services Research*, 12 (53), 1–8. [Viewed 5 October 2021]. Available from: https://bmchealthservres.biomedcentral.com/track/pdf/10.1186/1472-6963-12-53.pdf

Fazackerly, A. (2021) 'Studying history should not be only for the elite, say Academics', *The Guardian*. 1 May. [Viewed 30 July 2021]. Available from: https://www.theguardian.com/education/2021/may/01/studying-history-should-not-be-only-for-the-elite-say-academics

Fitzgerald, D. and Callard, F. (2014) 'Social science and neuroscience beyond interdisciplinarity: experimental entanglements', *Theory, Culture and Society*, 32 (1), pp. 3–32. [Viewed 5 October 2021]. Available from: https://journals.sagepub.com/doi/pdf/10.1177/0263276414537319

Gelbier, S. (2005) '125 years of developments in dentistry, 1880–2005. Part 6: general and specialist practice', *British Dental Journal*, 199(11), 10 December, pp. 746–750.

Gibson, B. et al. (2004a) 'Entangled identities and psychotropic substance use', *Sociology of Health and Illness*, 26(5), pp. 597–616. [Viewed 5 October 2021]. Available from: 10.1111/j.0141-9889.2004.00407.x

Gibson, B. et al. (2004b) 'Recovering drug users and oral health: a qualitative study', *Sociology of Health and Illness*, 26(5), pp. 1–20.

Gibson, B. (2008) 'Cultural history of the mouth and teeth', in: Pitts-Taylor, V. (ed.) *Cultural Encyclopaedia of the Body*. Westport: Greenwood Press, pp. 337–343.

Gibson, B. et al. (2019) 'Oral care as a life course project: a qualitative grounded theory study', *Gerodontology*, 36(1), pp. 8–17.

Hansen, B. (2004) 'Medical history for the masses: how American comic books celebrated heroes of medicine in the 1940s', *Bulletin of the History of Medicine*, 78(1), pp. 148–191.

Healthwatch. (2021a) 'Dental crisis is a social justice issue' [online]. *Healthwatch*. [Viewed 5 October 2021]. Available from: https://healthwatchreading.co.uk/news/2021-05-25/dental-crisis-social-justice-issue

Healthwatch. (2021b) 'Twin crisis of access and affordability calls for a radical rethink of NHS dentistry' [online]. *Healthwatch*, [Viewed 5 October 2021]. Available from: https://www.healthwatch.co.uk/news/2021-05-24/twin-crisis-access-and-affordability-calls-radical-rethink-nhs-dentistry

Horton, S. and Barker, J. C., (2009) '"Stains" on their self-discipline: public health, hygiene, and the disciplining of undocumented immigrant parents in the nation's internal borderlands', *American Ethnologist*, 36(4), pp. 784–798.

Horton, S. and Barker, J. C. (2010) 'Stigmatized biologies: examining the cumulative effects of oral health disparities for Mexican American farmworker children', *Medical Anthropology Quarterly*, 24(2), pp. 199–219.

Howley, L. et al. (2020) *The fundamental role of the arts and humanities in medical education*. Washington D. C.: Association of American Medical Colleges. [Viewed 6 October 2021]. Available from: https://store.aamc.org/downloadable/download/sample/sample_id/382/

Isenberg, A. C. (2014) 'Introduction: a new environmental history', in: Isenberg, ed. *The Oxford handbook of environmental history*. Oxford: Oxford University Press. pp. 1–22.

Jewson, N. (1976) 'The disappearance of the sick-man from medical cosmology, 1770–1870', *Sociology*, 10(2), pp. 225–244.

Jones, C. L. (2015) *The medical trade catalogue in Britain, 1870–1914*. Pittsburgh: University of Pittsburgh Press.

Kettle, J. et al. (2019) 'I didn't want to pass that onto my child, being afraid to go to the dentist': Making sense of oral health through narratives of connectedness over the life course, *Sociology of Health and Illness*, 41(4), pp. 658–672.

Kunzle, D. (1989) 'The art of pulling teeth in the seventeenth and nineteenth centuries: from public martyrdom to private nightmare and political struggle'. in: M. Feher et al. eds. *Fragments for a history of the human body, part 3*. Cambridge, Mass.: Zone. pp. 29–89.

Landecker H. (2016) 'Antibiotic resistance and the biology of history', *Body & Society*, 22(4), pp. 19–52.

*Life of Breath*. [Viewed 5 October 2021]. Available from: https://lifeofbreath.org/about/

Marshman, Z. et al. (2007) 'Seen but not heard: a systematic review of the place of the child in 21st century dental research', *International Journal of Paediatric Dentistry*, 17(5), pp. 320–327.

Marshman, Z. et al. (2015) 'Seen and heard: towards child participation in dental research', *International Journal of Paediatric Dentistry*, 25(5), pp. 375–382.

Marshman, Z. et al. (2020) 'Dental professionals' experiences of managing children with carious lesions in their primary teeth–a qualitative study within the FiCTION randomised controlled trial', *BMC Oral Health*, 20(1), pp. 1–16.

Nettleton, S. (1988) 'Protecting a vulnerable margin - towards an analysis of how the mouth came to be separated from the body', *Sociology of Health & Illness*, 10(2), pp. 156–169.

Nettleton, S. (1989) 'Power and the location of pain and fear in dentistry and the creation of a dental subject', *Social Science and Medicine*, 29(10), pp. 1183–1190.

Nettleton, S. (1991) 'Wisdom, diligence and teeth: discursive practices and the creation of mothers', *Sociology of Health & Illness*, 13(1), pp. 98–111.

Nettleton, S. (1992) *Power, pain and dentistry*. Buckingham: Open University Press.

Nettleton, S. (1994) 'Inventing mouths: disciplinary power and dentistry'. in: Jones, C. and Porter, R. (eds.) *Reassessing Foucault: power, medicine and the body*. London: Routledge.

Osborne, T. (2013) 'Inter that discipline. Interdisciplinarity: reconfigurations of the social and natural sciences', in: Barry A. and Born, G. (eds.) *Interdisciplinarity: reconfigurations of the social and natural sciences*. New York: Routledge, pp. 82–98.

Otto, M. (2017) *Teeth: the story of beauty, inequality, and the struggle for oral health in America*. New York, The New Press.

Porter, R. (1985) 'The patient's view: doing medical history from below', *Theory and Society*, 14(2), pp. 175–198.

Robinson, P. G., Acquah, S. and Gibson, B. (2005) 'Recovering drug users and oral health: a secondary analysis of qualitative data', *British Dental Journal*, 198, pp. 219–224.

Royal Historical Society. (24 May 2021) Statement on the recent closure of UK history departments [online] Royal Historical Society. [Viewed 6 October 2021]. Available from: https://royalhistsoc.org/news/rhs-statement-on-recent-uk-history-closures/#:~:text=RHS%20statement%20on%20the%20recent%20closure%20of%20UK, University%2C%20London%20South%20Bank%20University%20and%20Kingston%20University%29

Scott-Fordsmand H. (2020). 'Reversing the medical humanities', *Medical Humanities* [online]. [Viewed 6 October 2021]. Available from: 10.1136/medhum-2019-011745

Smyth Zahra, F. et al. (2018) 'Thinking outside the box for health and healthcare: humanities-based approaches to clinical learning', *Conference: Transform MedEd, Singapore. Imperial College London and Lee Kong Chian School of Medicine Singapore.*

Smyth Zahra, F. and Park, S. E. A. (2020) 'Dental education: contexts and trends', in: Nestle, D., Reedy, G., McKenna, L. and Gough, S. (eds.) *Clinical education for the health professions.* Singapore: Springer. pp. 1–13.

Thomas, J. A. (2014) 'History and biology in the anthropocene: problems of scale, problems of value', *American Historical Review*, 119(5), pp. 1587–1607.

Thompson, E. P. (1966) *The making of the English working class.* London: Vintage.

Tomes, N. (1990) 'The private side of public health: sanitary science, domestic hygiene and the germ theory, 1870–1900', *Bulletin of the History of Medicine*, 64(4), pp. 509–539.

Tomes, N. (1998) *The gospel of germs: men, women and the microbe in American life.* Harvard: Harvard University Press.

Ward, P. (2019) *The clean body: a modern history.* Kingston, ON: McGill-Queen's University Press.

Warren, L. et al. (2020) 'I've got lots of gaps, but I want to hang on to the ones that I have': the ageing body, oral health and stories of the mouth', *Ageing and Society*, 40, pp. 1244–1266.

Watt, R. G. et al. (2019) 'Ending the neglect of global oral health: time for radical action', *The Lancet*, 394(10194), pp. 261–262.

Watt, R. G. (2007) 'From victim blaming to upstream action: tackling the social determinants of oral health inequalities', *Community Dentistry and Oral Epidemiology*, 35(1), pp. 1–11.

Welshman, J. (1998) 'Dental health as a neglected issue in medical history: The school dental service in England and Wales, 1900–40', *Medical History*, 42(3), pp. 306–327.

Whitehead, A. and Woods, A. (2016) 'Introduction', in: Whitehead and Woods. (eds.) *The Edinburgh companion to the critical medical humanities.* Edinburgh: Edinburgh University Press. pp. 1–31.

# Part I

# Professionalism, ethics, and inequalities

# 2 Do dentists' views on professionalism include moral inclusiveness?

*Bonnie Yu, Abdulrahman Ghoneim, Herenia P. Lawrence, Michael Glogauer, and Carlos Quiñonez*

## Introduction

The professionalisation of dentistry in Canada can be traced back to the mid-nineteenth century, and it can be said that 'most if not all dentists practised as they do today, as health care practitioners in private settings, running sole-proprietorship, fee-for-service practices, with costs paid directly by the patient or a third party' (Quiñonez, 2021, p. 25). Even then, inequality in oral health and access to dental care was recognised, but there was little or no public infrastructure to respond (Quiñonez, 2021). Towards the late nineteenth and early twentieth centuries, the notion of the state bearing responsibilities towards the individual health of its citizens (the welfare state) became popular. Dentistry also involved itself in large public health movements, but its focus was 'on children, on hygiene, and on partnerships between charitable organizations and the profession' (Quiñonez, 2021, p. 29). It was already clear at this time that the profession had a predilection for basing its professional and social responsibility on their patients' capacity for individual responsibility; that is, the profession was willing to allocate care to those who could not be held responsible for their lot in life, such as children, but were less willing to do so for others (Quiñonez, 2021, p. 37).

Today, oral health-related inequity persists, with socially and economically marginalised populations carrying a disproportionate burden of oral disease and experiencing the greatest barriers to accessing dental care (Peres et al., 2019). Recognising the influence of social determinants on the health of low-income populations, the dental public health community has long advocated for integrated upstream and community-based approaches to deal with this inequity (Peres et al., 2019). An important question that remains unanswered though is how dentists in private practice perceive their duty to care for others. Indeed, where dentistry exists in a market environment, is addressing oral health-related inequity even a concern among practitioners?

People's scope of concern for others can be studied using the concepts of moral inclusion, moral community and moral inclusiveness (Morselli and Passini, 2012; Opotow, 1990; Schwartz, 2007). Moral inclusion is the application of moral

DOI: 10.4324/9781003047674-3

values, rules and considerations of fairness towards others (Opotow, 1990). Moral community has several definitions, and can be described as the group(s) whose well-being concerns us (Regan, 1983). More specifically, it is the group(s) of people to whom we apply moral inclusion. Moral community can also be described as those whose needs, interests or wellbeing we account for in our deliberations or social policies (Spohn, 1996; Warren, 1997). In turn, moral inclusiveness describes the breadth of one's moral community. Naturally, people extend moral inclusion to those they are close to, such as family or friends, or social groups they identify with, such as people who share the same gender, race, class, profession, religion or nationality (called their 'in-groups') (Schwartz, 2007; Spohn, 1996). People who only apply moral values to those they are close to, such as family and friends, are described as having a narrow moral community, or a low level of moral inclusiveness. Those who apply moral values to people who are different from themselves (or 'out-groups') are described as having a broad moral community, or a high level of moral inclusiveness (Morselli and Passini, 2012; Schwartz, 2007; Spohn, 1996). Theoretically, people's moral communities may span from only family and friends to all of society; but, for most, their moral communities fall somewhere in between (Spohn, 1996).

In Canada, dental care is not part of the national publicly funded health care system; dentistry is mostly privately financed, either through out-of-pocket payments or private insurance, with the small remainder supported by government (Quiñonez, 2021). It is within this context that we explore dentists' scope of concern for others. In this chapter, we briefly review the dental literature on professionalism and codes of ethics and codes of conduct for discussions of moral inclusion and moral inclusiveness. We then present the results of an exploratory study, which attempted to measure the moral inclusiveness of a random sample of dentists in the Province of Ontario, Canada's most populous province and the largest dental care market. The chapter concludes with a discussion on the implications of the study's findings. We contend that moral inclusiveness should be an integral part of dentists' professionalism, and that knowing the moral inclusiveness of dentists is important to tackling oral health-related inequity.

## Moral inclusion and moral inclusiveness in the dental literature

There has been extensive discussion in the dental literature on what constitutes professionalism, with most stipulating that dentists must act altruistically, putting patients' interests above their own (Bebeau, Born, and Ozar, 1993; Trathen and Gallagher, 2009; Welie, 2004; Zijlstra-Shaw, Roberts, and Robinson, 2013). There is also recognition that dentists should engage in shared decision-making with patients, using a patient-centred rather than biomedical approach to care (Apelian, Vergnes, and Bedos, 2020; Ozar and Sokol, 2002). These actions – applying fairness and accounting for others' needs – can be considered instances of moral inclusion.

With regard to moral inclusiveness, the literature describes dentists' duty towards the public at-large using the concepts of social responsibility and the social contract, but does not always explicitly state what this duty encompasses (Holden, 2016; Moeller and Quiñonez, 2020; Trathen and Gallagher, 2009; Zijlstra-Shaw, Roberts, and Robinson, 2013). The term social responsibility often refers to the profession's duty to address the health care needs of the public (Welie, 2012). Further, the social contract, which has been said to form the basis of professionalism, stipulates that when society grants doctors their professional status, in return, doctors are expected to put patients' interests above their own, address issues of societal concern, and be devoted to the public good (Cruess and Cruess, 2008).

Unlike models of professionalism, which tend to be more aspirational, codes of ethics and codes of conduct more formally capture how dentists ought to act (Trathen and Gallagher, 2009). Table 2.1 lists excerpts from codes of ethics that contain references to moral inclusion or moral inclusiveness. They are from the

*Table 2.1* Excerpts from codes of ethics for Ontario dentists which represent moral inclusion or moral inclusiveness

| CDA Principle | Excerpts from the CDA's Principles of Ethics | Relevant excerpts from the RCDSO Code of Ethics |
|---|---|---|
| Fairness | 'Be fair; treat all individuals, patients, and colleagues fairly, and practice in a just and equitable manner'. | 'Provide care with respect for human rights and dignity and without discrimination'. |
| Accountability | 'Act, first and foremost, for the benefit of, and in service to, the health of patients and the community'. | 'The paramount responsibility of a dentist is to the health and well-being of patients'. |
| Respect for autonomy | 'Respect the patient's right to choose; patients have the right to be fully informed and make choices for, and actively participate in, their care and pursue their personal values, beliefs and goals in achieving their optimal oral health'. | 'Respect the right of patients to be cared for by the dentist of their choice'. 'Obtain consent before proceeding with investigations or treatment'. |
| Duty to care | 'Provide care to, and promote the well-being of, all members of society; promote fair and reasonable access to quality oral health care without prejudice or discrimination, always regarding the patient as worthy of treatment'. | |
| Prevention | 'Prevent disease by encouraging healthful behaviour in individuals and society; promote health by addressing the broader contexts in which disease occurs'. | |

national dental association (Canadian Dental Association [CDA], 2015) and the regulator of dentists in Ontario (Royal College of Dental Surgeons of Ontario [RCDSO], 2020), where our study takes place.

Not surprising, most of the principles in the RCDSO code of ethics relate to one-on-one, dentist–patient interactions, as these are the interactions that regulatory bodies can objectively regulate. The CDA, not being in a regulatory role, has included principles that are more aspirational. Interestingly, the CDA's last two principles provide more clarity on dentists' responsibilities at the population level; they include ensuring access to care and support for the broader determinants of health.

Given the aforementioned context, dentists would be expected to exhibit high moral inclusiveness. However, the literature has documented dentists exhibiting the opposite: moral exclusion. Moral exclusion occurs to those who fall outside of the boundaries of fairness, and may be characterised by the following: (a) seeing those excluded as psychologically distant from and unconnected with oneself; (b) lacking constructive moral obligations toward those excluded; (c) viewing those excluded as nonentities, expendable and undeserving of fairness and community resources that could foster their well-being; and (d) approving of procedures and outcomes for those excluded that would be unacceptable for those inside the moral community (Opotow, Gerson, and Woodside, 2005). Moral exclusion's outcomes may range from severe, such as genocide and denial of basic human rights, to mild, such as unconcern or unawareness of others' needs (Opotow, 1990). Indeed, there are dentists who choose not to see individuals covered by government dental programmes, such as those receiving social assistance (Bedos et al., 2013, 2014), and the dentists who do see these individuals may 'signal the message, often inadvertently, that they would prefer not to have to treat such patients' (Burt and Eklund, 2005, p. 34). For example, dentists may re-book patients who have missed an appointment if they have private insurance but are less willing to do so for patients covered by public insurance, which invariably remunerates dentists at a lower rate (Bedos et al., 2013; Lévesque, Levine, and Bedos, 2015). Researchers have also shown that dentists tend to communicate and collaborate less on health care decisions with low-income patients (Verlinde et al., 2012; Willems et al., 2005) or may even disregard and not offer procedures that are complex or expensive, giving reasons such as a lack of remuneration from public programmes and patients' lack of self-care (Bedos et al., 2013; Redford and Gift, 1997). They instead perform what Bedos et al. (2013) call 'dentistry for the poor', or emergency dentistry or very basic care.

Ultimately, since any attempt to reduce oral health-related inequity will require the collective effort of the profession (Holden and Quiñonez, 2020; Moeller and Quiñonez, 2020; Welie and Rule, 2006), it seems reasonable that knowing and understanding the moral inclusiveness of dentists is important. This information can inform policy makers, dental educators, associations and regulators on policy strategies to address existing inequity. However, the moral inclusiveness of dentists as a group remains unknown.

## Measuring moral inclusiveness

The moral inclusiveness of dentists, or other health care professionals, has not been explored in any depth or quantified in the literature. Instead, researchers have indirectly measured dentists' moral inclusion while investigating other subject areas. For example, researchers have asked dentists if they believe in 'information giving' or allow 'patient influence' during treatment (Brennan and Spencer, 2005; Grembowski, Milgrom, and Fiset, 1991), which, again, in the context of shared decision-making, can arguably be considered aspects of moral inclusion. These studies correlated the responses to the above questions to information on dentists' clinical procedures. Other researchers have investigated the relationship between dentists' willingness to treat out-groups, specifically patients covered by public insurance, and dentist demographic characteristics. In these studies, dentists' willingness to treat patients with public insurance, measured as a 'yes/no' response, or as a high or low percentage of publicly insured patients in dentists' practices, was related to certain dentist demographic and practice characteristics (McKernan et al., 2015; Pourat et al., 2007; Quiñonez, Figueiredo, and Locker, 2009).

McKernan et al. (2015) used Likert-type scale questions to measure dentists' altruistic attitudes and their willingness to accept patients on Medicaid, an American public insurance programme for low-income children. Some of the Likert-type scale questions, such as 'Dentists have an ethical obligation to treat Medicaid patients', appeared to measure the breadth of dentists' moral communities. Agreeing with these altruistic statements was significantly associated with accepting Medicaid patients, after controlling for dentists' demographic characteristics.

As there appear to be no direct measures of moral inclusiveness in the health care professional literature, a review of sociology and psychology measures was conducted. Two scales are of note. Morselli and Passini (2012) created and validated the 'Inclusion/Exclusion of Other Groups Scale' (IEG) to measure respondents' moral communities. Moral inclusion was operationalised as a continuous variable, which could span from 'all out-groups included' to 'no out-group included'. Respondents were asked four Likert-type scale questions to gauge their willingness to accept members of other ethnic groups in their moral communities. The ethnic groups in question were of varying similarity to the Italian respondents. The sum of the responses yielded the IEG. The researchers found relationships between the IEG and other sociology and psychology scales; for example, the IEG was negatively correlated with scales that measure prejudice and authoritarian submission, and positively correlated with scales that measure support for democracy and democratic principles. In general, sex and age did not have significant relationships to the IEG.

Crimston et al.'s (2016) 'Moral Expansiveness Scale' (MES) was created to measure moral expansiveness, a concept that appears to be similar to moral inclusiveness. Moral expansiveness is defined as the breadth of entities deemed worthy of moral concern and treatment. A less morally expansive person restricts concern to those entities that are considered 'close' (e.g. their family), while a more morally expansive person extends care and consideration to more 'distant' entities (e.g. animals, non-sentient beings). Maximal moral expansiveness is demonstrated by granting the highest moral concern to all types of entities. In the study, respondents were asked to indicate their level of moral concern for several groups of people and entities. Included in the people category were in-groups (family, friend, somebody from the neighbourhood, citizen of the same country) and out-groups (foreign citizen, member of opposing political party, somebody with different religious beliefs). The four levels of concern spanned from 'These entities deserve no moral concern or standing', scored as '0' to 'These entities deserve the highest level of moral concern and standing … you have a moral obligation to ensure their welfare and feel a sense of personal responsibility for their treatment', scored as '3'. The sum of the responses yielded the MES. The researchers found that scoring high in the MES was correlated with scoring high on other scales, such as those measuring universalism values and the desire to base moral judgements on the consideration of the well-being of others and protecting them from harm.

## Do dentists' views on professionalism include moral inclusiveness?

In 2017, we conducted a study on the factors that may influence dentists' clinical decision-making. Data was collected via a 46-item, mail survey sent to a random sample of 3,201 general dentists in private practice in Ontario. Further methodological details of the study can be found in Yu et al. (2019). The three main categories of survey questions were about dentists' demographic and practice characteristics; business considerations; and professionalism and moral inclusiveness. Importantly, this was an exploratory study whose intent was not to create and validate a moral community scale but to provide insight into the beliefs and attitudes of dentists regarding their moral inclusiveness. The main research questions were: Do dentists support morally inclusive views? What is their level of moral inclusiveness? And what is associated with high moral inclusiveness?

Five Likert-type scale questions, previously validated in other studies to measure health care professional beliefs and attitudes, were used to measure dentists' views on moral inclusiveness (Table 2.2).

The first two questions tested if the dentist considered the patient to be in their moral community. The first was based on the idea that when a person has a sense of understanding with another, it is more likely that the person will place the other in their moral community (Opotow, 1990). The second was based on another definition for moral community: the group to whom one grants full and equal moral status (Warren, 1997). With respect to dentistry, someone who has full and equal moral status would arguably be an equal participant in treatment decisions (Ozar, 1985). The third, fourth and fifth questions measured the dentist's moral inclusiveness on a broad scale. The third asked if the dentist was

*Table 2.2* Dentists' level of agreement with the Likert-type scale questions on moral inclusiveness

| Likert-type scale question | Literature source | Percentage* | | |
|---|---|---|---|---|
| | | Strongly agree/agree | Strongly disagree/disagree | Not sure |
| It is important to understand a patient's culture and background in order to treat a patient's illness. (n = 1048) | (Krupat et al., 2000) worded in reverse | 75.3 | 11.1 | 13.6 |
| Patients should be treated as if they were partners with the dentist, equal in power and status. (n = 1043) | (Krupat et al., 2000) | 71.2 | 13.7 | 15.1 |
| That I provide an equally good standard of care whether working on publicly or privately insured patients is important to me. (n = 1053) | (Harris et al., 2014) | 98.0 | 1.1 | 0.9 |
| Reducing inequalities in oral health across the population is important to me. (n = 1041) | (Harris et al., 2014) | 79.5 | 5.4 | 15.2 |
| Dentists should lobby for dental benefits for the disadvantaged. (n = 1036) | (Bebeau et al., 1993) | 69.2 | 7.2 | 23.6 |

\* may not add up to 100 per cent due to rounding error.

willing to treat publicly insured patients (who can be considered an out-group) with the same consideration as privately insured patients (who can be considered an in-group). Burt and Eklund (2005) have argued that dentists in private practice tend to select for patients who are 'healthy, employed, dentally conscious, compliant, middle-class … [and] for whom accessibility to private care is rarely a problem and who can generally afford necessary treatment (frequently assisted by insurance)' (Burt and Eklund, 2005, p. 33) – essentially, the same socioeconomic status as the dentist. The fourth gauged whether the dentist's moral community included the whole population. The fifth referred to the idea that people will make sacrifices or act to ensure that the needs of those in their moral community are met (Opotow, 1990). 'Action' was represented by advocacy in this question.

To assess dentists' levels of moral inclusiveness, a 'moral community score' was developed. We conceptualised moral inclusiveness as the scope of people that dentists perceived they had a duty to care for. Thus, we asked respondents this Likert-type scale question: 'To which patient populations do you think you have a duty to care? Please state your level of agreement for each of the following groups'. Weights were applied to the dentists' Likert responses as follows. 'Disagree' and 'strongly disagree' were assigned a weight of '1' to represent the lowest level of moral inclusiveness. We also assigned 'not sure' a weight of '1', as we suspected that dentists, due to social desirability bias, would be more comfortable choosing this option rather than openly disagreeing. We further felt that it was unlikely that dentists, as health care professionals with experience treating low-income groups in dental school and in private practice, would not have any opinion on whether they should care for low-income groups. 'Agree' and 'strongly agree' were weighted as '2' and '3' to represent the high and highest levels of moral inclusiveness, respectively. Then, weights were applied to the six social groups: 'population at-large', 'all patients in my practice', 'low-income children', 'low-income adults', 'low-income seniors' and 'adults on social assistance'. The weights were meant to represent the dentist's level of moral inclusiveness but also to assess whether there may be 'clusters' of patients that respondents may have felt a strong duty to care for; for example, some respondents may have felt a strong duty to care for children and seniors, rather than adults. By definition, dentists who felt a duty to care for patient groups who were most different from themselves (out-groups) would be considered to have the highest level of moral inclusiveness. Thus, 'population at-large', 'low-income adults' and 'adults on social assistance' were assigned the highest weight of '3'. In contrast, 'all patients in my practice' was assigned a weight of '1', as these patients may be most similar or close to the dentist (in-group) (Burt and Eklund, 2005, p. 33). Though they are quite different from dentists, the low-income children and low-income senior groups were assigned the intermediate weight of '2', as the literature suggests that dentists and society consider these groups to be vulnerable and more 'deserving' of assistance (Quiñonez, 2021). Finally, the weights of the dentists' Likert responses were multiplied by the weights assigned to the six social groups. The sum of the six responses yielded the 'moral community score', with a minimum score of 14 and a maximum of 42. A higher score meant a broader moral community.

Questions on business considerations included an estimate of the percentage of different types of clinical procedures performed per week and Likert-type scale questions to assess dentists' perceptions about personal and market pressures, such as the size of student and practice loans and satisfaction with the level of busyness in their dental practices. Also, for a list of clinical procedures, we asked dentists to indicate their frequency of referral to other practitioners. We assigned scores of '1', '2', '3' and '4' to the Likert responses of 'never', 'occasionally', 'often' and 'always', respectively, and summed them to give the 'frequency of referral to other dentists score'. A higher score indicated a higher rate of referral. Further, we created a 'perception of other dentists' visual analogue scale to assess how respondents perceived other dentists, asking them to place an 'X' along a 100 mm line, with the two ends labelled as 'competitor' and 'colleague'.

We received 1,075 usable surveys, giving a response rate of 33.6 per cent. When compared to the membership records of the Ontario Dental Association, a voluntary professional organisation whose membership comprises 90 per cent

Table 2.3 Respondents' characteristics

| Demographic characteristic | Categories | n | Percentage | |
|---|---|---|---|---|
| | | | Survey sample | Ontario Dental Association members |
| Gender | Male | 700 | 65.5 | 62.0 |
| | Female | 369 | 34.5 | 38.0 |
| Age | 40 and younger | 154 | 14.4 | 29.0 |
| | 41 to 50 | 274 | 25.7 | 25.0 |
| | 51 to 60 | 325 | 30.4 | 22.0 |
| | 61 and older | 315 | 29.5 | 19.0 |
| Year of graduation | Before 1970 | 35 | 3.4 | 3.0 |
| | 1970–1979 | 184 | 17.8 | 11.0 |
| | 1980–1989 | 302 | 29.3 | 20.0 |
| | 1990–1999 | 296 | 28.7 | 22.0 |
| | 2000–2009 | 160 | 15.5 | 24.0 |
| | 2010–2016 | 55 | 5.3 | 20.0 |
| Place of initial dental training | Canadian dental school | 806 | 75.4 | 71.0 |
| | American dental school | 84 | 7.9 | 12.0 |
| | International dental school | 179 | 16.7 | 17.0 |
| Practice ownership | Owner/Partner | 777 | 73.3 | 66.0 |
| | Associate | 283 | 26.7 | 34.0 |

of dentists in Ontario, the respondents' demographic characteristics were aligned in terms of gender, place of initial dental training and practice ownership (Ontario Dental Association, 2020) (Table 2.3). However, a greater proportion of older than younger dentists responded to the survey.

Statistical analysis was conducted using SPSS version 23. Figure 2.1 shows the non-normal distribution of the moral community score, with a spike at the right, representing respondents who had the maximum score of '42'. The score was thus dichotomised at the median to produce 'broad' and 'narrow' moral community groups. Binary logistic regression was performed using demographic and practice characteristics and business consideration variables as the exposures and 'broad' moral community as the outcome. Variables that had significant relationships ($p \leq 0.05$) in binary logistic regression were then entered as a block into multivariable logistic regression to find those variables most strongly associated with the outcome.

As to our results, we found that the majority of dentists did agree with the Likert-type scale questions representing morally inclusive views (Table 2.2). The statement, 'That I provide an equally good standard of care whether working on publicly or privately insured patients is important to me', elicited the highest agreement by far, with 98 per cent of respondents agreeing or strongly agreeing. This may speak to the emphasis in dental education on providing predictable treatment outcomes, regardless of the patient's situation (Bedos et al., 2013; Lévesque, Levine, and Bedos, 2015). Further, in binary

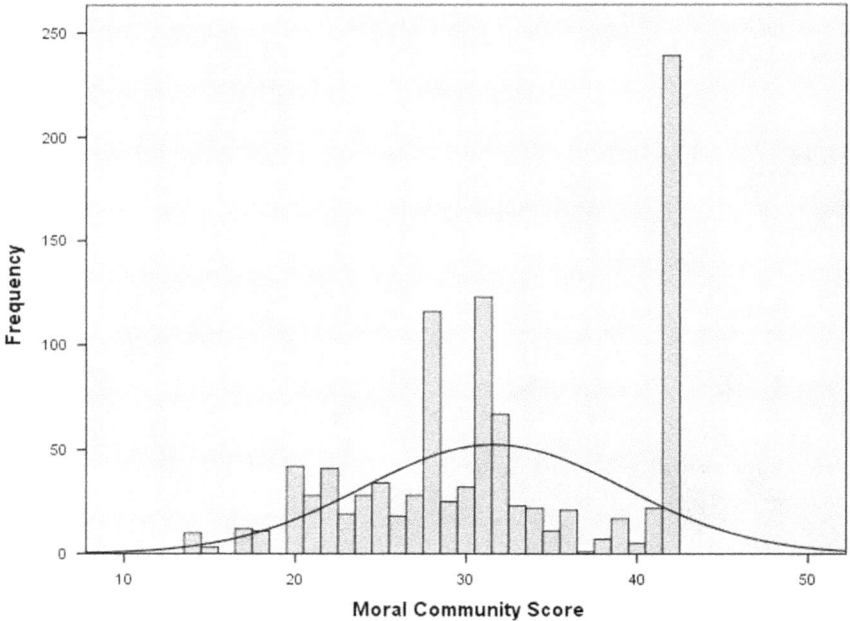

*Figure 2.1* Distribution of moral community scores.

logistic regression, we found that dentists who agreed or strongly agreed with morally inclusive values had increased odds of having a broad moral community than those who disagreed or strongly disagreed (Table 2.4).

We also found that dentists varied in their perceived duty to care for the six social groups; 94.7 per cent strongly agreed or agreed that they had a duty to care for all patients in their practices; 87.6 per cent for low-income children; 84.1 per cent population at-large; 82.3 per cent low-income seniors; 75.8 per cent low-income adults; and 68.9 per cent adults on social assistance. As for respondents' level of moral inclusiveness, we found that the most common moral community score was the maximum score of 42, given by 23.8 per cent of respondents (Figure 2.1). Further analysis was conducted to compare the demographic and practice characteristics of dentists who had the maximum score to the remaining respondents with lower scores. Bivariate analysis showed that there were generally no significant differences between the two groups. Thus, we proceeded to conduct statistical analysis using all the respondents' scores. After the moral community score was dichotomised at the median, we found that among 1,005 respondents, a small majority (57.5 per cent) had a broad moral community rather than a narrow one.

In terms of variables associated with having a broad moral community, we found associations with demographic characteristics, such as female gender and

*Table 2.4* Agreeing or strongly agreeing with Likert-type scale questions on moral inclusiveness and the odds of having a broad moral community

| Likert-type scale question | Odds ratio (95% CI) for broad moral community | p-value |
|---|---|---|
| It is important to understand a patient's culture and background in order to treat his/her illness. (n = 863) | 2.07 (1.38, 3.10) | <0.001 |
| Patients should be treated as if they were partners with the dentist, equal in power and status. (n = 846) | 1.55 (1.07, 2.23) | 0.021 |
| That I provide an equally good standard of care whether working on publicly or privately insured patients is important to me. (n = 994) | 3.65 (0.96, 13.84) | 0.057 |
| Reducing inequalities in oral health across the population is important to me. (n = 846) | 5.20 (2.79, 9.70) | <0.001 |
| Dentists should lobby for dental benefits for the disadvantaged. (n = 762) | 2.65 (1.62, 4.34) | <0.001 |

CI, confidence interval.

practising for less than ten years (Table 2.5). Other studies have reported women to be more patient-centred (Haidet et al., 2002; Hojat et al., 2001; Krupat et al., 2000) and more likely to accept poor patients (Medicaid and charity care) (Nicholson et al., 2015). As for the number of years in practice, studies have suggested that younger dentists may have received more instruction on ethics and patient-centred care in dental school (Gray, 2011; Ozar and Sokol, 2002). Further, older dentists, who are more likely to be practice owners and to be aware of the costs of running a business, may be more inclined to limit the number of low-income patients in their practices (Gordon and Batchelor, 2007; Quiñonez, Figueiredo, and Locker, 2009).

Additionally, variables measuring business considerations had significant relationships to moral community breadth (Table 2.5). In general, dentists who did not perceive competitive pressure from other practitioners, or who did not engage in actions that were associated with maximising income, were more likely to have broad moral communities. For example, perceiving little or no competitive pressure from neighbouring dental clinics, perceiving other dentists to be colleagues rather than competitors, referring at a higher frequency to other practitioners, and performing a lower percentage of treatment procedures per week were associated with increased odds of having a broad moral community (p<0.1).

Factors that did not have significant relationships to moral community breadth (p>0.1) included: location of practice (rural versus urban); place of initial training; hours spent in clinical practice; the share of patients who pay either by private insurance, public insurance or out-of-pocket; number of dentists in the practice; size of practice loans; age of practice; number of hygienists

Table 2.5 Logistic regression analyses for having a broad moral community

| Exposure variable | Bivariate | | Multivariable (n = 334) | |
|---|---|---|---|---|
| | Odds ratio (95% CI) | p | Odds ratio (95% CI) | p |
| Gender | | | | |
| Male (reference) | 1.0 | – | 1.0 | – |
| Female | 1.43 (1.09, 1.87) | 0.01 | 1.70 (1.02, 2.84) | 0.04 |
| Years of practice | | | | |
| 0–10 years | 1.56 (1.02, 2.40) | 0.04 | 1.57 (0.79, 3.15) | 0.20 |
| More than 10 years (reference) | 1.0 | – | 1.0 | – |
| Perception of student loans | | | | |
| Small (reference) | 1.0 | – | 1.0 | – |
| Medium | 1.67 (1.08, 2.57) | 0.02 | 1.64 (0.95, 2.84) | 0.08 |
| Large | 1.52 (0.97, 2.39) | 0.07 | 1.26 (0.69, 2.30) | 0.45 |
| Number of patients per day | | | | |
| 1–8 (reference) | 1.0 | – | 1.0 | – |
| 9 or more | 1.29 (1.01, 1.67) | 0.05 | 1.24 (0.77, 1.20) | 0.39 |
| Satisfaction with practice busyness | | | | |
| Very satisfied (reference) | 1.0 | – | 1.0 | – |
| Somewhat satisfied | 0.71 (0.52, 0.97) | 0.03 | 0.82 (0.46, 1.46) | 0.50 |
| Somewhat dissatisfied | 0.56 (0.38, 0.82) | <0.01 | 1.27 (0.62, 2.61) | 0.51 |
| Very dissatisfied | 0.85 (0.44, 1.64) | 0.62 | 1.75 (0.31, 5.77) | 0.36 |
| Percentage of treatment procedures per week[*] | | | | |
| 0–59% | 1.26 (0.98, 1.63) | 0.08 | – | – |
| 60–100% (reference) | 1.0 | – | – | – |
| Frequency of referral to other dentists score[*] | | | | |
| Low (reference) | 1.0 | – | 1.0 | – |
| High | 1.36 (1.03, 1.79) | 0.03 | 1.20 (0.74, 1.94) | 0.46 |
| Perception of other dentists | | | | |
| Competitor (reference) | 1.0 | – | 1.0 | – |
| Colleague | 1.58 (1.12, 2.23) | 0.01 | 2.17 (1.19, 3.98) | 0.01 |
| Perceived pressure from other dental practices | | | | |
| Medium/Large amount of pressure (reference) | 1.0 | – | 1.0 | – |
| Do not feel pressure/Small amount of pressure | 1.41 (1.08, 1.83) | 0.01 | 1.11 (0.62, 1.97) | 0.73 |

CI, confidence interval.
* continuous variable that was dichotomised at the median due to the lack of a normal distribution.

in the practice; number of hygienist hours; share of diagnostic and preventive procedures and elective procedures performed per week; whether the respondent was the primary income-earner in the household; number of dependents; and income.

In multivariable logistic regression, female gender and perceiving other dentists to be colleagues rather than competitors were most strongly associated with having a broad moral community. Interestingly, the 'perception of other dentists' variable can also be considered one which measures moral inclusiveness, as a dentist who believes other practitioners to be their colleagues would be demonstrating a willingness to include these others in their moral community.

## What does moral inclusiveness mean to the dental profession?

We set out to measure the moral inclusiveness of a representative sample of Ontario dentists and found that the majority of dentists did agree with morally inclusive values, and that those who agreed with morally inclusive values were more likely to have a broad moral community. However, congruent with Canadian literature, we found that the respondents showed bias against patients on social assistance (Bedos et al., 2013, 2014; Lévesque, Levine, and Bedos, 2015, 2016); while 94.7 per cent of respondents felt they had a duty to care for all patients in their practices, only 68.9 per cent felt they had a duty to care for adults on social assistance, the lowest percentage of all the social groups presented to dentists in our study. These findings, along with our respondents' lower agreement with the Likert-type scale questions 'Dentists should lobby for dental benefits for the disadvantaged' and 'Reducing inequalities in oral health across the population is important to me', suggest that dentists readily acknowledge a duty to care for the patients in their practices but are less supportive of the notion of providing care to groups who are not like themselves or the population broadly. One may further speculate that dentists may not recognise that the social contract includes a duty to look after the health of all of society.

More importantly, these findings lead to the question, 'Should moral inclusiveness be a part of dentists' professionalism?' We contend that the answer should be 'yes'. Researchers and the media have documented the public's perception that dentists are not acting altruistically with a resultant loss of public trust (Reid et al., 2014; Rule and Welie, 2009). Leaders in dentistry and researchers have consequently argued that the profession can regain the public's trust by re-affirming the social contract (Cruess and Cruess, 2008; Holden and Quiñonez, 2020; Moeller and Quiñonez, 2020). Central to the social contract is the dentist's responsibility to put patients' needs before their own and to act for the public good, two principles which embody moral inclusiveness. Indeed, if the dental profession is not seen as fulfilling their end of the social contract, then society may 'renegotiate' or at worse 'revoke' dentistry's professional status (Moeller and Quiñonez, 2020).

Recognising a duty to care for all patient groups may require dentists to reflect on their own biases. Qualitative studies have revealed the institutionalised views and misconceptions that dentists have about poverty and low-income patients (Bedos et al., 2013, 2014; Lévesque, Levine, and Bedos, 2015, 2016; Loignon et al., 2012). For example, researchers have found that dentists predominantly use a biomedical approach to care, though it fails to take into account the influence of the social determinants of health (Lévesque, Levine, and

Bedos, 2015; Peres et al., 2019). Patients who are unable to follow chair-side oral health advice due to lack of choice or personal capacity are met not with sympathy from dentists but disdain (Lévesque, Levine, and Bedos, 2015). Dentists may also categorise the poor into 'deserving' and 'non-deserving' and base their social responsibility on these categorisations (Lévesque, Levine, and Bedos, 2015; Loignon et al., 2012). It has been suggested that the discriminatory actions of health care professionals may arise from 'othering', a process that identifies those that are thought to be different from oneself or the mainstream (Johnson et al., 2004). Further, othering may be exacerbated by the power differential between dentists and poor patients (Otto, 2017). However, as members of a high-power group, dentists must understand the inequitable distributions of privilege and disadvantage within their society, and see how their individual actions may contribute to societal problems (Opotow, Gerson, and Woodside, 2005).

Whether moral inclusiveness, or professionalism for that matter, can be taught has been the subject of great debate and is beyond the scope of this chapter. However, if one believes professionalism to be a social construct, then the imparting of professionalism might best focus upon socialisation within an occupational setting rather than setting out to teach professionalism explicitly (Taylor, Grey, and Checkland, 2017). Furthermore, some have proposed that humanising people or helping a person gain a sense of understanding with another makes it more likely for a person to include the other in their moral community (Opotow, 1990). Testing this theory, one pilot course from McGill University in Canada has aimed to reduce dentist and their staff's reluctance to treat social assistance patients (Lévesque, Levine, and Bedos, 2016). By invoking personal stories of the poor and teaching about the social determinants of health, the course has shown modest changes in participants' attitudes towards low-income groups. However, it did have the unintended consequence of reinforcing some negative pre-existing views.

Ultimately, we envision morally inclusive dentists as those who understand that their duty to care for society at-large may go beyond their 'four clinic walls'. Sullivan (2005) has used the term 'civic professionalism' to refer to the movement in which individual physicians and the medical profession represent a force for good in society. Stevens (2001) further argues that the medical profession must fulfil its 'public roles' and be seen doing so in an exemplary fashion in order to gain public support for the concept of professionalism. For the dental profession, this may include actions to address oral health-related inequity. However, such initiatives require the skills of mobilising and working with governments to execute strategies at the population level (Halliday, 2011; Kuo et al., 2011). Recognising the need for such skills, the American medical profession has added political advocacy as a requirement for graduate medical education in paediatrics (Accreditation Council for Graduate Medical Education, 2020) and paediatric dentistry residency programmes have included advocacy instruction in their curricula (Vishnevetsky, Mirman, and Bhoopathi, 2018). While the profession of dentistry in Canada has not implemented such interventions, advocacy education could be considered as a means to fulfil (at least in part) dentists' responsibility for the health of the general public (Halliday, 2011; Kuo et al., 2011).

Further, while some have claimed that advocacy detracts from the doctor's primary work, which is to treat patients in their practices (Arnett, 2002; Huddle, 2011), others have argued that the social contract compels doctors to advocate (Girard-Pearlman Banack and Byrne, 2011; Welie, 2012). In essence, dentists, by virtue of their education, work, and status, and the privileges that these inhere, are ideally suited to become advocates in health (Rule and Welie, 2009; Vishnevetsky, Mirman, and Bhoopathi, 2018). As Girard-Pearlman Banack and Byrne (2011, p. 1065) explain, advocacy by doctors does not necessarily mean becoming politicians but can mean

> being sufficiently aware of the determinants of health, as well as problems and resources in the specific communities where their practices are located, to know when a situation requires them to become advocates for the individual or collective well-being of their patients.

Moreover, it is important to consider that governments, through their structuring and funding of health systems, can have a profound effect on professionalism, either by supporting or subverting professional healing roles and traditional values (Sullivan, 2005; also see Raskin, this volume). For example, structuring dentistry as separate from public health care systems can result in a lack of dentist participation and potentially the idea among dentists that they hold few responsibilities or even a role in the broader health care environment. Similarly, paying low fees, limiting the dental services that are covered and imposing complicated paperwork (common concerns among dentists) are known to result in a lack of dentist participation in public programmes (Borchgrevink, Snyder, and Gehshan, 2008; Quiñonez, Figueiredo, and Locker, 2009). As such, the profession needs members and their organised representation to advocate for structural and programme reform.

In addition, the relationship between business considerations and dentists' moral inclusiveness merits further investigation. Both the sociological (Crosby and Lubin, 1990; Opotow, 1990) and dental literature (Dharamsi, Pratt, and MacEntee, 2007; Harris et al., 2014; Harris and Holt, 2013; Öcek and Vatansever, 2014) have suggested that the breadth of one's moral community can be delimited by resource scarcity or economic pressures. For example, Harris and Holt (2013) found that their dentist-respondents prioritised the needs of their patients and the local community, rather than society as whole, explaining that their livelihoods depended on these close relationships. Furthermore, Dharamsi, Pratt and MacEntee (2007) found that dentists based their social responsibility not only on professionalism but on economic, political and structural factors as well. A greater understanding of the interplay between these factors on moral inclusiveness may aid in refining our study's measures.

Also, with regard to our unvalidated measures, we recognise the effect of social desirability on the distribution of the moral community score. We further acknowledge the controversy with using weights in measures (Evans, 1991). However, statistical analysis was done without applying the weights to the six social groups and was found to yield nearly identical results. Despite these limitations, our findings were mostly consistent with the literature or made inherent sense. Thus, our exploratory study may lay the preliminary groundwork for the development of a moral inclusiveness scale for dentists or other health care professionals, and for a greater exploration of these issues and their implications for such things as professionalism, tackling health-related inequities, and health care systems more generally.

To conclude, while some believe that doctors should only look after the health of their patients (Arnett, 2002; Huddle, 2011), we contend that dentists must also look after the health of the public at-large. The social contract compels the profession to do so, and if the profession is not seen as being morally inclusive, then dentists' professional status may be at risk (Holden and Quiñonez, 2020; Moeller and Quiñonez, 2020). In addition, dentists must understand the collective nature of professionalism (Welie and Rule, 2006). While the duty to look after the health of all of society is a daunting task, this may become much more manageable if each dentist assumes their fair share of the responsibility (Welie, 2012). Further, knowing and understanding dentists' moral inclusiveness is arguably an important consideration in strategies aimed at reducing oral health-related inequity, and for the success of public health programmes or policies. In the end, the challenge for dental educators, associations and regulators will be to facilitate in practitioners a 'willingness to go beyond the isolation of [narrowly] interpreting one's professional role in order to be connected to the concerns of other individuals and to the overall well-being of society' (Hershey, 1994, p. 33).

## References

Accreditation Council for Graduate Medical Education. (2020) 'ACGME Program Requirements for Graduate Medical Education in Pediatrics'. [Viewed 18 September 2020]. Available from: https://www.acgme.org/Portals/0/PFAssets/ProgramRequirements/320_Pediatrics_2020.pdf?ver=2020-06-29-162726-647

Apelian, N. et al. (2020) 'Is the dental profession ready for person-centred care?', *British Dental Journal*, 229(2), pp. 133–137.

Arnett, J. C. (2002) 'The medical professionalism project and its physician charter: new ethics for a political agenda', *Medical Sentinel*, 7(2), pp. 56–57. [Viewed 18 September 2020]. Available from: http://www.jpands.org/hacienda/arnett3.html

Bebeau, M. J., Born, D. O. and Ozar, D. T. (1993) 'Development of a professional role orientation inventory', *The Journal of the American College of Dentists*, 60(2), pp. 27–33.

Bedos, C. et al. (2013) 'How health professionals perceive and experience treating people on social assistance: a qualitative study among dentists in Montreal, Canada', *BMC Health Services Research*, 13(464), pp. 1–9.

Bedos, C. et al. (2014) 'Providing care to people on social assistance: how dentists in Montreal, Canada, respond to organisational, biomedical, and financial challenges', *BMC Health Services Research*, 14(472), pp. 1–9. [Viewed 18 September 2020]. Available from: http://www.ncbi.nlm.nih.gov/pubmed/25301021

Borchgrevink, A., Snyder, A. and Gehshan, S. (2008) *The effects of medicaid reimbursement rates on access to dental care*. Portland. [Viewed 18 September 2020]. Available from: https://nashp.org/wp-content/uploads/sites/default/files/CHCF_dental_rates.pdf

Brennan, D. S. and Spencer, A. J. (2005) 'The role of dentist, practice and patient factors in the provision of dental services', *Community Dentistry and Oral Epidemiology*, 33(3), pp. 181–195.

Burt, B. A. and Eklund, S. A. (2005) *Dentistry, dental practice, and the community*. St. Louis: Elsevier Saunders.

Canadian Dental Association. (2015) CDA *Principles of Ethics*. [Viewed 18 September 2020] Available from: https://www.cda-adc.ca/en/about/ethics/

Crimston, D., Bain, P. G., Hornsey, M. J. and Bastian, B. (2016) 'Moral expansiveness: examining variability in the extension of the moral world', *Journal of Personality and Social Psychology*, 109(12), pp. 1–18.

Crosby, F. J. and Lubin, E. P. (1990) 'Extending the moral community: logical and psychological dilemmas', *Journal of Social Issues*, 46(1), pp. 163–172.

Cruess, R. L. and Cruess., S. R. (2008) 'Expectations and obligations: professionalism and medicine's social contract with society', *Perspectives in Biology and Medicine*, 51(4), pp. 579–598.

Dharamsi, S., Pratt, D. D. and MacEntee, M. I. (2007) 'How dentists account for social responsibility: economic imperatives and professional obligations', *Journal of Dental Education*, 71(12), pp. 1583–1592.

Evans, M. G. (1991) 'The problem of analyzing multiplicative composites: interactions revisited', *American Psychologist*, 46(1), pp. 6–15.

Girard-Pearlman Banack, J. and Byrne, N. (2011) 'Do medical professionalism and medical education involve commitments to political advocacy? [Letter to the Editor]', *Academic Medicine*, 86(9), pp. 1064–1065.

Gordon, E. and Batchelor, P. (2007) 'A longitudinal study into changing ethical attitudes of newly-qualified dentists in South-East England', *Primary Dental Care*, 14(2), pp. 73–78.

Gray, J. B. (2011) 'From 'directing them' to 'it's up to them': the physician's perceived professional role in the physician–patient relationship', *Journal of Communication in Healthcare*, 4(4), pp. 281–288.

Grembowski, D., Milgrom, P. and Fiset, L. (1991) 'Dental decisionmaking and variation in dentist service rates', *Social Science & Medicine*, 32(3), pp. 287–294.

Haidet, Paul et al. (2002) 'Medical student attitudes toward the doctor–patient relationship', *Medical Education*, 36(6), pp. 568–574.

Halliday, M. (2011) 'Do medical professionalism and medical education involve commitments to political advocacy?' [Letter to the Editor], *Academic Medicine*, 86(9), pp. 1063.

Harris, R., Brown, S., Holt, R. and Perkins, E. (2014) 'Do institutional logics predict interpretation of contract rules at the dental chair-side?', *Social Science & Medicine*, 122, pp. 81–89.

Harris, R. and Holt, R. (2013) 'Interacting institutional logics in general dental practice', *Social Science & Medicine*, 94, pp. 63–70.

Hershey, G. H. (1994) 'Professors and professionals: higher education's role in developing ethical dentists', *Journal of the American College of Dentists*, 61(2), pp. 29–33.

Hojat, M. et al. (2001) 'The Jefferson Scale of physician empathy: development and preliminary psychometric data', *Educational and Psychological Measurement*, 61(2), pp. 349–365.

Holden, A. C. L. (2016) 'Self-regulation in dentistry and the social contract', *British Dental Journal*, 221(8), pp. 449–451.

Holden, A. C. L. and Quiñonez, C. (2020) 'The role of the dental professional association in the 21st century', *International Dental Journal*, 70, pp. 239–244.

Huddle, T. S. (2011) 'Medical professionalism and medical education should not involve commitments to political advocacy', *Academic Medicine*, 86(3), pp. 378–383.

Johnson, J. L. et al. (2004) 'Othering and being othered in the context of health care services', *Health Communication*, 16(2), pp. 253–271.

Krupat, E. et al. (2000) 'The practice orientations of physicians and patients: the effect of doctor–patient congruence on satisfaction', *Patient Education and Counseling*, 39(1), pp. 49–59.

Kuo, A. A. et al. (2011) 'Do medical professionalism and medical education involve commitments to political advocacy? [Letter to the Editor]', *Academic Medicine*, 86(9), pp. 1061–1062.

Lévesque, M., Levine, A. and Bedos, C. (2015) 'Ideological roadblocks to humanizing dentistry, an evaluative case study of a continuing education course on social determinants of health', *International Journal for Equity in Health*, 14(41), pp. 1–14.

Lévesque, M., Levine, A. and Bedos, C. (2016) 'Humanizing oral health care through continuing education on social determinants of health: evaluative case study of a Canadian private dental clinic', *Journal of Health Care for the Poor and Underserved*, 27(3), pp. 971–992.

Loignon, C. et al. (2012) 'How do dentists perceive poverty and people on social assistance? A qualitative study conducted in Montreal, Canada', *Journal of Dental Education*, 76(5), pp. 545–552.

McKernan, S. et al. (2015) 'The relationship between altruistic attitudes and dentists' Medicaid participation', *The Journal of the American Dental Association*, 146(1), pp. 34–41. e3.

Moeller, J. and Quiñonez, C. (2020) 'Dentistry's social contract is at risk', *The Journal of the American Dental Association*, 151(5), pp. 334–339.

Morselli, D. and Passini, S. (2012) 'Measuring moral inclusion: a validation of the inclusion/exclusion of other groups (IEG) scale', *LIVES Working Papers*, 14, pp. 1–18.

Nicholson, S. et al. (2015) 'The effect of education debt on dentists' career decisions', *Journal of the American Dental Association*, 146(11), pp. 800–807.

Öcek, Z. A. and Vatansever, K. (2014) 'Perceptions of Turkish dentists of their professional identity in a market-orientated system', *International Journal of Health Sciences*, 44(3), pp. 593–613.

Ontario Dental Association. (2020) 'About the ODA', [Viewed 18 September 2020]. Available from: https://oda.ca/about-the-oda

Opotow, S. (1990) 'Moral exclusion and injustice: an introduction', *Journal of Social Issues*, 46(1), pp. 1–20.

Opotow, S., Gerson, J. and Woodside, S. (2005) 'From moral exclusion to moral inclusion: theory for teaching peace', *Theory Into Practice*, 44(4), pp. 303–318.

Otto, M. (2017) *Teeth: the story of beauty, inequality, and the struggle for oral health in America*. New York: The New Press.

Ozar, D. T. (1985) 'Three models of professionalism and professional obligation in dentistry', *Journal of the American Dental Association*, 110(2), pp. 173–177.

Ozar, D. T. and Sokol, D. J. (2002) *Dental ethics at chairside: professional principles and practical applications*. Second. Washington D. C.: Georgetown University Press.

Peres, M. A. et al. (2019) 'Oral diseases: a global public health challenge', *The Lancet*, 394(10194), pp. 249–260.

Pourat, N., Roby, D. H., Wyn, R. and Marcus, M. (2007) 'Characteristics of dentists providing dental care to publicly insured patients', *Journal of Public Health Dentistry*, 67(4), pp. 208–216.

Quiñonez, C. (2021) *The politics of dental care in Canada*. Toronto: Canadian Scholars.

Quiñonez, C., Figueiredo, R. and Locker, D. (2009) 'Canadian dentists' opinions on publicly financed dental care', *Journal of Public Health Dentistry*, 69(2), pp. 64–73.

Redford, M. and Gift, H. C. (1997) 'Dentist-patient interactions in treatment decision-making: a qualitative study', *Journal of Dental Education*, 61(1), pp. 16–21.

Regan, T. (1983) *The case for animal rights*. Berkeley: University of California Press.

Reid, K. et al. (2014) 'A comparison of expectations and impressions of ethical characteristics of dentists: results of a community primary care survey', *Journal of the American Dental Association*, 145(8), pp. 829–834.

Royal College of Dental Surgeons of Ontario., (2020). *RCDSO Code of Ethics*. [Viewed 18 September 2020]. Available from: https://www.rcdso.org/en-ca/rcdso-members/your-responsibilities/code-of-ethics

Rule, J. T. and Welie, J. V. M. (2009) 'The dilemma of access to care: symptom of a systemic condition', *Dental Clinics of North America*, 53(3), pp. 421–433.

Schwartz, S. H. (2007) 'Universalism values and the inclusiveness of our moral universe', *Journal of Cross-Cultural Psychology*, 38(6), pp. 711–728.

Spohn, W. (1996) 'Who counts? Images shape our moral community', *Issues in Ethics*, 7(2), pp. 2–5. [Viewed 18 September 2020]. Available from: https://legacy.scu.edu/ethics/publications/iie/v7n2/spohn.html

Stevens, R. A. (2001) 'Public roles for the medical profession in the United States: beyond theories of decline and fall'. *The Milbank Quarterly*, 79(3), pp. 327–353.

Sullivan, W. M. (2005) *Work and integrity: the crisis and promise of professionalism in America*. Second. San Francisco: Jossey-Bass.

Taylor, C., Grey, N. J. A. and Checkland, K. (2017) 'Professionalism … It depends where you're standing', *British Dental Journal*, 222(11), pp. 889–892.

Trathen, A. and Gallagher, J. E. (2009) 'Dental professionalism: definitions and debate', *British Dental Journal*, 206(5), pp. 249–253.

Verlinde, E. et al. (2012) 'The social gradient in doctor-patient communication', *International Journal for Equity in Health*, 11(12), pp. 1–14.

Vishnevetsky, A., Mirman, J. and Bhoopathi, V. (2018) 'Effect of advocacy training during dental education on pediatric dentists' interest in advocating for community water fluoridation', *Journal of Dental Education*, 82(1), pp. 54–60.

Warren, M. A. (1997) *Moral status: obligations to persons and other living things*. Oxford: Clarendon Press.

Welie, J. V. M. (2004) 'Is dentistry a profession? Part 1. professionalism defined', *Journal of the Canadian Dental Association*, 70(8), pp. 529–532.

Welie, J. V. M. (2012) 'Social contract theory as a foundation of the social responsibilities of health professionals', *Medicine, Health Care and Philosophy*, 15(3), pp. 347–355.

Welie, J. V. M. and Rule, J. T. (2006) 'Overcoming isolationism: moral competencies, virtues and the importance of connectedness', in: Welie, J. V. M. (ed.) *Justice in oral health care*. Milwaukee: Marquette University Press. pp. 97–125.

Willems, S. et al. (2005) 'Socio-economic status of the patient and doctor–patient communication: does it make a difference?', *Patient Education and Counseling*, 56(2), pp. 139–146.

Yu, B. et al. (2019) 'Perceived professional roles and implications for clinical decision-making', *Journal of Public Health Dentistry*, 80(1), pp. 43–50.

Zijlstra-Shaw, S., Roberts, T. E. and Robinson, P. G. (2013) 'Perceptions of professionalism in dentistry – a qualitative study', *British Dental Journal*, 215(E18), pp. 1–6.

# 3 Designing healthy smiles

*Rizwana Lala*

The dental profession often defines cosmetic dentistry as 'unessential' treatments pursued by people solely to improve their appearance despite looking 'normal'. Contradictorily, this unessential healthcare is sometimes described as treatments to make people look 'normal' (Nuffield Council on Bioethics, 2017; Department of Health, 2012; Dental Council of New Zealand, 2009). In other words, cosmetic dentistry is concerned with contested beauty norms. Understanding cosmetic dentistry in this sense, as an aesthetic practice to achieve the normative beauty ideal, leads to the question of how this ideal is negotiated, defined and propagated.

Teeth and mouth modifications to improve appearance have a long and diverse history from wide-ranging practices such as inlays fashioned in teeth by the Olmecs in Mexico, going as far back as 1400 B.C. (Tapia et al., 2002); Japanese women blackening their teeth in the Tokugawa period (seventeenth century to nineteenth century A.D.) (Ring, 1992), to current whitening and straightening trends. However, what is unique about cosmetic dentistry today is that it is undertaken by registered healthcare professionals in clinical and quasi-clinical environments (Nuffield Council on Bioethics, 2017; Department of Health, 2012). This gives the practice a distinctive legitimacy that works towards masking the potential negative consequences for patients and society at large.

This chapter examines how beauty treatments provided as healthcare causes symbolic damage to healthcare systems and violates people's autonomy over their bodies.[1] The cosmetic dentistry journey of a patient named Janette, quotes from dentists, patients and members of the public, and excerpts from the *Dentists Act 1984* (the principal legislation that currently governs UK dentistry), highlights how the institutionally legitimated status of dentists as educated, healthcare professionals produces symbolic power which works towards shaping what is considered a beautiful and even a normal smile. This constructed perception of a normal smile is at odds with the diverse smile and face appearances that exist in a plural society. This mismatch is fuelling the demand for beauty treatments in private dentistry. Moreover, the increasing provision of private care limits access to NHS dentistry and the value attached to its provision.

DOI: 10.4324/9781003047674-4

## Janette's journey

Scrolling down her Instagram feed, Janette saw a new post from Dr James titled 'Smile Tweaks' with before and after photographs of smiles. The after photograph was brilliant white, toothy and framed with fleshy red-lipsticked borders. The post had 452 'likes' and described how the naturally beautiful smile was designed with just simple re-contouring of the teeth with composite bonding[2] and some non-surgical tweaks – tweakments[3] – to the lips. Janette scrolled down the 43 comments, some of which were from other cosmetic dentists she followed on Instagram – 'wow', 'beautiful', 'quality', 'so natural' and so forth.

The Instagram profile of a well-groomed, bespectacled 'Dr James BDS MFDS RCSEd MJDF RCS Eng – Award Nominated Dental Surgeon, Cosmetic Dentist, Cosmetic Dentistry Trainer' had over 20,000 followers. Thumbing down his posts, Janette saw before and after pictures of smiles Dr James had 'designed' as well as photographs of Dr James with his wife confidently smiling at their Hollywood-style wedding, extravagant honeymoon and family holidays.

Below Dr James' profile, Janette clicked the monikered hyperlink, www. drjamesedwards.co.uk and was taken to pages showing Dr James' awards for his cosmetic dental designs. These designs had featured in magazines Janette read. She browsed the gallery of before and after photographs, patient videos and testimonies. There were photographs of white, gleaming laughter of Dr James' patients and family, some of which were already familiar to her from Instagram. A range of treatments were offered to design the perfect 'smile zone': composite bonding, veneers, Invisalign,[4] non-surgical facial tweaks and skincare.

Prompted by the various finance options displayed on the website, Janette clicked on the online booking form for her free consultation with Dr James. For this, Janette had travelled to an unfamiliar part of Britain. The American accent of Google maps informed her she had arrived at her destination – the Dental Health and Beauty Spa – located on a quiet suburban street in a beautiful Victorian house. The white-wooden framed windows had the pink of orchids peeping through the glass. The Dental Health and Beauty spa was inviting – comfortable, not clinical.

Janette walked up the steps to ring the buzzer adjacent to familiar media logos: *BBC, Daily Mail, Marie Claire* – all of which she had already seen whilst browsing Dr James' website. The buzzer was answered by a plummy but friendly feminine voice. Janette spoke into the metal block about her appointment and with the cue of the buzz, she pushed the door open. She walked up to the receptionist who told her to take a seat on one of the cream upholstered sofas. The surroundings were very different from Janette's usual NHS practice. Blasting Radio 2 was substituted with calming music, polypropylene canteen chairs with comfortable sofas, toothpaste and toothbrush with Obagi creams, sunscreens, moisturisers, eye creams and serum boosters.

## The beautiful smile in messages

Janette's journey to the Dental Health and Beauty Spa was paved with messages in various media: magazines, Instagram, photographs, websites, finance and appointment forms, 'Dr' James' qualification letters and awards, YouTube videos of patient testimonies, the practice plaque. These media messages market cosmetic treatments, products and dentists themselves. As Janette's journey progressed, her experiences and these messages highlighted the contrasts between conventional dentistry – for routine care and care for pain – and cosmetic dentistry for beauty.

Smith (2005) describes how messages in various media such as Instagram, qualification certificates and websites can be significant symbols. Significant symbols are when the creator and the observer of the message understand it as the same thing (Smith, 2005; Mead, 1934). So, Dr James created his website and practice plaque to show his smile designs had featured in *Marie Claire*, knowing that observers of the *Marie Claire* logo would interpret his smile designs as beautiful. He sandwiches his name with the title Dr and qualification letters on Instagram to show his followers, including Janette, that he is a highly trained and educated health professional. Dr James is creating messages that are intended to be interpreted in specific ways. That is, a beautiful smile is one with straight, white teeth framed with certain facial features and dentists with abundant Instagram followers, titles, letters after their name, awards, glamorous and hence, 'successful' lifestyles, are highly skilled at undertaking cosmetic treatments. Moreover, expensive skincare products like Obagi sold at cosmetic dental practices are effective, and practices that have their NHS logo replaced with those of *Marie Claire* provide superior 'healthcare'. This does not mean that readers of the messages do not have their own interpretations, but the very notion of a misinterpretation is based on the assumption of what ought to have been understood (Smith, 2005).

People's individual activities are relational to wider institutions. Thus, Dr James writing press releases of his work and using his qualification titles, Janette reading magazines and perusing Instagram are related to institutions like print, digital and social media as well as healthcare and education institutions. These individual activities and their wider institutional relationships play co-ordinated roles in influencing people's interpretation of the beautiful or normal smile. However, this norm is often very narrow.

A UK study examined the photographs of front teeth in magazines aimed at 9–16-year-old girls. The findings showed a very narrow range of teeth shades used in the magazines when compared with the shade spectrum found in young girls and women in real life. Three-quarters of the teeth images had shades that were whiter than those found in nature. Therefore, the magazines portrayed an unrealistic representation of teeth to children and young girls (Chadwick, Cage, and Playle, 2007). Another study of magazines targeting teenage girls also found the images did not reasonably reflect the positions of teenagers' teeth (Mattick, Gordon, and Gillgrass, 2004). This unrealistic representation of teeth in the media has prompted some dentists, like Richard to suggest that media images create unrealistic demands for cosmetic dentistry.

> *The Only Way is Essex, Love Island, Keeping up with the Kardashians* all these shows are having a massive impact because when the patients come into me and they say to me they want this treatment, they come in and they've had their lips done and have had a lot of Botox and these are young patients. Patients who are in their twenties, these are not patients in their fifties, they've had Botox done, they've had lip fillers done and then they want their teeth done. And when they say they want their teeth done, they don't only want teeth whitening, they're asking for veneers and they're not looking for shades of (B1)[5] they're looking for shades of ultra-white shades which almost look ridiculous but that's what they're asking for. And I ask them 'why do you want that?' They frequently quote these programs: Love Island, The only way is Essex, The Kardashians and others that's what they're asking for.
>
> (Richard: UK General Dental Council Registered Dentist)

The evidence from UK magazines and Richard's quote highlight how institutions, such as the media, and individuals are in relationships with one another. These relationships work towards reproducing, reinforcing and propagating specific smile ideals.

Social media, in particular, can pervasively target people who show even the slightest interest in cosmetic dentistry as described by Avatel.

> That's being presented to me via Instagram rather than me having to search online for cosmetic dentistry.
>
> (Avatel: person considering cosmetic dental treatments)

The relational nature of individual and institutional activities is increasing the prevalence of a narrow, normative ideal of the straight, white smile. But the role of dentists and dental institutions in reproducing, reinforcing and propagating beauty ideals is of particular interest because dentists' knowledge and status are institutionally and medically legitimated. Therefore, healthcare professionals – now inclusive of cosmetic dentists – can exercise symbolic power in a way that is not available to beauty practitioners (Bourdieu, 1989, 1991, 1993, 2000). However, cosmetic dentistry, like all clinical treatments, is not risk-free and these risks create tensions and contradictions within healthcare systems.

## Cosmetic dentistry – the contradiction of beauty in healthcare

Within the UK legislative framework, healthcare, including dentistry, is concerned with the treatment of disease, disorder and injury (Care Quality Commission, 2019; Great Britain, Health and Social Care Act 2008; Great Britain, The Health and Social Care Act (Regulated Activities) Regulations 2014). As such, cosmetic dentistry is regarded as 'unessential'. Nonetheless, dentistry is also concerned with appearance as shown by Simon's quote.

> Now, we all know that in medicine we do loads of things that are to do with patients' well-being, self-esteem, etc … And we do a lot. We do loads. You can still do crowns and veneers on the NHS when … what are they for? I mean, crowns, is it just to improve the appearance? I'm sure a lot were put on just for that reason.
>
> (Simon: Senior postgraduate trainer of dentists and
> GDC registered specialist in Orthodontics)

This is not just Simon's or an individual dentist's perception. The General Dental Council (GDC) mandates UK dental schools teach students about aesthetics demonstrated by the learning outcome given here:

> Restore the dentition using the principle of minimal intervention, maintaining function and aesthetics.
>
> (Preparing for Practice: General Dental Council, 2015 - page 90)

Moreover, a whole dental specialty, orthodontics, is largely concerned with treatments for appearance; not only on teeth but also the whole face (Nuffield Council on Bioethics, 2017). Orthodontic treatments often take years, and like most healthcare interventions carry risks of bodily harm. These physical harms to people's bodies such as damage to teeth caused by medical interventions are termed 'clinical iatrogenesis' (Illich, 1976).

Despite the physical harms, orthodontic treatments are often undertaken on adults and children and funded by the UK taxpayer (provided on the NHS) to make people's teeth and face look 'normal'. Simon, a specialist orthodontist describes orthodontics as just giving people a relatively normal appearance.

> And we are just trying to put … ensure that those patients have a relatively normal dentofacial appearance, to make them look normal, in the normal range.
>
> (Simon: Senior postgraduate trainer of dentists and
> GDC registered specialist in Orthodontics)

Simon recognises that orthodontics and by extension, dentistry have always been concerned with treating the whole face and not looking at teeth in isolation.

> As a consultant orthodontist, I am involved in treating patients with significant skeletal discrepancies. Dentofacial appearance is one phrase that's used within my specialty or within the profession. Absolutely, I understand that you can talk about the whole face as well as talking about the teeth.
>
> (Simon: Senior postgraduate trainer of dentists and
> GDC registered specialist in Orthodontics)

So, dental professionals are educated and trained to assess and determine if a person's teeth and face are 'normal'. If someone's appearance falls outside the institutionally defined range of normal, the dental profession labels them as having a 'significant dentofacial discrepancy' – or a disorder warranting a medical intervention. Therefore, treatments that are solely to improve appearance shift from being unessential to essential – in other words they veer from beauty to healthcare. It has been argued that by defining and propagating normal dental and face standards, dentistry has contributed to creating a narrow Euro-centric range of desirable looks. And this narrow range was created because it was in dentists' financial interests (Picard, 2009; Hunt, 1998).

## The business of dentistry

Healthcare and cosmetic treatments are big business. The UK healthcare system funds 'essential' treatments. In order to access this funding, dentists and orthodontists may label people's appearance as abnormal. Nonetheless, over the past decade, the NHS dental budget has remained relatively static at £3.5bn (GDPC Exec, 2019; British Dental Association, 2019; Armstrong, 2018; NHS England, 2014). Therefore, additional income for dentists has to largely come from unessential treatments, or cosmetic dentistry.

Janette's journey shows how cosmetic dentists use digital and conventional media to increase the uptake of cosmetic dentistry. However, Janette's journey is not solitary. Increasing demand for cosmetic dentistry is an organised professional strategy. The British Academy of Cosmetic Dentistry (BACD) encourages dentists to actively offer cosmetic dentistry by placing posters and leaflets in surgeries and place adverts in magazines (Mintel Custom Solutions, 2006, 2007). Dentists' trade union, the British Dental Association (BDA) produces courses, events and marketing literature to support dentists to encourage the uptake of cosmetic treatments by patients (British Dental Association, 2012). The GDC recognises that dentists market treatments and therefore has produced advertising guidance documents for them to follow (GDC 2016, 2013b, 2013a, 2013c, 2012).

However, in the cosmetic market, beauticians are situated as direct competitors to dentists. Thus, dentists create messages – significant symbols – to mark out their superior healthcare training. Janette's journey is interspersed with many messages entered by Dr James signifying his dental training and professional status such as titles, qualifications and grand job descriptions. These significant symbols found in Janette's personal story are tied to the wider institutional relations that legitimate dentists' training and work towards influencing her choices. Nonetheless, there are disjunctures or mismatches between these messages – the authoritative representations of dental training – and the actual cosmetic training of dentists.

## Dentists' cosmetic training – the disjunctures

Throughout her journey, Janette repeatedly read: 'Dr James BDS MFDS RCSEd MJDF RCS Eng – Award Nominated Dental Surgeon, Cosmetic Dentist, Cosmetic Dentistry Trainer'. Instagram, Dr James' website, the practice plaque, his award certificates are just a few places where Janette was exposed to the significant symbols attesting Dr James' training. These significant symbols are read not only by Janette but also by Dr James' 20,000 Instagram followers and the umpteen followers of the people who like, share and comment on his posts.

The title Dr is particularly significant in coordinating people's perception that dentists are highly trained to undertake cosmetic dentistry. This perception also works towards relegating the training of beauticians who traditionally provide cosmetic treatments, which is notable from Avatel and Tasnim's quotes.

> I would be much more inclined to go to a dentist rather than a beautician because I don't think I would trust their training … I would go to a dentist and I'd try to go to as reputable a dentist as possible. And a specialist in tooth whitening, probably.
>
> (Avatel: Member of the public)

> Well as Botox wise, I wouldn't go to a salon or something like that, I would go to like doctors and dentist doctors and those who are qualified, a specialist like. I'd go to one of them to do it … Beauticians does it yeah, but I wouldn't trust going to beautician. I will go to someone proper who really did the course and know what they are doing, I would not go to beautician.
>
> (Tasnim: Member of the public)

Despite dentists like Dr James using the title Dr to signify their 'dentist doctor' training to gain a competitive advantage in the cosmetic dentistry market, the *Dentists Act 1984* forbids dentists from using the title.

> A degree or licence in dentistry granted by a dental authority shall not confer any right or title to be registered under the Medical Act 1983, nor to assume any name, title or designation implying that the holder of the degree or licence is by law recognised as a practitioner or licentiate in medicine or general surgery.
>
> (Section 7: Dentists Act 1984)

Along the same vein, Dr James' Instagram profile description — 'Award Nominated Dental Surgeon, Cosmetic Dentist, Cosmetic Dentistry Trainer' – also contravenes the *Dentists Act 1984* because it is not limited to the descriptions 'dentist', 'dental surgeon' or 'dental practitioner' which is what the legislation specifically requires.

Use of titles and descriptions - A registered dentist shall by virtue of being registered be entitled to take and use the description of dentist, dental surgeon or dental practitioner.

(Section 26 [1]: Dentists Act 1984).

The *Dentists Act 1984* gives powers to the GDC to regulate dentistry through statutory oversight of education, training, dentists' registration, professional standards and fitness to practise. All UK dentists, in order to practise, must meet the GDC's educational requirements and be placed on its dentists' register. In the event of poor practice, the GDC assess dentists' fitness to practise which can result in professionals being removed from the GDC register, and, therefore, unable to practise (General Dental Council, 2019).

None of Dr James qualifications signalled by the letters BDS MFDS RCSEd MJDF RCS Eng include any cosmetic dentistry training. The BDS or Bachelor of Dental Surgery is the primary, undergraduate dental qualification with oversight from the GDC. *Preparing for Practice* is the document that lists all the learning outcomes that UK dental schools must teach and assess for their students to be awarded the BDS and subsequently be registered with the GDC to undertake the 'practice of dentistry'. However, none of the learning outcomes for dentists in *Preparing for Practice* relate to cosmetic dentistry with the terms teeth whitening, Botox, fillers, injectables, cosmetic and beauty absent (General Dental Council, 2015).

The MFDS and MJDF are qualifications awarded after two years in clinical practice and only reinforce basic undergraduate BDS education. Mirroring *Preparing for Practice*, teeth whitening, Botox, fillers, injectables or cosmetic are absent from the MFDS and MJDF syllabuses. The MFDS syllabus specifically states that the qualification is not a specialist examination and does not relate to specialist skills (The Royal College of Surgeons of Edinburgh & The Royal College of Physicians and Surgeons of Glasgow, 2018; Faculty of General Dental Practice (UK) & Faculty of Dental Surgery of the Royal College of Surgeons of England, 2018).

It is important, furthermore, to remember that the MFDS is not a specialist examination and that the level of knowledge expected in any area of the syllabus will not exceed that which would be expected of a dentist who has two years' experience of clinical dental practice.

(Paragraph 20.3, MFDS Regulations, Syllabus, 2018)

Some of Dr James' postnominal letters simply refer to the institutions that awarded the qualification; Royal College of Surgeons Edinburgh (RCSEd) and Royal College of Surgeons England (RCS Eng).

We see that Janette, Avatel and Tasnim's local experiences and perceptions of 'specialist' cosmetic dentistry are influenced by reading the qualification letters that signify cosmetic dentists' education which are awarded and legitimated by institutions such as the GDC, universities and Royal Colleges.

Nonetheless, there is a disjuncture between public perceptions of cosmetic dentists' training in beauty and dentists' actual training.

Despite the GDC's statutory role in regulating dentists and enforcing the *Dentists Act 1984*, we observe that the GDC allows dentists to use the title Dr, which is in breach of the Act. This is in spite of the GDC's own research showing an overwhelming public feeling that dentists who do not hold a medical degree or doctorate should not be allowed to use the title 'Dr' because they felt this was highly misleading. Seventy-three per cent of the participants in the GDC commissioned research felt action should take against dentists falsely using the title 'Dr', with some even stating these dentists should be struck off the register (Costley and Fawcett, 2010). Nonetheless, guidance with respect to the use or misuse of titles is currently absent from any of the GDC's professional standards guideline documents for dentists (General Dental Council, 2013a, 2013b). The BDA defends dentists' right to use 'Dr' and is pressing for the law – the *Dentists Act 1984* – to be changed (British Dental Association, 2013).

As the book's introduction by Jones and Gibson demonstrates, the contentious use of titles and problematic advertising by dentists emerged with the processes of the professionalisation of dentistry. Despite the fact that dental advertising was considered unprofessional and unethical, thus legislatively prohibited throughout the nineteenth century, contemporary dental and medical literature demonstrates that advertising by dentists was widespread. It was only in 1997 that the GDC's position on advertising by dentists started to relax (General Dental Council, 1997) in response to pressure from various bodies, including the Office of Fair Trading (Basker, 2006).

Avatel and Tasmin's assumptions that they would seek a 'specialist' in tooth whitening or cosmetic dentistry demonstrates why the use of titles by dentists is contentious. Currently, cosmetic dentistry is not a GDC speciality; therefore, the GDC does not regulate the training and education of cosmetic dentists (General Dental Council, 2019a). The GDC regulations state that dentists should not use the term 'specialist' if they are not on the specialist register; however, there is no restriction on using the term 'cosmetic dentist' which may imply specialist training.

From Janette's story we see that people act in response to the significant symbols that are introduced by some cosmetic dentists in their advertising practices. In particular, people seek cosmetic dentistry specifically from dentists because they assume that they are highly regulated and trained to undertake the treatments. This assumption also works towards undermining beauticians.

I guess I would assume that dentists' surgeries, whether public or private, will be regulated by some kind of overarching dental ethos. I don't really know. But anything that you could buy publicly [internet, beauticians] would not be.

(Avatel: Member of the public).

Despite these assumptions; first, we can see from Dr James' profile that he may not have specific training in cosmetic dentistry or beauty and second, beauticians can train for years for many possible qualifications (NVQ, BTEC, HND[6], etc.) to carry out cosmetic treatments. This training can include the study of anatomy and physiology, first aid and health and safety. However, just like cosmetic dentists, beauticians' training may or may not include some treatments they provide, such as filler injections (Department of Health, 2012). In other words, akin to cosmetic dentists, beauticians' training in cosmetics is unregulated.

In addition to the disjuncture seen between cosmetic dentists' training and public perceptions and expectations, dentists' symbolic capital[7] and power, by virtue of the recognition of the title Dr, and their educational status, allows them to charge higher prices than beauticians. Craig described how cosmetic dentistry is expensive, but he chooses to go to a dentist; 'someone who is qualified', rather than a beautician. Francesca, who is Craig's cosmetic dentist, is all too aware of the higher prices she charges when compared with beauticians.

> The cost does affect me a little bit … You know, somebody who's qualified, but it is expensive.
>
> (Craig: Cosmetic Dentistry Patient)

> The younger ones want to have their lips puffy and I don't do masses of that because I'm not the cheapest person … I probably get more of that middle-aged group because I'm a bit more expensive.
>
> (Francesca- UK GDC registered dentist)

We can see that cosmetic dentists' symbolic capital is converted into economic capital in the form of higher charges, thus higher profit margins. This polarisation of capital results in cosmetic dentists having heightened economic and symbolic resources to express and prescribe a legitimate view (Bourdieu, 1989, 2000, 2001). This view is the ideal of the straight, white smile with particular facial features which is reproduced through individual and institutional messages found in Instagram before and after photographs, magazines and marketing literatures.

As well as the disjuncture between cosmetic dentists' professional training and people's expectations, the significant symbols or marketing of cosmetic dentistry leads to another disjuncture; the beautiful, glamorous images of cosmetic dentistry and most people's unglamorous lived experiences of visiting the dentist.

## Glamorous beauty in healthcare

Janette's journey shows how cosmetic dentists on Instagram present a glamorous, beauty side of cosmetic dentistry that can overshadow the health and even the messy painful elements of healthcare. At the private Dental Health and Beauty Spa, the beauty messages outshine those surrounding dental health, with toothbrushes and toothpastes replaced with the expensive Obagi award-winning 'medical' skincare range (Obagi, 2020).

Tamara described this disjuncture, arguing that the beauty focus of cosmetic dentistry places dentists and dentistry within the beauty industry, rather than healthcare.

> Makes me realise how pervasive the expectation to have white teeth is, and how trends surrounding it are driven by social media gimmicks rather than the less glam side of dentistry ... It's almost as if dentists are a separate thing ... like teeth is part of the beauty industry rather than the health industry.
> (Tamara – Cosmetic Dentistry Patient's Diary)

The focus on beauty in dentistry is also leading to tensions within the profession. Despite the recognition that dentistry is concerned with the appearance of the face and teeth, some dentists, including orthodontists like Simon, disagree with smile tweakments with Botox and fillers.

> I think when you come onto enhancement of facial features, so things around Botox, fillers and these sorts of things, I have a significant amount of concern about this being seen as part of dentistry. I was shocked to see an article in the BDJ[8] last year which almost led me to think about resigning again, which was purely about the use of Botox to change facial aesthetics and nothing to do with dentistry.
> (Simon: Senior postgraduate trainer of dentists and GDC registered specialist in Orthodontics)

> I don't consider it [Botox and fillers] to be dentistry, no. But it is done frequently by dentists and is done frequently in conjunction with dental procedures and is now being seen almost as a whole package of lips, fillers, Botox and teeth but it doesn't sit comfortably with me.
> (Richard: UK General Dental Council Registered Dentist)

These quotes show that changes to social norms do not occur uniformly. Some institutions and individuals within dentistry have been more responsive and accepting of change which is creating tensions (Webb, 2002; Bourdieu, 2001). And although treatments to improve the face have long been part of dentistry, dental institutions largely consider dental practice to be healthcare. Thus, facial aesthetics or the further encroachment of beauty practices into dental practice/healthcare is causing disagreements over the values of dentistry. Nonetheless, the social practices and values within dentistry are changing. These changes have potential impacts for individuals and society.

## Social impacts

The institutional legitimation of cosmetic dentistry and its uptake have four key social consequences. First, as described, cosmetic dentistry is not risk-free. Clinical iatrogenesis or the physical harms caused by dental treatments are common. These range from pain, swelling, infection, damage to the teeth and gums short- and long-term failures of treatments that require remedial care. Teeth in particular are hard tissues; once they are drilled, they do not heal – the damage is permanent. Thus, the before and after pictures Janette saw on Instagram hide the messy failures – the damaging and unhealable facets of cosmetic dentistry.

> They'll only post their good ones … that's terrible to me … I think it's absolutely awful that we think, you know, you've done a before and after, can you show me that patient in 10 years? In five years? So they've got some beautiful veneers, well, if they'd had orthodontics and a bit of bleaching … can we see them in 10 years and see what the periodontal condition[9] is, etc.?
>
> (Simon: Senior postgraduate trainer of dentists and GDC registered specialist in Orthodontics)

Second, these failures have impacts on the NHS. The NHS often provides remedial care for failures and sub-standard cosmetic treatments provided in the private sector (Nuffield Council on Bioethics, 2017, 2018). Not only this, the focus away from dental health towards beauty, with the concurrent loss of dental health prevention messages may increase dental health treatment needs. Specifically, dentists focusing on private beauty treatments can create workforce shortages within the NHS and timely dental care access problems. Thus, the provision of private beauty treatments by healthcare professionals can divert healthcare and personnel resources away from the NHS.

Third, the practice of cosmetic dentistry is not a neutral exercise, it does symbolic damage to the NHS. Despite the remedial care provided by the NHS in response to cosmetic treatment failures, the value patients attach to private dental care can work towards relegating the value they attach to the NHS. Janette drew unfavourable comparisons of her NHS dental care relative to the choices and care she received at the Dental Health and Beauty Spa. Cosmetic dentists often argue that private dental practice allows them to give patients wider treatment choices – choices that are unavailable on the NHS. These private choices can make people feel limited within the NHS as seen by Elsie's quote:

> I have had NHS treatment before and I'm not saying that they don't do a good job. But here I just feel you are more well looked after, and things are tailored to your needs. They go through 101 different options with you and I just think that … it's just made me feel comfortable and I can trust.
>
> (Elsie: Cosmetic Dentistry Patient)

In some respects, choice is plentiful in cosmetic dentistry. As Elsie said, there are a 101 options. But the 101 options are only a tiny fraction of the continually expanding cosmetic dental market. The vastness of the market makes it difficult for the public to make informed choices independently; therefore, people rely on gatekeepers – dentists – to offer the appropriate choices. However, cosmetic dentists have a vested financial interest in the uptake of cosmetic dentistry. This conflict of interest has the potential to constrain choice, particularly the choice to decline treatments.

Third, as an extension of orthodontics, treatments provided by cosmetic dentists to create straight, ultra-white teeth with additional Botox and fillers to create the coveted 'beautiful' smile may further shift and narrow the 'range' of what is professionally defined as 'normal'. This new normal may have the effect of creating more 'significant dentofacial discrepancies' that require healthcare interventions. Therefore, social practices, such as the practice of cosmetic dentistry, and social norms, such as a normal smile, do not just appear, but they have a history that is related to both individual and institutional activities (Smith, 2005; Bourdieu, 1993, 2000).

Tamara presciently describes how messages in the media with the complicity of the dental profession is narrowing the range of normal so that everyone has 'the same face'.

> This other trap of like being bombarded with these images of, it's literally everyone on Instagram has got the same face. They've had the same fillers, they've had the same dental treatment. They've had the same kind of work done everywhere. So it's really hard to not just start to kind of see that as 'that's what you must look like.'
>
> (Tamara: Cosmetic Dentistry Patient)

Quotes from patients and dentists indicate that there is already a shift towards a narrower ideal of 'normal' leading to calls for cosmetic dentistry to be provided on the NHS.

> Not everyone can afford to come private. I mean, it's expensive. I do think it should be more readily available for people at a more affordable cost for people.
>
> (Elsie: Cosmetic Dentistry Patient)

> I would like to see, obviously, more NHS resources for cosmetic procedures.
>
> (Richard: UK General Dental Council Registered Dentist)

Thus, this narrow, normative smile ideal paradoxically uses the notion of choice to limit free choice and curtail any possibilities that are broader than the endorsed norm (Bauman, 2005). This absence of choices – what type of smile to have and who to go to for treatments – disproportionately affects those who cannot afford cosmetic dentistry as described by Elsie and also curtails the choices of diverse communities who may hold different views of beauty that do not conform to Euro-centric beauty norms. As examples, women have traditionally sought beauty care from other women (beauticians) and Black people have sought treatments within their own communities. Nonetheless, despite taking on the diverse practice of beautifying the smile, dentists are often reluctant to provide treatments that veer from the straight white smile as seen from Zahra's views on gold teeth:

> My personal view is that I think it can take away from the beauty of the smile to have gold teeth. That's my personal view. When I'm asked, I've been asked maybe two or three times in my career to place a gold anterior tooth and I struggled with them, ethically, because I felt that if the person likes it now because it's on trend or their friends have something like it or they're copying a certain look, they may regret it in years to come and it's a permanent change that I'm not necessarily comfortable doing.
>
> (Zahra: Cosmetic Dentist, Facial Aesthetician, Facial Aesthetics Trainer)

Dentistry and the facial cosmetic industry poses difficult questions about racism and identity. Anti-semitic references to a 'Jewish nose' in plastic surgery date as far back 1892 (Haiken, 2000: Roberts, 1892). Reports have suggested that in the early twentieth century, white orthodontists offered Black American children a more European, or more bluntly a white profile (Picard, 2009). Indeed, the 'need' for orthodontic treatment in the UK, hence its availability on the NHS, is largely based on the professionally defined parameters of normal appearance that have been developed based on what a tiny group of white dental academics considered to be aesthetically acceptable – the Index of Orthodontic Treatment Need (IOTN) (Brook and Shaw, 1989). According to the UK dental profession's metrics (IOTN), a third of British children have an unacceptable smile in need of orthodontic treatment on the NHS. Interestingly, because publicly funded orthodontic care for a third of American children would be socially unacceptable, a different metric, the Dental Aesthetic Index (DAI) is used to assess treatment eligibility in public programmes. The DAI is a mathematical calculation of orthodontic treatment need developed using a mere 200 teeth photographs of children in New York state (Jenny and Cons, 1996). This practice of measuring Black and brown people and classifying them as 'abnormal' and in need of improvement is a form of enduring colonialism (Smith, 2012). Therefore, cosmetic dental practice and its broader orthodontics legacy reinforce and reproduce racism and racist divisions that intersect with gendered and class hierarchies.

Finally, these class, gender and racist hierarchies bring into view the social harms caused by the propagation of cosmetic dentistry which Illich (1976) described as social iatrogenesis. Illich (1976) also described cultural iatrogenesis – which in this case is the dental profession's culpability in undermining people's ability to accept diverse smiles. These social and cultural harms are evident with the propagation of narrow beauty ideals which can potentially discriminate against people who cannot afford cosmetic dentistry, those who do not conform to Euro-centric beauty ideals and people with obvious facial disfigurements.

## Conclusion

There is a long, diverse tradition of humans modifying their bodies and mouth. Within contemporary cosmetic dentistry, the body has been reduced to a commodity by healthcare professionals and institutions. Therefore, people's autonomy to modify their bodies is restricted by sitting in relation to the interests of dentists and the wider cosmetics industry. The restriction of body autonomy presents itself as the absence of wide choices and the obfuscation of beauty practices as healthcare. In particular, dentists' symbolic capital has been used to negotiate, define and propagate a very narrow smile ideal. Ultimately, the constrained choices result in the absence of diverse smiles which can create and exacerbate social and cultural harms such as racial, gendered, disablist and class inequalities. This sits alongside the symbolic damage to publicly funded healthcare and the movement of public sector dental resources into the private beauty industry, which further deepens the existing dental health and access inequalities.

## Notes

1 The data in this chapter was collated between 2018 and 2019 for a PhD study – An Institutional Ethnography of Cosmetic Dentistry – with ethical approval from the University of Sheffield's Research Ethics Committee.
2 Composite bonding is when white filling material is used to re-shape front teeth.
3 'Tweakments' include botulinum toxin (Botox) and filler injections and facial chemical peels.
4 Invisalign are clear braces used to straighten teeth.
5 B1 is the whitest shades on the dentists' shade guide and one of the whitest shades to occur in in naturally in teeth.
6 An NVQ is a National Vocational Qualification which is a work-based way of learning. Business Technology and Education Council (BTEC) provides a way to learn through practical work and study. An HND is the Higher National Diploma, a two-year qualification equivalent to two years at university.
7 Symbolic capital is social recognition, often due to the accumulation of other forms of capital such as cultural capital, and often manifest in a non-monetary asset such as an award or an honour. Cultural capital is a form of value attached to the material or immaterial representations of knowledge, skill and taste. For example, the value attached to dentists' university degrees (Bourdieu, 1989, 1991, 2000).
8 *BDJ* is the *British Dental Journal*, a bimonthly publication produced by the BDA and circulated to all its members.
9 Periodontal condition refers to the health of the gums.

## References

Armstrong, M. (2018) '5 Things Dentists Need to Know about the NHS Funding Pledge'. [online]. *British Dental Association*. [Viewed 9 January 2020]. Available from: https://bda. org/news-centre/blog/5-things-dentists-need-to-know-about-the-nhs-funding-pledge

Basker, R. (2006) *General dental council - The first 50 years*. London: GDC Gazette.

Bauman, Z. (2005) *Work, consumerism and the new poor*. 2nd ed. Maidenhead: Open University Press.

Bourdieu, P. (1989) 'Social space and symbolic power', *Sociological Theory* [online], 7(1), pp. 4–25. [Viewed 23 December 2019]. Available from: doi:10.2307/202060

Bourdieu, P. (1993) 'Structures, habitus, power: basis for a theory of symbolic power', in: Dirks, N. B., Eley, G., and Ortner, S. B. (eds.) *Culture / power / history: a reader in contemporary social theory*. Princeton, N.J: Princeton University Press, pp. 155–199.

Bourdieu, P. (2000) *Distinction: a social critique of the judgement of taste*. London: Routledge.

Bourdieu, P. (2001) *Masculine domination*. Cambridge: Cambridge Polity.

Brook, P. H. & Shaw, W. C. (1989) 'The development of an index of orthodontic treatment priority', *European Journal of Orthodontics* [online], 11(3), pp. 309–320. [Viewed 6 September 2021]. Available from: 10.1093/oxfordjournals.ejo.a035999

British Dental Association. (2012) *BDA advice – marketing*. London: British Dental Association.

British Dental Association., (2013) *BDA advice – title 'Dr'*. London: British Dental Association.

British Dental Association., (2019). 'NHS dentistry: £12 slashed: care for every man, woman and child in England since 2010', *British Dental Association* [online]. [Viewed 18 December 2019]. Available from: https://www.the-dentist.co.uk/content/news/bda-statement-12-slashed-from-care-for-every-man-woman-and-child-in-england-since-2010

Care Quality Commission., (2019). 'Treatment of disease, disorder, or injury', *Care Quality Commission*. [online]. [Viewed 12 January 2020]. Available from: https://www.cqc.org.uk/guidance-providers/registration/treatment-disease-disorder-or-injury

Chadwick, B., Cage, B. and Playle, R. (2007) 'Do teenage magazines give a genuine view of tooth colour?', *British Dental Journal* [online], 203(5), pp. E9. [Viewed 18 January 2020]. Available from: doi: 10.1038/bdj.2007.680

Costley, N. and Fawcett, J. (2010) *GDC: Public attitudes research report*. [online]. Edinburgh, London: George Street Research. [Viewed 20 February 2020]. Available from: https://www.gdc-uk.org/docs/default-source/research/gdc-public-attitudes-to-standards-for-dental-professionals.pdf?sfvrsn=a614b23c_2

Dental Council of New Zealand., (2009) *Cosmetic dentistry practice standard*. Auckland: Dental Council of New Zealand.

Department of Health., (2012) *Review of the regulations of cosmetic interventions: call for evidence* [online]. London: Department of Health. [Viewed 11 September 2019]. Available from: https://www.gov.uk/government/publications/review-of-the-regulation-of-cosmetic-interventions-call-for-evidence

Faculty of General Dental Practice (UK) & Faculty of Dental Surgery of the Royal College of Surgeons of England., (2018) 'Membership of the Joint Dental Faculties (MJDF) Examination Syllabus [online]', *Royal College of Surgeons*. [Viewed 8 July 2019]. Available from: http://www.mjdf.org.uk/wp-content/uploads/2018/02/MJDF-Syllabus-for-candidates.pdf

GDPC Exec., (2019) '5 things you need to know about NHS dental charges [online]', *British Dental Association*. [Viewed 9 January 2020]. Available from: https://bda.org/news-centre/blog/5-things-you-need-to-know-about-nhs-charges

General Dental Council., (1997) *Maintaining standards*. London: General Dental Council.

General Dental Council., (2012) *Principles of ethical advertising* [online]. London: General Dental Council. [Viewed 9 December 2019]. Available from: https://www.valident.co.uk/wp-content/uploads/2012/06/Ethical-advertising-statement-Jan-2012.pdf

General Dental Council., (2013a) *Standards for the dental team* [online]. London: General Dental Council. [Viewed 30 November 2017]. Available from: https://www.gdc-uk.org/professionals/standards/team

General Dental Council., (2013b). *Guidance on advertising* [online]. London: General Dental Council. [Viewed 5 May 2019]. Available from: https://www.gdc-uk.org/api/files/Guidance%20on%20advertising%20(Sept%202013).pdf

General Dental Council., (2013c) *Advertising checklist* [online]. London: General Dental Council. [Viewed 3 February 2020]. Available from: https://standards.gdc-uk.org/Assets/pdf/Advertising%20Checklist.pdf

General Dental Council., (2015) *Preparing for practice* [online]. London: General Dental Council. [Viewed 19 March 2019]. Available from: https://www.gdc-uk.org/docs/default-source/quality-assurance/preparing-for-practice-(revised-2015).pdf?sfvrsn=81d58c49_2

General Dental Council., (2016) *Guidance on using social media* [online]. London: General Dental Council. [Viewed 19 March 2019]. Available from: https://www.gdc-uk.org/docs/default-source/principle-4/guidance-on-using-social-media.pdf?sfvrsn=abf03a63_2

General Dental Council., (2019) *Fitness to practise* [online]. London: General Dental Council. [Viewed 20 January 2020]. Available from: https://www.gdc-uk.org/about-us/what-we-do/fitness-to-practise

General Dental Council. (2019a) Specialist Lists[online]. London: General Dental Council. [Viewed 11 January 2020]. Available from: https://www.gdc-uk.org/registration/your-registration/specialist-lists

Great Britain., (1984) *Dentists Act 1984*. c.24 [online]. London: The Stationary Office. [Viewed 15 March 2019]. Available from: https://www.legislation.gov.uk/ukpga/1984/24

Great Britain., (2008) *The Health and Social Care Act 2008 (Regulated Activities) Regulations 2014* SI 2008/2936 [online]. London: The Stationery Office. [Viewed 11 September 2019]. Available from: https://www.legislation.gov.uk/ukdsi/2014/9780111117613/contents

Haiken, E. (2000) 'The making of the modern face: cosmetic surgery', *Social Research*, 67(1), pp. 81–97.

Hunt, E. (1998) *Oral history: how Americans got their straight, white teeth*. Ph.D. thesis, University of Pennsylvania. [Viewed 11 January 2020]. Available from: https://repository.upenn.edu/dissertations/AAI3073084/

Illich, I. (1976) *Limits to medicine: medical nemesis: the expropriation of health*. London: Boyars.

Jenkins, R. (1996) *Social identity*. London: Routledge.

Jenny, J. and Cons, N. C. (1996) 'Comparing and contrasting two orthodontic indices, the Index of Orthodontic Treatment Need and the Dental Aesthetic Index', *American Journal of Orthodontics and Dentofacial Orthopaedics*, [online], 110(4), pp. 410–416. [Viewed 30 September 2021]. Available from 10.1016/S0889-5406(96)70044-6

LaingBuisson., (2019) 'Dentistry market report - 5th edition [online]', *LaingBuisson*. [Viewed 31 May 2019]. Available from: https://www.laingbuisson.com/shop/dentistry

Mattick, C. R., Gordon, P. H. and Gillgrass, T. J. (2004) 'Smile aesthetics and malocclusion in UK teenage magazines assessed using the Index of Orthodontic Treatment

Need' (IOTN)', *Journal of Orthodontics* [online], 31(1), pp. 17–19. [Viewed 18 January 2019]. Available from: doi: 10.1179/146531204225011373

Mead, G. H. (1934) *Mind, self, and society: the standpoint of a social behaviorist.* Chicago: University of Chicago Press.

Mintel Consulting. (2006) *British Academy of cosmetic dentistry survey.* London: Mintel Group.

Mintel Custom Solution. (2007) *British Academy of cosmetic dentistry survey.* London: Mintel Group.

NHS England., (2014) *Improving dental care and oral health – a call to action* [online]. Leeds: NHS England. [Viewed 9 February 2020]. Available from: https://www.england.nhs.uk/wp-content/uploads/2014/02/imp-dent-care.pdf

NHS England., (2019) *The review body on doctors' & dentists' remuneration* [online]. Leeds: NHS. [Viewed 12 January 2020]. Available from: https://www.england.nhs.uk/wp-content/uploads/2019/03/nhs-england-evidence-to-the-ddrb-gps-dentists.pdf

Nuffield Council on Bioethics., (2017) 'Cosmetic procedures: ethical issues [online]', *Nuffield Council on Bioethics.* [Viewed 18 December 2019]. Available from: https://nuffieldbioethics.org/wp-content/uploads/Cosmetic-procedures-full-report.pdf

Nuffield Council on Bioethics., (2018) 'Cosmetic procedures: ethical issues - one year on [online]', *Nuffield Council on Bioethics.* [Viewed 18 December 2019]. Available from: http://nuffieldbioethics.org/wp-content/uploads/Cosmetic-procedures-one-year-on.pdf

Obagi., (2020) 'Obagi skincare products [online]', *Obagi.* [Viewed 4 August 2020]. Available from: https://www.skinstation.co.uk/obagi-skin-care-products?gclid=EAIaIQobChMInOzYiNXi6QIVj-vtCh0UYAXREAAYASAAEgIluPD_BwE

Picard, A. (2009) *Making the American mouth. Dentists and public health in the twentieth Century.* New Jersey: Rutgers University Press.

Ring, M. E. (1992) *Dentistry: an illustrated history.* New York: Harry N. Abrams, Inc.

Roberts, J. B. (1892) 'The cosmetic surgery of the nose', *JAMA. The Journal of the American Medical Association,* 19(8), pp. 231–233.

Royal College of Surgeons of Edinburgh & The Royal College of Physicians and Surgeons of Glasgow., (2018) 'Diploma of membership of the Faculty of Dental Surgery (MFDS) regulations [online]', *Royal College of Surgeons.* [Viewed 8 July 2019]. Available from: https://rcpsg.ac.uk/documents/examinations/dentistry/mfds/368-mfds-regulations-syllabus/file

Smith, D. E. (2005) *Institutional ethnography: a sociology for people.* Walnut Creek, CA: AltaMira Press.

Smith, L.T. (2012) *Decolonizing methodologies.* 2nd ed. London: Zed Books.

Tapia, J. L., Suresh, L., Plata, M. and Aguirre, A. (2002) 'Ancient esthetic dentistry in Mesoamerica', *The Alpha Omegan,* 95(4), pp. 21–24.

Webb, J. (2002) *Understanding Bourdieu.* London: SAGE.

# 4 Feminism, pipelines and gender myths: interrogating gender equality and inclusion in dentistry

*Patricia Neville*

## Introduction

Historically dentistry developed as a male-dominated profession (Chia-Chun et al., 2010; see also chapters by Holden and Carstairs in this volume). Though the historical record mentions individual women practising a form of dental care until the medieval period, the extraction of carious teeth by barbers and blacksmiths from the sixteenth century onwards effectively closed off dental care to women positing that it required a physical strength assumed lacking in women (Ring, 1985; Ortiz and Diaz de Kuri, 2001; Loevy and Kowitz, 2002). This masculinist logic persisted into the nineteenth century when dentistry became a recognised profession and formal programme of study. Dr George Baker, writing in 1865, proclaimed that women did not possess the 'mental and physical equipment of the highest order' to become dentists (Baker, 1865). Despite these claims, women were eventually accepted into British dental schools with Lilian Lindsey graduating as the first UK female dentist in 1895, followed in 1912 by women being accepted into the Royal College of Surgeons in England (Lala and Thompson, 2020; Stewart and Drummond, 2000).

Since the 1970s, there has been a steady increase in the number of women entering the profession. For instance, in 2010, 46.6 per cent of dental students in the United States were female (Ioannidou, D'souza and MacDougall, 2014). This grew to 50 per cent in 2015 (Feldman, 2015, p.S14). In the Asia sub-continent, 50–60 per cent of Indian dental students were female in 2006 (Parkash et al., 2006). The increased participation of women in dentistry has also been recorded in Europe. In 2013, 63 per cent of dental students and 49 per cent of registered dentists in the EU/EEA were female (Council of European Dentists, 2015, p.33, p.39). According to the General Dental Council (UK), parity was achieved between male and female dental students in 2011/12 (Pacey, 2014). By 2018, 63 per cent of UK dental graduates were female (Evans, 2018). It is now estimated that 50 per cent of the global dental workforce under the age of 35 are female (Ivanoff et al., 2018). These university and workplace statistics indicate that dentistry has undergone a process of feminisation (Gross and Schafer, 2011; Adams, 2005; Brocklehurst and Tickle, 2012) namely, a numerical increase in women in the dental profession (Riska, 2008).

DOI: 10.4324/9781003047674-5

This process of feminisation has also been found in medicine (Riska, 2008, 2011; Heru, 2005) and veterinary science (e.g. Chieffo, Kelly and Ferguson, 2008; Women in the veterinary profession 2014, Treanor, 2016).

For some, the changing gender composition of the profession of dentistry signifies that the masculinist nature of dentistry (Adams, 2005) has been reversed and that gender equality has been achieved in the profession. The increased representation of women in the profession, both as students and practitioners, could indicate that dentistry does not suffer from the 'leaky pipeline' common to most STEM disciplines (Blickenstaff, 2005). Also, research in the United States has claimed that dentistry has become more welcoming and accepting of the women entering the profession (Rosenberg, Cucchiara and Helpin, 1998). Such pronouncements about the gender inclusivity of dentistry are echoed in individual motivations for pursuing a career in dentistry. One of the leading reasons why both genders are attracted to dentistry is its perceived flexibility and amenable work-life balance vis-a-vis other healthcare professions like medicine (Scarbecz and Ross, 2003; Du Toit et al., 2014; Waylen et al., 2017). This is supported by the finding that female dentists are more likely to work part-time and take career breaks than their male counterparts (Ayers et al., 2008, p. 347). In their sum, these findings could be interpreted as evidence that dentistry is an inclusive and progressive profession.

Feminist and sociological scholarship warns against conflating the numerical increase of women into the dental profession with the assumption that dentistry is an equal opportunities profession. In particular, they contend that the process of feminisation can be a complicated one and does not automatically ensure the successful integration of women into the profession (e.g. Riska, 2008, pp. 4–5; Bolton and Muzio, 2008). For instance, there has been a rise in studies documenting the prevalence of sexual harassment in dental surgery and dental hygiene education since the 1990s (e.g. Webster et al., 1999; Garbin et al., 2010; Ivanoff et al., 2018; Zarkowski, 2018; Zurayki et al., 2019). In addition, the high incidence of women working part-time in dental practice is itself a recognition that work-life balance is difficult to attain in this profession rather than an indication of the opposite (Macerollo, 2008, p.125).

Despite such feminist pronouncements, it is striking how a perception of dentistry as an inclusive, meritocratic and family-friendly profession has established itself as a taken for granted 'fact' among young and aspiring dental professionals (e.g. Scarbecz and Ross, 2003; Du Toit et al., 2014; Waylen et al., 2017). While this ideology is prominent within and outside the dental profession, it has been rarely reflected upon or acknowledged by the dental profession. It is the aim of this chapter to study this ideology. It contends that a gender myth operates in dentistry that works to 'obscure', 'cover up' or 'disappear' contrary or inconvenient facts (Lye, 1999) about the gendered nature of dentistry. This 'gender myth' asserts the belief that women's increased access to education automatically leads to personal choice and personal power in their dental career, regardless of any structural factors and cultural constraints (Rao and Sweetman, 2014, p.6). Such a gender myth is dangerous to both the profession and its members as it perpetuates an unproblematic world view of the dental profession and obscures the extent to which gender is an active constituent of the day-to-day working lives of dentists and the organisation of the profession itself. As a result, the prevalence of sexism and sexual harassment within the profession, as well as the vertical and horizontal segregation that women encounter that 'block' their progression through the dental pipeline, hides in plain sight and evades critical attention. This 'silencing' of gender discrimination is also damaging for those victimised by sexism and gender discrimination because it means that they are forced to face this experience alone, possibly blaming themselves for personal wrongdoing rather than seeing it as a structural issue of the profession.

Feminist analysis allows us to catalogue the different faces of gender inequality in the dental profession as well as ascertain the scale of the inequalities (Ahmed, 2015, pp.10–11). By naming and documenting instances of gender discrimination within the dental profession, the chapter contributes to a larger feminist project of critiquing healthcare as a patriarchal institution (e.g. Ehrenreich and English, 1988; Oakley, 1980 cited in Riska, 2001), with a gendered construction of healthcare work (e.g. Witz, 1992; Davies, 1996; Riska, 2001) and a masculinist work culture (see De Simone and Scano, 2017). Such a gendered analysis of dentistry also complements the seminal work of sociologist Adams (2000, 2005, 2010) on the role women play in the historical development of dentistry. This chapter will bear witness to the gendered/patriarchal experiences of women in the dental profession and signpost ways in which the profession must change to be more inclusive to all its members.

## Using feminism to navigate the dental pipeline

According to the 'critical mass' theory of change, 'the presence of a sufficient number of women brings about qualitative improvement in conditions and accelerates the dynamics of change' (Lagesen, 2007, p.71). Advocates of this theory assume that once the critical mass of women has been achieved, a process of change will be triggered 'automatically' culminating in the full integration of women into the profession (Lagesen, 2007, p.71). However, feminists are keen to highlight that such an interpretation of feminisation is simplistic and naïve. They maintain that the process of feminisation is paradoxical, creating opportunities for women but also gender imbalances within the profession (Bolton and Muzio, 2008), such as the possible 're-segregation of the profession' as 'women's work' and with it a devaluation of its social status, or the 'ghettoisation' of women within the profession (Riska, 2008, pp. 4–5). This section takes the more complicated interpretation of feminisation as its starting point and will use the feminist tool of the 'pipeline' to examine whether there is gender-based change and inclusion for women in dentistry.

The concept of the 'pipeline' was first coined by Berryman (1983) to convey the challenges women face in pursuing a career in science, a profession where they have traditionally been under-represented. The model contests the popular assumption that people progress seamlessly through their career of choice, from first establishing an initial desire to become a scientist, to attending and graduating college and then achieving full employment. This pipeline model identifies 'blockages' (Berryman, 1983, p.5) at a number of key junctures which prevent women progressing in the scientific professions. In her initial theorising, Berryman focused on how the educational experience of women at primary and secondary school level can adversely influence college and career choices later in life. This could include teaching staff discouraging female students from pursuing an interest in mathematics or science, or by school curricula design that limit or undermine female students' opportunities to study these subjects. This 'early educational pipeline' (Berryman, 1983, p.5) was presented as the first obstacle or 'leak' that women need to overcome in order to develop an interest and career in the sciences. Cronin and Roger (1999) identify three further stages to the pipeline: access, participation in higher education and career progression. Together, these four stages offer us a framework for investigating whether a profession can be considered inclusive. We will now interrogate the scholarship conducted on two key theoretical stages – access and participation in higher education and the career progression – in order to ascertain whether women can commence and maintain a career in dentistry.

### Access and participation in higher education

Dentistry is widely considered to be a valued profession to enter, either as an undergraduate or postgraduate qualification. As a result, dental school selection is very competitive with applicants required to demonstrate scientific acumen and overall academic excellence (Adams, 2005, p.76) Despite such high admissions criteria, dental school enrolment and completion figures suggest an interesting pattern. For instance, in the UK from 2007 to 2014, the number of women applying for and being accepted into dental surgery programmes increased. Niven et al. (2013, p.119) found that 58 per cent of applicants for the five-year dental degree programmes, 59 per cent of the four-year dental programmes and 67 per cent of the 3-year/six-year dental programmes in 2007–2008 were female. In their five-year analysis of UK UCAS applications to dentistry from 2010 to 2014, Gallagher et al. (2017, p.187) found that females were more likely to be offered and accept a place in dentistry than men, with on average 60/40 split (p. 183). This trend is mirrored in many other countries such as the United States, Canada, Bulgaria, Ireland, Germany and Sweden (Blanton, 2006; Adams, 2005; Ioannidou, D'souza and MacDougall, 2014; Gross and Schäefer, 2011; Neville, 2016) where women make up more than half of the dental student body as well as the dental workforce.

The over-representation of female applications to dental schools would appear to signal that the structural barriers that may have traditionally blocked women's access through the 'educational pipeline' (Berryman, 1983) into dentistry have become movable. This steady flow of women into the profession can be taken to indicate that dentistry does not suffer from the 'leaky pipeline' common to most STEM disciplines (Blickenstaff, 2005) on the point of access and participation in higher education.

### Career progression

The next question to consider is, what impact does a steady influx of women into dentistry have on the profession, their working lives and career prospects? The traditional pipeline model contends that women can experience a further narrowing of the pipeline at the career progression stage. This 'narrowing' represents pressure points in women's career which can cause them to 'fall out' of the profession altogether or have their efforts restricted by being shoehorned into specific types of work and conditions. Common examples of pressure points include the decision to have children, the number of actual children and other family responsibilities (Bennett, 2011, p. 151). Two processes sustain and underpin these pressures – horizontal and vertical segregation. Horizontal segregation refers to the process whereby women and men are clustered into specific job types or roles. This practice appears to be informed by gender stereotyping and sexism (Riska, 2008, p.4). Vertical segregation is concerned with the position of women in relation to power, status and control in their profession. It assumes that women have less power and influence than men in determining their career trajectory and that their ability to attain positions of power, prestige and status is inhibited by such mechanisms as gender discrimination and glass ceilings (Riska, 2008).

There are different ways of measuring/evidencing the extent of horizontal sex segregation in dentistry. First, studies report that women are over-represented in special care dentistry, paediatric dentistry, dental public health and dental education and under-represented in oral maxillofacial surgery and endodontics (e.g. Adams, 2005; McKay and Quiñonez, 2012; Pacey, 2014; Dental Schools Council, 2013). This mirrors a trend observed in medicine where there are less women in the surgical and more prestigious specialisms (Riska, 2001 cited in Adams, 2005, p. 78). Second, a gendered work pattern has been identified with male dentists working more hours and taking less career breaks than women (Pacey, 2014, p.4). Female dentists are more likely to work part-time (Ayers et al., 2008, p.347; Pacey, 2014, p.4), as associates or in hospitals (Ayers et al, 2008, p.348) and are less likely to own their own dental practices (Newton, Thorogood and Gibbons, 2000 cited in Ayers et al., 2008, p. 348; Adams, 2005; McKay and Quiñonez, 2012, p.3). For instance, in the United States, 20 per cent of female dentists work less than 30 hours a week, 36 per cent of dental practice owners are female compared with 53 per cent of male dentists, and 41 per cent of women work as associates compared to 28 per cent of men (Dringer, Phipps and Carsel, 2013 cited in Feldman, 2015, p.315).

It would be easy to explain these known occupational trends as nothing more than the expression of personal choice; however, feminists would counter this to argue that gender stereotyping and structural issues are in fact at play. Gender stereotyping alludes to the presumption that men and women have different skill sets because of their gender. As a result, women are assumed to have a natural affinity to work with children, the elderly and other vulnerable groups. This gender essentialism resonates in dentistry as the popular assumption that women have better empathy and communication skills than their male dental counterparts (McKay and Quiñonez, 2012, p.4). There is also the perception that female dentists are less likely to rush a patient, be more caring and spend more time with their patients than male counterparts (McKay and Quiñonez, 2012, p.4). Despite the populism of this belief, there is no evidence that women have better communication and empathy skills than men; it has been found that women and men express themselves differently (e.g. Tannen, 1995; Kendall and Tannen, 2015).

The gendered pattern of work described earlier reveals that female dentists, like most formally employed women, occupy a non-linear or non-continuous career path with having children identified as the leading contributor for these changes in their work patterns (Newton, Thorogood and Gibbons 2000; Ayers et al., 2008, p.349). Female dentists are more likely to work part-time and take career breaks than their male counterparts (Ayers et al., 2008, p.347). The most popular reason women take a career break is to care for children, whereas men use it as an opportunity to find a new job, to pursue further studies or out of personal choice (Ayers et al., 2008, p.348). Most women take on postgraduate training before children (60.7 per cent) compared with men (34.3 per cent) (Ayers et al., 2008). A woman's choice of speciality is also determined by location and proximity to family (McKay and Quiñonez, 2012, p.4). A further implication of this gendered work pattern is the fact that women prefer to be in salaried positions, either in clinics or universities. This desire for a salaried position helps to offset the financial stress of self-employment and lends security to maternity leave provisions (De Wet, Truter and Ligthelm 1997; Newton, Thorogood and Gibbons 2000 cited in Ayers et al., 2008, p. 348).

Furthermore, this gendered pattern of working also reveals the existence of a gender pay gap in dentistry. Since women are more likely to work less hours and be salaried compared to male dentists, they record a significant loss in earnings vis a vis their male counterparts. Research in the United States in the 1990s put this gender wage gap at approximately 78 per cent of male counterparts' incomes (Adams, 2005, p.76). In 2014, the gap was 74 per cent (*New York Times* April 23, 2014 cited in Feldman, 2015, p.316). In the UK, the gender pay gap for NHS contracted dentists is smaller at 17 per cent (NHS Digital, 2021 cited in www.bda.org, Lala and Thompson, 2020). Nevertheless, the mean average taxable income for self-employed primary care physicians (from NHS and private dentistry by gender) was over £80,000 for men and under £60,000 for women (NHS Digital report on NHS Earnings and Expenses Estimates 2015/16). Clearly, female dentists earn less than their male counterparts. The material difference between men and women's earning power has an impact on women's financial independence and pension planning. Another telling indicator of women's lack of control over their financial future is their under-representation as practice owners. Female dentists are more likely to be 'performer-only' dentists (90 per cent) than their male colleagues (72 per cent) (NHS Digital report on NHS Earnings and Expenses Estimates 2015/16). In the UK, while 49 per cent of NHS dentists are female, only 9 per cent are practice owners. This compares with the 18 per cent of male dentist practice owners with NHS contracts (NHS Digital Data cited in www.bda.org).

Vertical sex segregation attends to the position and status of women within the profession. Failure to acknowledge the contribution made by women suggests an organisational and professional culture that could be 'chilly' towards women (Blickenstaff, 2005, p.376), as well as obviously discriminatory and patriarchal. In the remainder of this section, we will attend to two examples: the glass ceiling in academic dentistry and the prevalence of sexism and harassment, both in dental schools and in the profession itself to ascertain the level of power, influence and status women have within dentistry.

A sectoral analysis of staffing levels in UK dental academia reveals that the process of feminisation has transformed the dental academy. Between 2004 and 2016, UK dentistry witnessed a substantive increase of 104.1 per cent in the number of women working as clinical academics compared to an increase of 7.6 per cent in male clinical academics (Dental Schools Council, 2017, p.17). This was represented in a headcount of 562 men and 426 women. This report claims that while 'most of the overall expansion of the academic workforce has therefore been of women' (Dental Schools Council, 2017, p.17), there was still a higher proportion of men at senior grades (Dental Schools Council, 2017, p.17) with only 21.2 per cent of professors in dentistry being female. There were only two female Dental Deans in the UK in 2015 (Whelton and Wardman, 2015, p. S10). This continues a trend seen internationally. In 2006, only 18 per cent of dental deans in the US were female. By 2019, it had risen slightly to 20.8 per cent (Li et al., 2019).

Why is there an under-representation of female dental academics in positions of leadership (Blanton, 2006)? Feminist scholarship posits that patriarchal work practices and misogynistic ethos impose a glass ceiling, or 'that invisible barrier to advancement that women face at the top level of the workplace' (Bertrand, 2018). This includes the practice of academic sexism whereby a discipline fails to recognise women's contribution to the field, by failing to cite the work of women, or when the physical appearance of female faculty is mentioned in staff and teaching evaluations (Ahmed, 2015). In addition, others claim that the 'job design' of academia (i.e. teaching, research and scholarship) is inflexible when trying to juggle work and family responsibilities (see Bertrand, 2018). Female career academics have been found to devote less time to research after they have children (Misra et al., 2012) compared to male counterparts (Misra et al., 2012). Relatedly, more women have difficulty with playing the 'corporate game' of higher education compared to their male counterparts with women spending more time on college administrative tasks and committees than their male colleagues (Misra et al., 2012). Such activities, though clear examples of good citizenship, rank as being of 'low promotability' (Babock et al., 2017) from a career progression perspective.

Academic dentistry is also hallmarked by similar patterns. There is a lack of positive female role models in academic dentistry. It has been noted that there is a tendency for less dental conferences to have female speakers (www.biaswatchneuro.com cited in Faber, 2017, p.1). In a study of 68 major dental journals, only 14.8 per cent of their editorial board members were women (Ioannidou and Rosania, 2015). Only 3 out of 38 editors-in-chief of a North American oral health journal are female (Li et al., 2019). UK dental professional associations struggle to attain gender parity in the composition of their official Boards, despite the growing number of women in the profession (O'Brien et al., 2020).

Research publications are a commonly understood marker of academic activity as well as being a key component in determining ones eligibility for progression and promotion. It has been found that female dental academics produce less academic outputs than their male counterparts and spend more time on administration and teaching than research (Whelton and Wardman, 2015; Albino et al., 2019). A study by Nesbitt et al. (2003 cited in McKay and Quiñonez, 2012, p.4) reported that while female dental academics do the same hours as male counterparts, the men had more administrative support, office space and protected research time than women. These studies indicate the existence of an unconscious bias towards women's work in academic dentistry (D'silva et al., 2019).

Sexism, according to Ahmed (2015), is a 'problem' that invades all aspects of women's professional lives. This 'problem' can take many different forms: as barriers to career progression (Biggs et al., 2018), being treated differently to your male colleagues (Powell and Sang, 2015), having your performance and ability measured against 'false aspirations/ideals' or stereotyping of what is expected of women (Calder-Rowe and Gavey, 2016) or a fear of unwanted physical contact (McLaughlin et al., 2017). In their sum, sexism amounts to a wide range of discriminatory practices against women simply because they are women. Sexism and sexual harassment exist at every stage of the dental pipeline – as a student, in the dental workplace and finally at the level of professional bodies.

Sexual harassment has been recorded in dental schools since the 1990s (e.g. Webster et al., 1999; Garbin et al., 2010; Ivanoff et al., 2018). The first transnational survey of female dental students and their perception of gender bias and harassment reported that 6 per cent of US and Brazilian students had been a victim of sexual assault, of which 4 per cent identified their aggressor as a male dental student (Ivanoff et al., 2018). Another study found that 15 per cent of the Brazilian respondents were sexually harassed by a patient, relative of a patient or a professional. Overall 25.4 per cent witnessed sexual harassment in dental schools (Garbin et al., 2010). This sexual harassment can also occur online, as exemplified by the Dalhousie University scandal (Hunter et al., 2015) when 13 male dental students were suspended from their programme amid claims that they had created a 'Class of DDS 2015 Gentlemen' Facebook account containing misogynistic statements about their female colleagues and 'gendered hate speech' (Jane, 2017, p.2).

The dental workplace is not immune to sexual harassment. In their survey of female maxillofacial surgical residents, Zurayki et al. (2019) found that 96 per cent of the respondents (*n* = 67) experienced at least one form of sexual harassment and gender harassment. Fifty-two per cent had unwanted sexual attention and 61 per cent said they had no training on how to respond to harassment and gender bias. These studies call for the need for training on how to respond to harassment and gender bias in everyday interactions (Garbin et al., 2010; Ivanoff et al., 2018; Zurayki et al., 2019).

Sexism also appears to be part of the profession itself. In 2019, the British Dental Association (BDA) was openly criticised for the marketing style adopted by one of the orthodontic companies exhibiting at their British Dental Conference and Dentistry Show. One source described the sight of three women wearing clear PVC raincoats over revealing dresses and stiletto heels as something reminiscent of 1990s 'laddish culture' (Thompson 2019 cited in Lala and Thompson, 2020) and wholly inappropriate for such a professional platform. The use of 'booth babes' (BBC News, 2019) at a professional show registered as a particularly tone-deaf move by the BDA. Though not then in breach of the Advertising Standards Authority (ASA) and the Committee of Advertising Practice because of the use of potent gender stereotypes, it did result in over 400 critical comments being posted on the Facebook page of the event (Lala and Thompson, 2020). These responses represent both a 'calling out' of the sexism of the event as well as holding the BDA to account for their actions.

## Discussion and recommendations

The aforementioned evidence strikes at the heart of the gender myth of dentistry as an equal opportunities' profession. What should dentistry do to address these issues? A multi-pronged approach is needed due to the multifaceted nature of this inequality. Here are some suggested recommendations.

First, there needs to be more widespread recognition that dentistry is a patriarchal institution, underpinned by misogyny, gender stereotyping and sexism. This recognition needs to be matched by the will to tackle these biases at an individual and institutional level. Including content on gender and sexism as part of the undergraduate curriculum would be a good starting point from which to build individual awareness of how gender impacts on oral health but also the vertical and horizontal segregation of the profession and the importance of work-life balance in the profession. Sexual harassment training and bystander training should be offered to both student and faculty. Though all universities have a sexual harassment policy, it would be important that the Dental School Council, the body that oversees dental education in the UK, puts its support behind a sector wide sexual harassment and acceptable behaviours policy.

Second, whether female dentists pursue a clinical career or an academic career, the work culture of both share many masculinist values. Both are premised on an 'ideal' professional worker who is single-minded, independent, unfettered by caring responsibilities and able to work long hours and be flexible to move to pursue further opportunities and achieve career goals. While there is a backlash against this 'toxic' work culture in academia (e.g. Dumitrescu, 2019), profound structural and policy changes will be needed to remove the glass ceiling in dental academia. This includes reconfiguring productivity and markers of esteem as not something that can only be measured quantitatively in terms of research outputs, but one that also recognises and values contributions to academic citizenship and communities of practice. Many equality and diversity scholars point to the success of the Athena Swan Award scheme as an encouraging sign of gender based sectoral change. Athena SWAN statistics reveal that all UK Dental Schools have fully engaged with this gender equality initiative with most of UK Dental Schools awarded Silver Athena SWAN awards, demonstrating evidence of good gender-based institutional practices. However, the Athena SWAN award scheme has become so successful in UK higher education that Athena SWAN is now treated as a 'proper noun' rather than an acronym (Cafferty et al., 2016) leading some to query whether the process has become a tick box exercise since success at a Silver award status is a condition of securing NIHR funding (Bhopal and Henderson, 2019). One of the aims of the Athena Swan award scheme is to facilitate the sharing of good gender-based practice, however, the way in which the scheme is administered doesn't readily allow for this to happen. More networking events on the topic of gender inclusive practices in dental schools are needed to raise awareness and best practice in the sector.

Third, the preference for part-time work has implications for the future staffing of public health services (Brocklehurst and Tickle, 2012, p.343). Within general dental practice, the feminisation of the dental workforce demands creating more flexi-working arrangements not only to support returning women after maternity or parental leave but also with regard to specialist training. The transition to work after a period of leave can be challenging and mentoring may be a beneficial form of support at this time. Most specialist training must be completed full-time within a set number of years. This emphasis on full-time study means women can find themselves in the difficult position of delaying having children, postponing their studies or giving up on career aspirations. Establishing a flexible training pathway, one that can accommodate pauses and periods of leave, will help increase the attractiveness of specialising.

Fourth, the lack of representation of women in positions of authority means that the dental profession is under-utilising the skills and talent coming into the field. It also resonates as a social justice issue (Bertrand, 2017, p.4). Efforts have been made by specialist groups to celebrate the contribution of women in dentistry by creating annual prizes as well as special issue and journals celebrating their scholarship and academic impact (e.g. Afshari et al., 2017; Ioannidou et al., 2019; D'silva, Herrer, and Mina, 2019). While such competitions and publications help to increase the cultural visibility of female dental academics, their ability to effect actual change is questionable. It might be time for UK dentistry to employ affirmative action and creating gender quotas for leadership posts/professorships.

## Conclusion

Current student enrolment rates and workplace statistics appear to confirm that the future of dentistry is female. While many commentators may look upon this development as evidence that dentistry is a gender inclusive profession, this chapter finds little evidence to support this claim. Using a variety of feminist tools of analysis, such as the pipeline model and the processes of vertical and horizontal sex segregation, the career trajectory of women in dentistry appears to be non-continuous and prone to individual, structural and` institutional pressures the further along the pipeline they travelled. The evidence suggests that while women have largely overcome the issue with access (pending grades and selection criteria), their opportunities to progress in the career upon qualification would appear to be constrained by a number of key pressures points: the decision to have children, the caring implications of having children and the sexism and patriarchal work culture they work in. Together, these challenges force women to manoeuvre creatively within their profession, by electing to work part-time, or seek out secure salaried positions, such as teaching and hospital jobs. However, on the issue of promotions and positions of leadership, there would appear to be more immovable structures in place to curtail progression.

It is important to state that the issues faced by women outlined here are not the exclusive preserve of dentistry; in fact, they are experienced by all women working in the formal economy. Nevertheless, it is important to name and catalogue these gender-related issues in dentistry because of the prevalence of a gender myth which openly propagates the belief that dentistry is an equal opportunities profession.

## References

Adams, T. L. (2000) *A Dentist and a gentleman: gender and the rise of dentistry in Ontario.* Toronto: University of Toronto Press.

Adams, T. L. (2005) 'Feminization of professions. The case of women in dentistry', *Canadian Journal of Sociology*, 30(1), pp. 71–94.

Adams, T. L. (2010) 'Gender and feminization in health care professions', *Sociology Compass*, 4(7), pp. 454–465.

Advance H. E. (March 2020) 'The future of the Athena SWAN. The report of the Athena SWAN charter review independent steering group for Advance HE [online]', [Viewed 29 September 2021]. Available from: https://www.advance-he.ac.uk/knowledge-hub/review-athena-swan-charter-report-and-appendices

Afshari, F., Chia-Chun Yuan, J. and Sukotjo, G. (2017) 'Women in prosthodontics: a brief look at pioneers, leaders and inspirers', *Journal of Prosthodontics*, 26, pp. 351–358.

Ahmed, S. (2015) 'Introduction: sexism – a problem with a name', *New Formations*, 86, pp. 5–13.

Albino, J., Teles, F. and Cohen, L. K. (2019) 'Commentary: challenges and opportunities for women in dental research', *Advances in Dental Research*, 30(3), pp. 119–123.

Ayers, K. M. S., Thomson, W. M., Rich, A. M. and Newton, J. T. (2008) 'Gender differences in dentists' working practices and job satisfaction', *Journal of Dentistry*, 36, pp. 343–350.

Babock, L., Recalde, M. P., Westerlund, L. and Weingart, L. (2017) 'Gender differences in accepting and receiving requests for tasks with low promotability', *American Economic Review*, 707(3), pp. 714–747.

Baker, G. T. (1865) 'Dental surgery – should females practice it?', *Dental Times*, 3, pp. 152–155.

BBC News., (2019) 'Booth babes' cause controversy at business show [online]. 17 May. [Viewed 13 October 2021]. Available from: www.bbc.co.uk/news/business-48313132

Bennett, C. (2011) 'Beyond the leaky pipeline: consolidating understanding and incorporating new research about women's science careers in the UK', *Brussels Economic Review*, 54(2/3), pp. 149–176.

Berryman, S. (1983) *Who will do science? Trends, and their causes in minority and female representation among holders of advanced degrees in science and mathematics.* New York: Rockefeller Foundation.

Bertrand, M. (2018) 'The glass ceiling', *Becker Friedman Institute for Research in Economics. Working Paper No 2018-19*, 47, [Viewed 13 October 2021]. Available from: DOI: 10.2139/ssrn.3191467

Bhopal, K. and Henderson, H. (2019) 'Competing inequalities: gender versus race in higher education institutions in the UK', *Educational Review* [online]. Available from: 10.1080/00131911.2019.1642305

Biggs, J., Hawley, P. H. and Biernat, M. (2018) 'The academic conference as a chilly climate for women: effects of gender representation on experiences of sexism, coping responses and career intentions', *Sex Role*, 78(5-6), pp. 394–408.

Blanton, P. (2006) 'Women in dentistry: negotiating the move to leadership', *Journal of Dental Education*, 20(11), pp. 38–40.

Blickenstaff, J. C. (2005) 'Women and science careers: leaky pipeline or gender filter?', *Gender and Education*, 17(4), pp. 369–386.

Bolton, S. and Muzio, D. (2008) 'The paradoxical processes of feminization in the professions: the case of established, aspiring and semi-professions', *Work, Employment & Society*, 22(2), pp. 281–299.

Brocklehurst, P. and Tickle, M. (2012) 'Planning a dental workforce for the future for the National Health Service in the United Kingdom: what factors should be accounted for?', *Health Education Journal*, 71(3), pp. 340–349.

Caffrey, L., Wyatt, D., Fudge, N., Mattingley, H., Williamson, C. and McKevitt, C. (2016) Gender equity programmes in academic medicine: a realist evaluation approach to Athena SWAN processes, *BMJ Open*, 6, e012090.

Calder-Rowe, O. (2015) 'The choreography of everyday sexism: reworking sexism in interactions', *New Formations*, 86, pp. 89–105.

Calder-Rowe, O. and Gavey, N. (2016) 'Making sense of everyday sexism: young people and the gendered contours of sexism', *Womens Studies International Forum*, 55, pp. 1–9.

Chia-Chun Yan, J. et al. (2010) 'Gender trends in dental leadership and academics: a twenty-two-year observation', *Journal of Dental Education*, 74(4), pp. 372–380.

Chieffo, C., Kelly, A. M. and Ferguson, J. (2008) 'Trends in gender, employment, salary, and debt of graduates of US veterinary medical schools and colleges', *Journal of American Veterinary Medicine Association*, 233(6), pp. 910–917.

Council of European Dentists.m (2015) *Manual of dental practice 2015.* Edition 5.1 [online]. [Viewed 26 January 2017]. Available from: http://www.cedentists.eu/library/eu-manual.html

Cronin, C. andRoger, A. (1999) 'Theorizing progress: Women in science, engineering and technology in higher education', *Journal of Research in Science Teaching*, 36(6), 637–661.

Davies, C. (1996) 'The sociology of professions and the profession of gender', *Sociology*, 30, pp. 661–678.

D'silva, N. J., Herrer, S. S. and Mina, M. (2019) 'Women recipients of IADR Distinguished Scientists Awards', *Advances in Dental Research*, 30(3), pp. 85–94.

De Simone, S. and Scano, C. (2017) 'Discourses of sameness, unbalance and influence: dominant gender order in medicine', *Journal of Gender Studies* [online], 27(8), pp. 914–927. [Viewed 21 July 2017]. Available from: 10.1080/09589236.2017.1357541

Dental Schools Council., (2013) *A survey of staffing levels of clinical academics dentists in UK dental schools as at 31 July 2012.* London: Dental Student Council.

Dental Schools Council., (2015) *A survey of staffing levels of clinical academics dentists in UK dental schools as at 31 July 2014.* London: Dental Student Council.

Dental Schools Council., (July 2017) *Survey of dental clinical academics staff levels 2017.* London: Dental Schools Council.

Du Toit, J., Hanin, S., Montalli, V. and Govender, U. (2014) 'Dental students' motivations for their career choice: an international investigative report', *Journal of Dental Education*, 78(4), pp. 605–613.

Dumitrescu, I. (2019) 'Ten rules for succeeding in academia through upward toxicity', *Times Higher Education* [online], [Viewed 13 October 2021]. Available from: https://www.timeshighereducation.com/opinion/ten-rules-succeeding-academia-through-upward-toxicity?fbclid=IwAR1JbklaPAW9T4pKaSqiA3anGLsLZlgUv09o5KevDihfLTukROzOTCRJvAY

Ehrenreich, B. and English, E. (1988) *For her own good: 150 years of experts advice to women.* New York: Anchor Press.

Evans, S. (2018) *Report on UK dental market: percentage of female dentists set to increase* [online]. Dentistry.co.uk. [Viewed 13 October 2021]. Available from: https://dentistry.co.uk/2018/10/26/report-uk-dental-market-percentage-female-dentists-set-increase/

Faber, J. (2017) 'A call to promote gender equality in dentistry', *Journal of the World Federation of Orthodontists*, 6(1), 1.

Feldman, C. A. (2015) 'Attaining and sustaining leadership for US women in dentistry', *Journal of Dental Education.* Special Supplement, 79(5), pp. S 13–S 17.

Gallagher, J. E., Calvert, A., Niven, V. and Cabot, L. (2017) 'Do high tuition fees make a difference? Characteristics of applicants to UK medical and dental schools before and after the introduction of high tuition fees in 2012', *British Dental Journal*, 222(3), pp. 181–190.

Garbin, C. A., Zina, L. G., Garbin, A. J. and Moimaz, S. A. (2010) 'Sexual harassment in dentistry: prevalence in dental school', *Journal of Applied Oral Sciences*, 18(5), pp. 447–452.

Gross, D. and Schafer, G. (2011) 'Feminization' in German dentistry. Career paths and opportunities. A gender comparison', *Womens Studies International Forum*, 34, pp. 130–139.

Heru, A. M. (2005) 'Pink-collar medicine: Women and the future of medicine', *Gender Issues*, 20, doi: 10.1007/s12147-005-0008-0

Hunter, K., Maxwell, E. and Brunger, F. (2015) 'Misogyny in health professions? An analysis of the Dalhousie dentistry scandal', *Bioéthique Online* [online], 1. [Viewed 13 October 2021]. Available from: doi:10.7202/1035508ar

Ioannidou, E., D'souza, R. N. and MacDougall, M. J. (2014) 'Gender equity in dental academics: gains and current challenges', *Journal of Dental Research*, 93(1), pp. 5–7.

Ioannidou, E. and Rosania, A. (2015) 'Under-representation of women on dental journal editorial boards', *PLoS ONE* [online], 10(1). [Viewed 13 October 2021]. Available from: pp. e0116630, doi: 10.1371/journal.pone.0116630

Ioannidou, E., Letra, A. M., Shaddox, L., Telas, F., Aijboye, S., Ryan, M., Fox, C. H., Tiwari, T. and D'souza, R. N. (2019) 'Empowering women researchers in the new century: IADR's strategic direction', *Advances in Dental Research*, 30(3), pp. 69–77.

Ivanoff, C. S., Luan, D. M., Hottel, T. L., Andonov, B., Ricci Volpato, L. E., Kumar, R. R. and Scarbecz, M. (2018) 'An international study of female dental students' perceptions about gender bias and sexual misconduct at four dental schools', *Journal of Dental Education*, 82(10), pp. 1022–1035.

Jane, E. A. (2017) *Misogyny online. A short (and brutish) history*. Los Angeles: Sage.

Kendall, S. and Tannen, D. (2015) 'Discourse and gender', in: Tannen, D., Hamilton, H. E. and Schriffin, D. (eds.) *The handbook of discourse analysis*, Second Edition. New York: John Wiley and Sons. pp. 639–660.

Lagesen, V. A. (2007) 'The strength in numbers: strategies to include women into computer science', *Social Studies of Science*, 37910, pp. 67–92.

Lala, R. and Thompson, W. (2020) 'An equal world is an enabled world'; Equality in the dental profession', *BDJ in Practice*, 33(2), pp. 17–19.

Loevy, H. T. and Kowitz, A. A. (2002) 'Women dentistry. Hobbs and after', *Journal of the History of Dentistry*, 50, pp. 123–130.

Li, J., de Souza, R., Esfandiari, S. and Feine, J. (2019) 'Have women broken the glass ceiling in North American dental leadership?', *Advances in Dental Research*, 30(3), pp. 78–84.

Lincoln, A. E. (2010) 'The shifting supply of men and women to occupations: feminization in veterinary education', *Social Forces*, 88(5), pp. 1969–1998.

Lye, J. (1997) Ideology: A brief guide. https://academic.uprm.edu/laviles/id218.htm. date accessed 31/3/22

Macerollo, A. (2008) 'The power of masculinity in the legal profession: women lawyers and identity formation', *Windsor Review of Legal and Social Issues*, 25(121).

McKay, J. C. and Quiñonez, C. (2012) 'The feminization of dentistry: implications for the profession', *Journal of Canadian Dental Association*, 78, c1, pp. 1/7–7/7.

McLaughlin, H., Uggen, C. and Blackstone, A. (2017) 'The economic and career effects of sexual harassment of working women', *Gender & Society*, 31(3), pp. 333–358.

Misra, J., Hickes Lundquist, J. and Templar, A. (2012) 'Gender, work time and care responsibilities among faculty', *Sociological Forum*, 27(2), pp. 300–323.

Neville, P. (2016) 'An observational analysis of recent female dental enrolment figures in the Republic of Ireland', *European Journal of Dental Education*, 21(4), pp. 235–239.

NHS Digital (19 August 2021) Dental earnings and estimates 2019/20. https://digital.nhs.uk/ data - and - information/publications/statistical/dental - earnings -and-expenses-estimates/2019-20

Niven, V., Cabot, L. B. and Gallagher, J. E. (2013) 'Widening participation – a comparison of characteristics of successful UK applicants to the five-year and four-year dental programmes in 2007 and 2008', *British Dental Journal*, 214(3), pp. 117–122.

O'Brien, K., Ahmad, M., Harrhy, L., McCaul, L., Stevens, C. and Baker, S. (2020) 'There is a gender imbalance on the UK dental boards'. Kevin O'Brien ortho blog [online], 16 December 2020. [Viewed 13 October 2021]. Available from: https://kevinobrienorthoblog.com/balance-boards/

Oakley, A. (1990) *Women confined: towards a sociology of childbirth*. Oxford: Martin Robertson.

Ortiz, R. M. G. and Diaz de Kuri, M. (2001) 'Women in dentistry', *Journal of the History of Dentistry*, 49, pp. 37–41.

Pacey, L. (2014) 'Have women changed the dental workforce?', *British Dental Journal*, 216(Jan), pp. 4–5.

Parkash, H., Mathur, V. P., Duggal, R. and Jhuraney, B. (2006) 'Dental workforce issues: a global concern', *Journal of Dental Education*, 70(11), pp. 22–26.

Powell, A., and Sang, K. J. (2015) 'Everyday experiences of racism in male dominated professions: a Bourdieusian perspective', *Sociology*, 49(5), pp. 919–931.

Rao, N. and Sweetman, C. (2014) 'Introduction to gender and education', *Gender and Development*, 22(1), pp. 1–12.

Ring, M. E. (1985) *Dentistry. An illustrated history*. New York: Harry N Abrams Inc.

Riska, E. (2001) 'Health professions and occupations', in: Cockerham, W. C. (ed.) *The Blackwell Companion to Medical Sociology*. London: Blackwell Publishers Ltd, pp. 144–158.

Riska, E. (2008) 'The feminization thesis: discourses on gender and medicine', *NORA-Nordic Journal of Feminist and Gender Research*, 16(1), pp. 3–18.

Riska, E. (2011) 'Gender and medical careers', *Maturitas*, 68, pp. 264–267.

Rosenberg, H. M., Cucchiara, A. J. and Helpin, M. L. (1998) 'Dental students' attitudes to gender roles', *Social Science & Medicine*, 47(11), pp. 1877–1880.

Scarbecz, M. and Ross, J. A. (2003) 'Gender differences in first year dental studies motivation to attend dental school', *Journal of Dental Education*, 66(8), pp. 952–961.

Stewart, F. M. J. and Drummond, J. R. (2000) 'Women and the world of dentistry', *British Dental Journal*, 188, pp. 7–8.

Tannen, D. (1995) 'The power of talk: who gets heard and why', *Harvard Business Review*, 73(5), pp. 138–148.

Tiwari, T. et al. (2019) 'Gender inequalities in the dental workforce: global perspectives', *Advances in Dental Research*, 30(3), pp. 60–68.

Treanor, L. (2016) 'Why aren't more veterinary practices owned or led by women?', *Veterinary Record*. October, 22, pp. 406–407.

Waylen, A., Benyan, P., Barnes, O. and Neville, P. (2017) 'Can an examination of student motivations for studying dentistry inform us about gender and BME differences in academic dental careers?', *British Dental Journal*, 222(1), pp. 13–15.

Webster, D. B., Smith, T. A., Marshall, E. O., Seaver, D. C., Szelunga, M. A. and Illich, T. T. (1999) 'Dental students' sexual harassment experiences and attitudes', *Journal of Dental Education*, 63(9), pp. 665–672.

Whelton, H. and Wardman, M. J. (2015) 'The landscape for women leaders in dental education. Research and practice', *Journal of Dental Education*. Special Supplement. Supporting Women's Development in Dentistry, pp. S7–S12.

Witz, A. (1992) *Professions and patriarchy*. London: Routledge.

Women in the Veterinary Profession. (2014) 'Gender statistics about veterinary surgeons in the UK', *Vet Futures*. London, UK: Royal College of Veterinary Surgeons.

Zarkowski, P. (2018) 'Simply stated: harassment and gender bias are unacceptable', *Journal of Dental Education*, 82(10), pp. 1015–1016.
Zurayki, L. F. Cheung, K. L., Zemplenyi, M., Burke, A. and Dillion, J. K. (2019) 'Perceptions of sexual harassment in oral and maxillofacial surgery training and practice', *Journal of Oral and Maxillofacial Surgery*, 77(12), pp. 2377–2385.

# Part II

# Cultural representations of the mouth and teeth

# 5 Toothy tales: dentures in the writings of H. Rider Haggard and Rudyard Kipling

*Ryan Sweet*

In his 1965 work *Rabelais and His World*, literary theorist Mikhail Bakhtin contends that the mouth plays a central role in the aesthetics of one of the most enduring modern artistic modes, the grotesque:

> The most important of all human features for the grotesque is the mouth. It dominates all else. The grotesque face is actually reduced to the gaping mouth; the other features are only a frame encasing this wide-open bodily abyss. (p. 317)

For Bakhtin, the image of the gaping mouth is all-consuming, a metaphor for the abyss that all other bodily features merely frame. The mouth is vital according to Bakhtin as it is within this space that 'the confines between bodies and between the body and the world are overcome' (1965, p. 317). Given the importance Bakhtin places on the mouth, it is surprising that this topic remains under-researched in literary studies. In the few papers that address this topic in nineteenth-century literature, teeth tend to be analysed for their metaphorical meaning in broader arguments that connect imagery with other social themes. For example, regarding the 'feline'-toothed villain James Carker from Charles Dickens's *Dombey and Son* (1846–48, p. 198), Robert Clark declares that his teeth signify 'both a sexual and an economic rapacity' (1984, p. 79); James E. Marlow considers them as an apt symbol for 'cannibalistic England' (1994, p. 93); and Gail Turley Houston contends that Carker's mouth represents 'unrestrained acquisition—hostile takeovers as well as corporate and corporal raids' (1994, p. 98; Carlyle Tarr, 2017, p. 135 n. 85). Though fascinating, these readings do not tell us much about how teeth were viewed socially in Victorian Britain. More recently, a select number of studies address this issue, considering imaginaries of teeth metonymically. Clayton Carlyle Tarr reads nineteenth-century portrayals of long, white, uniform teeth (including Carker's) in context with the professionalisation of dentistry, ultimately arguing that teeth of this kind 'signalled the threat of degeneration' (2017, p. 113). Adopting a similar approach, Andrea Goulet's 2017 article 'Tooth Decay: Edgar Allan Poe and the Neuro-déca"dent" isme of Villiers and Huysmans' argues that 'tooth-rot' ... becomes revalued as part of a modern aesthetic sensibility, a refined reaction

DOI: 10.4324/9781003047674-7

against the effects of American consumerism and base materiality' (2017, p. 198). In her analysis, imaginaries of teeth rot are read contiguously alongside transnational discourses of dentistry, neuropathology, consumerism, and aesthetics. The following draws from Carlyle Tarr's and Goulet's approaches but considers how teeth, specifically false ones (which have seen even less scholarly attention), can be read as metonym, metaphor, *and* comic prop. Unlike previous studies, I show that teeth perform multiple affective roles in particular late nineteenth- and early twentieth-century imperial writings.

Specifically, this chapter investigates the rich use of false teeth in the late-nineteenth- and early twentieth-century works of H. Rider Haggard and Rudyard Kipling. By re-examining depictions that have until now been read in ways that have overlooked key dental, biographical and cultural contexts, this chapter provides a new approach to reading teeth in literature. It argues that Haggard's and Kipling's works provided metonymic commentaries on the fit and functionality of false teeth while utilising their symbolic flexibility as devices to perform a variety of roles, stimulating comedy, personal reflection, and grotesque intrigue. An important role concerns how false teeth were deployed as metaphors to interrogate anxieties about the perceived ailing condition of Britain's colonial forces.

Imaginaries of false teeth have been neglected in studies of the long nineteenth century for three key reasons. First, as Guy Woodforde (one of few historians to write about the history of false teeth) explains, 'laboured attempts at a natural appearance' alongside post-Regency sentimentalities meant that though false teeth were common among the middle classes in nineteenth-century Britain, propriety forbade any mention of them (1968, p. 2–3). As a result, dentures appeared infrequently in Victorian fiction—though Carlyle Tarr's article and my 2017 essay '"Get the best article in the market": Prostheses for Women in Nineteenth-Century Literature and Commerce' reveal some notable exceptions (Sweet, 2017). Second, false teeth (as one might expect) were often imagined in comical ways and, as Bob Nicholson points out, even the best work in the field is often underpinned by assumptions about the oppressive seriousness of the Victorians (2012, p. 35). As a result, Victorian humour remains an under-researched area. Third, and related to the previous point, the mouth has been viewed as a relatively insignificant topic, mirroring the extent to which oral health has been neglected socially on a global scale (Watt et al., 2019). The focus of literary studies is, after all, often a reflection of what society views as important. The following analysis shows that representations of artificial teeth are worth our attention: they reveal attitudes to health, aesthetic standards, technology, social institutions, and nationhood; they also expose the power of the mouth as a symbol of cultural conformity/difference, physical fitness and selfhood. Like David Scott's contribution to this collection (Chapter 6), this essay gives overdue attention to the language and metaphors of the mouth, specifically those related to dentures.

## Grotesque humour

Haggard's Captain Good from *King Solomon's Mines* (1885) is arguably the most famous and visible denture user in Victorian literature. While Woodforde asserts that 'one might read a whole library of Victorian novels without learning that anyone's teeth were artificial' (1968, p. 3), Haggard's work is an exception. Indeed, Good's immaculate artificial teeth are prominent aesthetically and in terms of Haggard's plot. One could, in fact, consider them an early example of unrealistically perfect teeth—representations of which in contemporary media are the focus of Rizwana Lala's analysis in Chapter 3. Good, a former Royal Navy officer, who 'had been turned out of her Majesty's employ with the barren honour of a commander's rank, because it was impossible that he should be promoted', is revealed as a user of 'two beautiful sets' of false teeth (Haggard, 1885, p. 13). Throughout the imperial adventure novel, which sees Good, the narrator-protagonist Allan Quatermain and the aristocrat Sir Henry Curtis travel to Southern Africa to find the latter's estranged brother, Good's teeth are recognised for appearing in 'perfect order' (p. 44). Their appearances matches the former Navy lieutenant's stereotypically pristine toilette: Quatermain re- marks that Good 'looked the neatest man I ever had to do with in the wild- erness' (p. 44). Good's teeth go on to hold a significant (albeit comic) role in the story as his nervous tick of 'dragging the top set down and allowing them to fly back to his jaw with a snap' bewilders a group of Kukuanaland warriors holding Good and his comrades hostage, leading them to believe that the Western men are 'wizards' (pp. 85, 88). The confusion and misplaced awe generated by this encounter saves the adventurers' lives. This infamous scene has been read by contemporary literary critics as an example of ethnocentrism (Patteson, 1978, p. 113; Kestner, 2010, p. 67)—revealing of a Western arrogance that mocks non-Westerners for having unenlightened approaches to technology—but such a reading only tells part of the story regarding the aesthetic and contextual significance of Good's teeth. In his 2007 introduction to the Penguin Classics edition of *King Solomon's Mines*, Robert Hampson provides a helpful but somewhat limiting reading of Good:

> Good is 'of a susceptible nature' ... but this becomes the sentimental counterpart to the comic presentation of his character. Otherwise, his character is little more than a neatness of dress, a fixed eyeglass and a set of false teeth, and it is dramatized through his being positioned as the butt of various humiliations[.] (p. xxviii)

Hampson is correct that Good's artificial teeth are character-defining and that he is a figure of fun, but this representation also encodes both a slapstick mockery of English Navy Officers and a comic exploitation of the potential offered by particular prosthetic technologies. Good is by no means a complex and highly developed character but his depiction is significant as it exposes nineteenth-century attitudes to both Navy officers and spring-fixed upper- and lower-plate dentures.

Another work of British imperial fiction that draws from the humorous capacity of false teeth—albeit in a much darker and more symbolic way—is Kipling's, 1904 short story 'Mrs. Bathurst'. This mysterious and dense literary work contains within a frame narrative (of four men gossiping and drinking beer at Simon's Town, South Africa) a story about a false-teeth-using warrant rank officer of the Royal Navy, called Vickery, who falls in love with the keeper of 'a little hotel at Hauraki—near Auckland' (Kipling, 1904, p. 389). While moored in Cape Town one Christmas, eighteen months before his pension is due, Vickery becomes obsessed with a travelling circus's cinematograph film of 'the Plymouth Express arrivin' at Paddin'ton' as he believes it shows his beloved looking for him (p. 395). Vickery's obsession leads him to watch the film six consecutive nights before he is granted leave to travel to Bloemfontein 'to take over some Navy ammunition left in the fort' (p. 387). Vickery uses this opportunity to travel to Worcester, the circus's next destination, so that he can see the film a further time. During this trip, he goes AWOL. He is later found charred along with another man after being struck by lightning in a teak forest. He is ultimately identified by his false teeth, which remain intact following his death: 'That's what they really were, you see—charcoal. They fell to bits when we tried to shift'em. The man who was standin' up had the false teeth. I saw'em shinin' against the black' (p. 407). Again exemplifying the affective richness of false teeth, Kipling's short story uses grotesque humour and literary allusion to provide a contextual commentary on partial denture plates while exploiting false teeth as a character-defining synecdoche and a metaphor for human–machine integration. Together *King Solomon's Mines* and 'Mrs. Bathurst' show the potent roles that teeth play in the literary imagination.

In Haggard's novel, the neatness, whiteness, and artificiality of Good's dentures aptly represent his character and, by extension, caricature the typical late-Victorian Navy officer. Good's teeth are described as 'beautiful', 'in perfect order', and 'lovely' (pp. 13, 44, 86). Quatermain, who reveals himself as a false teeth user as well, laments that Good's teeth have often caused him to break the tenth commandment: 'Thou shalt not covet … anything that is thy neighbour's' (Exodus 20:17). To appreciate the imaginary of Good's teeth contextually, one must note that Royal Navy officers' uniforms, which were standardised in the 1880s and 1890s, communicated 'upper-middle-class masculine qualities of patriotism, leadership ability and self-discipline' (Colville, 2003, p. 115). Good's attentiveness to personal hygiene and maintaining a neat appearance, which is represented by his 'perfect' dentures, certainly matches the qualities of self-discipline and patriotism promoted by real-life officers' uniforms. But Haggard makes a mockery of these ideals when Good ironically becomes heralded for appearing superhuman by the people of Kukuanaland. It is initially Good's nervous pulling down of his top set that arrests his captors' attention, but they are ultimately convinced of his magic after Quatermain instructs Good to remove and replace his dentures entirely:

'Open your mouth', I said to Good, who promptly curled up his lips and grinned at the old gentleman like an angry dog, revealing to his astonished gaze two thin red lines of gum as utterly innocent of ivories as a new-born elephant. The audience gasped.

'Where are his teeth?' they shouted; 'with our eyes we saw them'.

Turning his head slowly and with a gesture of ineffable contempt, Good swept his hand across his mouth. Then he grinned again, and lo, there were two rows of lovely teeth.

Now the young man who had flung the knife threw himself down on the grass and gave vent to a prolonged howl of terror; and as for the old gentleman, his knees knocked together with fear.

'I see that ye are spirits', he said falteringly. (p. 86)

The surprising and extreme reaction of the Kukuanaland people, who, according to the novel's condescending and derogatory ethnocentric logic, are 'as utterly innocent of ivories as a new-born elephant' (p. 86), creates part of the comedy of this scene. But this extreme reaction works in tandem with the slapstick grotesqueness and social impropriety of a former Royal Navy officer exposing his bare gums. The problematic animal simile used to describe the Kukuanaland gentleman is paired with an also degrading animalistic comparison of Good as he exposes his gums—he 'curled up his lips and grinned at the old gentleman like an angry dog'—though note how the Westerner is compared to a domesticated nonhuman associated with 'faithfulness, sagacity, and self-sacrifice' in the Victorian imagination (Esmail, 2014, p. 19), while the man from Kukuanaland is compared to not only a wild and exotic animal but a new-born one at that.

The demeaning comparison of Good is nonetheless significant as it emphasises just how uncouth it was to remove one's false teeth publicly in such a manner, a move made even more shocking as it is performed by an individual tied to the presentational standards of the Royal Navy. As Woodforde notes, 'In ordinary polite society, propriety forbade any mention of false teeth' (1968, p. 2). He explains,

> By about 1840 laboured attempts at a natural appearance had brought false teeth into the category of the modern male toupee: however blatantly artificial, and loose, they had to be passed off as the work of Nature; however inconvenient for eating, they stayed in at meals. (1968, p. 1)

Regarding the expected appearance of navy officers, Colville observes that 'Pride in the self, and pride in the navy and its traditions, were treated as interchangeable concepts' (2003, p. 124). Furthermore, we must also note that cleanliness was instilled into navy men as a matter of the upmost importance in the nineteenth century (Smith, 2018). Though no longer officially serving with the navy, given how closely Good's character is tied to the institution, the vulgarity and uncleanliness of removing one's teeth in public appears doubly shocking (and thus incongruously humorous) when we consider the extent to which navy men's attention to their appearance was seen to represent their attachment to the institution and pride in good sanitation—both to maintain appearances and to protect their comrades from contagious diseases. As Elise Juzda Smith writes, at the time Haggard was writing, 'personal presentation now appeared as a visible symbol of enhanced naval discipline' (2018, p. 190). Good's act certainly represents a breach of self-discipline, but it is one with unexpected and amusing consequences, which endure: the humorous results of the scene are extended as Good is forced to maintain the half-dressed appearance that he exhibits when ambushed by the Kukuanaland men—with half of his face shaven and no trousers—to stay in character as a '[Son] of the Stars' (p. 97). Alongside the incongruous humour caused by this scene is a satirical jab at the navy as an institution. As I will return to later, there is a suggestion that appearances were being favoured over substance.

Complicating Haggard's depiction, Good's false teeth, though comically rendered, are represented as useful—and not just because of the impression that they give to the people of Kukuanaland. Earlier, they are shown to be functional in a more regular sense. On the white men's treacherous journey to Kukuanaland, which requires them to cross the forty leagues of desert between Kalukawe River and the mountain range Sheba's Breasts, they are saved from dehydration after stumbling across a patch of wild melons. Upon finding these, Good appears to have no trouble devouring 'about six' using his dentures. As Quatermain reports, within seconds of discovering the fruit, Good 'had his false teeth fixed in one' (p. 70). Later in their journey, in another act of famished desperation, Good makes short work of raw meat from an alpine antelope known locally as an 'Inco' (pp. 78 –79). In both scenes, there is an irony and dark humour to the white men's (and especially Good's) savage eating habits. Contextually, the comedy is heightened by the knowledge that false teeth often failed at mealtimes. As Woodforde observes, 'Actual teeth were often so ill-arranged that even a close-fitting denture was at once dislodged on chewing' (1968, p. 74). He also explains that 'Victorian false teeth, more than anything else, lay behind the Victorian custom of eating in bedrooms just before dinner. It was a custom which insured against disaster at the table' (1968, p. 4). Though contextual knowledge of false teeth's usual deficiencies may have added to these scenes, building comic tension about a dental mishap likely to occur, Good's teeth hold up well. Haggard thus exploits false teeth's comic potential without diminishing their functionality, mirroring his personal experiences with dentures, which I will return to towards the end of this chapter.

Contrasting Haggard's rather jovial depiction of Good, in Kipling's short story, there is an uneasiness regarding the permanency of Vickery's teeth, which not only remain intact but 'shinin'' after this violent death. This mood resonates with several earlier representations of prosthetic body parts, which figure as enduring mementos following the death of their users. For example, in

Robert Williams Buchanan's 'Lady Letitia's Lilliput Hand' (1862), the eponymous protagonist is memorialised following her death by her 'Lilliput Hand', a dainty and perfectly formed prosthetic. Furthermore, H. G. Wells's *The Food of the Gods and How It Came to Earth*, which was published just a few months before 'Mrs. Bathurst' in May 1904, features a glass eye, which is the only remnant of an elderly farmer named Mr Skinner after he is eaten by a giant rat. In each of these imaginaries, there is an unsettling permanency to the prosthetic body part, which stands uncomfortably alongside the comparative fragility of the human condition. Metonymically, the prostheses stand as exemplars of a trade that has developed hugely over the course of a century. Metaphorically, the prostheses represent how mankind's obsessive attention to its creations can lead to them outlasting or even replacing human beings. In the case of Vickery, the grotesque image of his charred corpse contrasting his white dentures focalises the mouth in line with Bakhtin's observations about the prominence of this feature in relation to the grotesque. Indeed, the freakishness of Vickery as a character becomes synecdochally represented by this final image of his prominent teeth.

Earlier in the short story, Vickery's teeth exacerbate his oddness as a character. For a start, unlike Captain Good's dentures, Vickery's are noticeable for the wrong reasons: they are loose, meaning that they cause a repetitive clicking sound. This noise is so prominent that Vickery is known by the nickname 'Click'. In Nicholas Daly's analysis of 'Mrs. Bathurst', he claims that the clicking noise is 'evidently meant to remind the reader of that made by a projector' (2004, p. 74), thereby sonically linking Vickery to the novel technology fuelling his obsession. However, we can also read this depiction as a literal critique of partial denture plates, which were, at the time Kipling was writing, 'inclined to be so loose and uncomfortable that most people refused to wear them' (Woodforde, 1968, p. 79). Like many contemporary real-life partial plates, his is certainly not closely fitting, hence the infamous sound it produces. Unlike Haggard's complementary presentation of spring-fixed dentures in *King Solomon's Mines*, metonymically the depiction of Vickery's false teeth provides a subtle critique of partial plates. His dentures not only fail to enable him to pass as someone with a full set of teeth but draw attention to his prosthesis use to the extent that his name and identity are reduced to the very noise that they produce: 'Click'. Metaphorically, the loose-fitting prosthesis transmogrifies a navy officer into a grotesque human-machine hybrid.

As well as critiquing partial plates and forewarning the spectre of human-machine integration—aspects that contrast Haggard's imaginary of dentures—Vickery's artificial teeth add to his unsettling nature. For instance, Pyecroft, the man who tells the story of 'Click's' obsessive visits to the travelling circus, describes the first time he watched 'the Western Mail came in to Paddin'ton' (p. 419) with Vickery by focussing on the grotesque image of his mouth: 'Vickery touched me on the knee again. He was clickin' his four false teeth with his jaw down like an enteric at the last kick' (p. 398). Here, Vickery's clicking makes audible his excited and nervous state while his mouth appears like an enteric (typhoid or paratyphoid) fever patient on the cusp of death. This morbid image foreshadows 'Click's' grisly death, which comes as an unlikely consequence of his fixated pursuit of the cinematograph projection. Pyecroft is so disturbed by Vickery that he notes his relief upon realising his death: 'Well, I don't know how you feel about it … but'avin' seen'is face for five consecutive nights on end, I'm inclined to finish what's left of the beer an' thank Gawd he's dead!' (p. 408).

The prosthesis user's obsessive quest in pursuit of an infamous but almost mythical being, which ultimately leads to his undoing, links him intertextually with Herman Melville's Captain Ahab (1851). However, *Moby-Dick* is not the only novel that his depiction recalls. His disturbing persona also links him to earlier predatory male characters known for their prominent teeth, including Sir Francis Varney from James Malcolm Rymer's *Varney the Vampire; or, the Feast of Blood* (1845–1847), Carker from Dickens's *Dombey and Son*, and the eponymous anti-hero of Bram Stoker's *Dracula* (1897). Of course, predominantly these representations feature the Gothic trope of the vampiric fang, though John Sutherland has speculated that Carker's gnashers are likely artificial: 'Carker's "glistening" teeth, in the mouth of a 40-year-old man, and their astonishing "regularity and whiteness", are surely too good to be true. They must be porcelain, we suspect' (1999, p. 84). In the case of Vickery, it is not so much the shape or whiteness of his teeth that make him appear disconcerting. Rather, it is the chattering sound that they produce that underscores his unsettling depiction. His clicking teeth speak for him in a ghoulish way, expressing his angst and overstimulated nervous excitement.

## Imperial concerns

While there are clear differences in the way that false teeth are imagined in Haggard's and Kipling's writings, ingrained in both is an anxiety regarding the dwindling condition of Britain's imperial forces. Infamously, Britain's failings in the Boer War stimulated fears of national decline, which were ratified by the Interdepartmental Committee on Physical Deterioration's damning report. This was published in July 1904, just a couple of months before 'Mrs. Bathurst' first appeared in *Windsor Magazine* in England and the *Metropolitan Magazine* in America. The report revealed 'widespread physical weakness among the working class' (Gilbert, 1965, p. 144). More specific to oral health, the Army Medical Department Report for the Year 1903 revealed that of 69,553 men inspected 4,400 were not accepted due to 'loss or decay of many teeth' (Medical Division, War Office, 1905, p. 43). As Helen Strong notes in Chapter 9 of this collection, this issue remained prevalent during World War One. While Good and Vickery are depicted as navy officers of the middle class, rather than soldiers of the working classes, for both characters, false teeth are insignias of unfitness. Good, for instance, lacks preparedness for battle due to the complexity of his toilette—which he only gets away with due to the unfamiliarity of his foes to the wonders of modern technology. On the other hand, Vickery's troubled nature and frailty as a character are aptly captured by the continual chattering of his dentures. The vanity of both men, as represented by their false teeth use, is also opened to critique as they each fall in love with women who, at the time of publication, would have been considered unsuitable: Good falls in love with a Kukuanaland servant, who cares for him after he is badly injured in battle (another scene that underscores his weakness as an imperial warrior); Vickery, of course, becomes obsessively attached to not merely a woman of low social status on the other side of the world, but, more specifically, the image of that woman as represented by the cinematograph (highlighting his fragile mental state and anticipating a kind of techno-sexual dystopia). Reading these works as critiques of Britain's military and national fitness aligns with the authors' publicly stated concerns about maintaining colonial control. As Andrew Rutherford notes in his introduction to the Oxford World Classics collection *War Stories and Poems* (1990), Kipling's stories about the Boer War presented dismay at the inefficiency shown at many levels throughout the Army while his works between this conflict and World War One warned of Britain's need to prepare itself for Armageddon (pp. xii, xix–xx). In Haggard's *Diary of an African Journey*, on the other hand, which he wrote during his return to South Africa as a diplomat in 1914, he noted a conversation with a Royal Navy captain in which they discussed 'the falling off in the quality of the young Englishmen of all classes who take to the sea nowadays and especially of the officers' (2000, p. 277). This conversation brings into focus how Haggard's depiction of Good almost thirty years earlier anticipated later anxieties about the military in decline. In both *King Solomon's Mines* and 'Mrs. Bathurst', we can read false teeth as a metaphor of an empire that presented itself as well formed and intact but behind the veneer was weakened and unhealthy.

## Personal experience

Other personal factors affecting Haggard's and Kipling's representations of false teeth concern their real-life experiences with dentures and dental problems. We learn from their letters and autobiographical writings that both Haggard and Kipling were false teeth users: Kipling from at least 1897 (when he was in his early thirties) and Haggard from at least 1914 (when he was in his late fifties), though one suspects the latter lost his teeth earlier than this—archaeological studies of nineteenth-century London reveal very high levels of tooth decay in middle- and upper-class population groups across all ages (Whittaker, 1993; Henderson et al., 2013). Indeed, one wonders whether the following comments about Good's dentures in *King Solomon's Mines* come from the fictional narrator or the author himself: 'he had two beautiful sets that have often, my own being none the best caused me to break the tenth commandment. But I am anticipating' (p. 13). This metafictional moment, read in context with the contemporary prevalence of dental carries and Haggard's later open writing about false teeth use, suggests that his imaginary of Good's highly finished dentures may have stood in contrast with his own, or at least the ones he anticipated wearing. We know for sure that Haggard was acquainted with dentures from an early age. In the first volume of his autobiography *The Days of My Life* (published posthumously in 1926), he recounted a comical scene from a childhood family trip up the Rhine that involved his mother's maid racing to retrieve his father's false teeth from 'a mile or more away' just as their steamer was about to depart (1926, ch. 1). This early exposure to the practical realities and comical potentiality of false teeth use may well have contributed to Haggard's depiction of Good's denture use.

Kipling, on the other hand, was a false teeth user several years before the publication of 'Mrs. Bathurst'. His letters reveal that he suffered terribly from toothache in the winter of 1896–1897, leading him to spend extensive periods 'in the embraces of the local dentist' (1896, p. 273). Kipling wrote openly with characteristic imagination and dark humour about his dental woes. For instance, in a letter to writer and editor Ripley Hitchcock on 17 January 1897, Kipling remarked, 'my constant occupation is going to the dentist: for my teeth miss the dry air of Vermont and like cherubim and seraphim "continually do cry"' (1897b, p. 282). Having recently moved to England from Vermont, here Kipling rationalised his toothache while providing a combination of simile, personification, and allusion to the hymn '*Te Deum Laudamus*' to emphasise hyperbolically how strongly his teeth were communicating their ill state—in the context of the hymn, cry means exclaim rather than weep (Church of England, 1662, p. 51). By June 1897, Kipling used false teeth. In another light-hearted letter to his doctor, James M. Conland, Kipling provided an account of attending a navy steam trial of a 30-knot torpedo boat in which he recounted, 'I felt my false teeth shaking in my head!' (1897a, p. 300). The vibrations of this experience were long-lived: Kipling noted that it took two days to get the 'jumps' out of his legs (1897a, p. 301). Such an experience provided a precedent for Kipling's depiction of Vickery's rattling false teeth, which can be read in this context to represent not only a nervous disposition but a body reeling from the shocks of steam-powered sailing.

As teeth took on a comical and curious role in Haggard's earlier fiction, in his 1914 *Diary of an African Journey*, they became symbols of deep reflection and lament. After passing Cape Gardafui, a headland in Somalia, Haggard recounted a sorrowful dental incident: 'I had two teeth taken out by the doctor this morning. They have been my companions for half a century but the best of friends must part! They looked very lonely lying there upon the table' (2000, p. 274). It is notable that Haggard took time to describe dental details such as this in a work otherwise focussed on African affairs and the author's often regretful reflection on his personal achievements. Haggard exposes here a vulnerability similar to the experiences of those 'having work done' in Barry Gibson, Jennifer Kettle, and Lorna Warren's essay (Chapter 11). The loneliness projected onto Haggard's personified, extracted teeth resonates with the regret he expressed as he said farewell to Africa and considered the broader impact of his life's work:

It is impossible for me to avoid contrasting the feelings with which I leave [South Africa] now that I have grown old, with those with which I bade goodbye to its shores in 1881 while I was young. Then life was before me and I had hopes and ambitions. Now life is practically behind me with its many failures and its few successes. Now I have, I think, no ambitions left and my only hope is that I may end my days in peace and remain of some slight services to my country and others till the last. (2000, p. 241)

Despite this very different tone and treatment of teeth, Haggard recorded with some of his usual slapstick humour two incidents involving his dentures. First, the top plate of his recently fitted false teeth was crushed by the iron lid of a washbasin, requiring him to use an 'old temporary set', which 'the dentist wanted to destroy' (2000, p. 76). Second, one morning Haggard awoke to find his servant, Mazooku, who he had been reunited with after nearly forty years, 'in the act of consigning [his] wretched false teeth to everlasting oblivion' (2000, p. 180). Haggard noted that Mazooku 'did not know the use of or recognise' his false teeth (2000, p. 180), recalling the confusion caused by Good's dentures in *King Solomon's Mines*. That Haggard included these incidents in his diary, which he intended for publication, shows how false teeth remained humorous and symbolically rich devices in his imagination as well as an aspect of his identity that he did not wish to hide from public scrutiny.

## Conclusion

Building on the work of Carlyle Tarr and Goulet, this chapter has shown that in literary studies as in medicine, you learn a lot by turning attention to the mouth. For Haggard and Kipling, dentures served multiple purposes, operating as metaphor, metonym, and comic prop. In their writings, false teeth are symbols of technological sophistication (in the case of Good's performance in front of the hostile soldiers of Kukuanaland), human–machine hybridity (in the case of Vickery's clicking and lightning-proof teeth), and dwindling imperial might (as in *King Soloman's Mines* and 'Mrs. Bathurst'). Metonymically, these imaginaries function as commentaries on dental prostheses that were surprisingly useful (as with Good), poorly fitted (as with Vickery's partial plates), or representative of unpleasant yet also at times sentimental personal experiences (as evident in *King Solomon's Mines* and 'Mrs. Bathurst' when these works are read in context with Haggard's and Kipling's personal writings). For both writers, artificial teeth were potent comic props: for Haggard as a hilarious focal point of slipstick mishaps and social misfortunes; for Kipling as a grotesque synecdoche for an odd and curious character. As this chapter has shown, in literary writings, false teeth are rich and pliable devices that reveal much about issues of communication (not just verbal), social expectations, and anxieties regarding health (physical and mental) at various scales: individual, institutional, and national. This conclusion begs the question: to what extent are these observations true for earlier and more

modern imaginaries of dentures—in literature, film, and other cultural arte-
facts? I urge scholars working in cognate fields to find the answers.

## References

Bakhtin, M. (1965) *Rabelais and his world*. Translated by Iswolsky, H. Bloomington:
Indiana University Press, pp. 1984.
Buchanan, R. W. (1862) 'Lady Letitia's Lilliput hand', *Temple Bar*, 4 and 5, pp. 551–569.
Carlyle Tarr, C. (2017) 'Long in the tooth: dental degeneracy and the Savage mouth',
*Gothic Studies*, 19(1), pp. 113–136.
Church of England., (1662) '*Te Deum laudamus*', in: Church of England. *The book of
common prayer*. London: Eyre & Spottiswoode, 1892. pp. 51–52.
Clark, R. (1984) 'Riddling the family firm: the sexual economy in Dombey and Son',
*ELH*, 51(1), pp. 69–84.
Colville, Q. (2003) 'Jack Tar and the gentleman officer: the role of uniform in shaping
the class- and gender-related identities of British naval personnel, 1930–1931',
*Transactions of the Royal Historical Society*, 13, pp. 105–129.
Daly, N. (2004) *Literature, technology, and modernity, 1860–2000*. Cambridge: Cambridge
University Press.
Dickens, C. (1846–1848) *Dombey and son*. Edited by Sanders, A. London: Penguin,
pp. 2002.
Esmail, J. (2014) 'The little dog is only a stage property': the blind man's dog in Victorian
culture', *Victorian Review*, 40(1), pp. 18–23.
Gilbert, B. B. (1965) 'Health and politics: the British physical deterioration report of
1904', *Bulletin of the History of Medicine*, 39(2), pp. 143–153.
Goulet, A. (2017) 'Tooth decay: Edgar Allan Poe and the Neuro-déca'dent' isme of
Villiers and Huysmans', *Nineteenth-Century French Studies*, 45(3), pp. 198–218.
Great Britain., (1904) *Report of the inter-departmental committee on physical deterioration*.
London: His Majesty's Stationary Office.
Haggard, H. R. (1885) *King Solomon's mines*. Edited by Hampson, R. New York: Penguin,
pp. 2007.
Haggard, H. R. (1926) *The days of my life*. Edited by Longman, C. J. [Viewed: 16 February
2021]. Available from: http://www.gutenberg.net.au/ebooks03/0300131.txt.
Haggard, H. R. (2000) *Diary of an African journey*. Edited by Coan, S. New York: New
York University Press.
Hampson, R. (2007) 'Introduction', in: Haggard, H. R. (ed.) *King Solomon's mines*. Edited
by Hampson, R. New York: Penguin, pp. xiii–xxxiv.
Henderson, M., Miles, A., Walker, D., Connell, B. and Wroe-Brown, R. (2013) '*He being
dead yet speaketh': excavations at three post-medieval burial grounds in Tower Hamlets, East
London, 2004–10*. London: Museum of London Archaeology.
Kestner, J. A. (2010) *Masculinities in British adventure fiction, 1880–1915*. Burlington:
Ashgate.
Kipling, R. (1896) 'To James M. Conland, 8–24 November', in: Kipling, R. *The Letters of
Rudyard Kipling*. Edited by Pinney, T. Vol. 2 of 6. Iowa City: University of Iowa Press,
1990. pp. 272–275.
Kipling, R. (1897a) 'To James M. Conland', 1 June. in: Kipling, R. *The Letters of Rudyard
Kipling*. Edited by Pinney, T. Vol. 2 of 6. Iowa City: University of Iowa Press, 1990.
pp. 298–303.

Kipling, R. (1897b) 'To Ripley Hitchcock', 17 January. in: Kipling, R. *The Letters of Rudyard Kipling*. Edited by Pinney, T. Vol. 2 of 6. Iowa City: University of Iowa Press, 1990. pp. 282–283.

Kipling, R. (1904) 'Mrs. Bathurst', in: Kipling, R. (ed.) *Traffics and discoveries*. New York: Charles Scribner's Sons, 1909. pp. 377–408.

Marlow, J. E. (1994) *Charles Dickens: the uses of time*. Cranbury: Associated University Press.

Medical Division, War Office., (1905) *Army medical department report for the year 1903*. London: His Majesty's Stationary Office.

Melville, H. (1851) *Moby-Dick*. London: Penguin, 2012.

Nicholson, B. (2012) 'Jonathan's Jokes', *Media History*, 18(1), pp. 33–49.

Patteson, R. F. (1978) "King Solomon's mines": imperialism and narrative structure', *The Journal of Narrative Technique*, 8(2), pp. 112–123.

Rutherford, A. (1990). 'Introduction', in: Kipling, R. *War stories and poems*. Edited by Rutherford, A. Oxford: Oxford University Press, 2009.

Rymer, J. M. (1845–1847) *Varney the vampire; or, the feast of blood*. London: E. Lloyd, 1847.

Smith, E. J. (2018) 'Cleanse or die': British naval hygiene in the age of steam, 1840–1900', *Medical History*, 62(2), pp. 177–198.

Stoker, B. (1897) *Dracula*. Edited by Hindle, M. London: Penguin, 2004.

Sutherland, J. (1999) *Who betrays Elizabeth Bennet?* Oxford: Oxford University Press.

Turley Houston, G. (1994) *Consuming fictions: gender, class, and hunger in Dickens's novels*. Carbondale: Southern Illinois University Press.

Watt, R. G. et al. (2019) 'Ending the neglect of global oral health: time for radical action', *The Lancet*, 394(10194), pp. 261–272.

Wells, H. G. (1904) *The food of the gods and how it came to earth*. London: Thomas Nelson and Sons, 1909.

Whittaker, D. K. (1993) 'Oral health', in: Molleson, T., Cox, M., and Waldron, A. H. (eds.) *The Spitalfields project: The middling sort. Volume 2: The anthropology CBA research report 86*. York: Council for British Archaeology, pp. 49–65.

Woodforde, J. (1968) *The strange story of false teeth*. London: Routledge & Kegan Paul.

# 6 Metaphors in the mouth: on dental fitness and iatronormativity

*David Scott*

## Fitness as metaphor

'We pass through a gorge, emerge into daylight, and behold a glass dish and hear a voice saying, "Rinse the mouth. Rinse the mouth," while a trickle of warm blood runs from between the lips'.[1] Tooth extraction is an ordeal, that is, in the original sense of the word. It is a trial by which we subscribe to a new trajectory through life, and – perhaps less sublime a state – the indubitable signifier of an impending societal condition: that of edentulism (toothlessness). A few years before writing this passage, the author Virginia Woolf had recounted in a letter to a friend, the artist Duncan Grant, her recollection of 'a terrifically exciting and somehow sexual dream' on waking from a general anaesthetic at the dentist's surgery – a dream which, unsurprisingly, found its way into her literary musings. Woolf was no stranger to tooth loss, and she resumed this theme once more in her essay *On Being Ill*, a personal exploration of illness's conspicuous absence from classic literature. She attributes this lacuna to the 'poverty of the language', opining that 'the merest schoolgirl, when she falls in love, has Shakespeare, Donne, Keats to speak her mind for her; but let a sufferer try to describe a pain in his head to a doctor and language at once runs dry' (2012 [1926], p. 34). The mouth *as* a metaphor has, since then, been considered by numerous other writers in the fields of sociology, anthropology and literary studies (Sweet, this volume);[2] however, an explicit attention to the language and metaphors *of* the mouth remains comparatively overdue.

One example of these oral metaphors is the normative judgement known colloquially as 'dental fitness' (Rogers, 1989). It is a routine practice, albeit seldom mentioned in print, for individuals awaiting cardiac surgery to be referred to dental surgeons for a declaration of dental fitness in advance of their scheduled surgery. According to the account given by cardiologists and cardiothoracic surgeons, this preparatory step is a safeguard designed to pre-empt the potentially life-threatening diagnosis of infective endocarditis: a complication that on rare occasions can result from cardiac surgery. From the pathological viewpoint, infective endocarditis comprises a localised form of inflammation that afflicts the inner lining (endocardium) of the heart's muscular wall; a condition attributed to the presence of harmful micro-organisms, such as

DOI: 10.4324/9781003047674-8

streptococci of the oral cavity, adhering and proliferating on the heart surface. The biomechanical theory would indicate, for this reason, that teeth of poor prognosis – in other words, those liable to develop inflammatory lesions surrounding the apex of the root – are able to act as focal points of infection, thus seeding bacteria from the mouth into the bloodstream. Consequently, these infective foci may mediate a route through the circulatory system for pathogens to gather along the vulnerable post-operative heart tissue.

Platelets and fibrin, components of the blood clotting cascade that takes place during and in the immediate aftermath of cardiac surgery, together form a meshwork called a thrombus (or 'vegetation') which can shield invasive microbes from the body's natural defence system. The accumulation of these vegetations displays a marked tendency to contribute towards necrosis of the underlying heart tissue, which typically affects the valves of the heart. Furthermore, since the thrombus can gradually enlarge and become increasingly friable, thrombotic pieces may detach themselves in the shape of emboli: fragments which can disseminate to other major bodily organs, such as the brain or kidneys, and potentially occlude their blood supply (infarction). This, then, is the primary means by which infective endocarditis can affect its systemic and often life-threatening sequelae on patients. However, notwithstanding its robustly mechanistic coherence, any solely biomechanical account would neglect to consider the social significance of supposed infective foci, and therefore fail to situate therapeutic practices as being necessarily constituted by the semantic associations attached to these practices. It is through the normative judgements of medical practice that these tacitly shared meanings begin to intermesh with, and reconstitute, the biomechanical rationale.

Dental fitness, as a normative judgement, refers to the desired state of pre-operative suitability for cardiac surgery that is believed to minimise the risk of infective endocarditis (Isaac et al., 2017). In typical practice, it commonly means that the dental surgeon must sign a letter of declaration stating that dental fitness has been achieved; either that, or advise the postponement of cardiac surgery until the necessary measures have been taken to render the patient dentally fit. The declaration is subsequently applied by cardiologists and cardiothoracic surgeons as a benchmark against which to judge candidates on their surgical readiness; yet, the accomplishment of dental fitness and its wherewithal is largely left to the discretion of individual dental surgeons. Moreover, once this therapeutic practice of establishing dental fitness has been enveloped within the exigencies of everyday work, it frequently entails the extraction of teeth considered to be of poor prognosis. This incurs, more precisely, the removal of teeth that would normally have been expected to survive for a significantly longer period of time had they not been extracted so prematurely. Thus, these teeth of poor prognosis are effectively being removed for a social prophylactic as much as they are for a biomechanical cause.

However, what is perhaps even more striking here, especially when you consider the consequent burden of responsibility placed on dental surgeons, is the unfortunate dearth of clinical guidelines on which criteria ought to be used to establish dental fitness, and to what extent surgical interventions should be undertaken to achieve it. In fact, this ambiguous tension may have contributed to a variable interpretation between individual dental surgeons on what dental fitness actually means, with the potential for such decisions to become challenging and even, at times, overwhelming for the dental surgeon (Pantiora, 2017). It should come as little surprise, then, to imagine that dental surgeons, in the absence of clinical guidelines, should develop their own idiosyncratic routines and rituals with the aim of establishing a heightened level of idealised dental health. Tooth extraction with the intent to achieve dental fitness can therefore be seen to assume the role of a dramaturgical act: a performance that functions symbolically as a ritual of purification and anticipates the embodied conflict of cardiac surgery.

Ritualised practices of removing human teeth with the intent to establish a heightened state of purity have notable precedents, both historical and anthropological. Take, for instance, *ilhamba* – a 'hunter's tooth' among the indigenous Ndembu people of Zambia – a tooth that is ceremonially 'drawn' from the sick person's body in a public ritual that seeks to resolve community tensions and conflict. As portrayed by the anthropologist Victor Turner, 'the Ndembu "doctor" sees his task less as curing an individual patient than as remedying the ills of a corporate group. The sickness of a patient is mainly a sign that "'something is rotten" in the corporate body' (Turner, 1967, p. 392). This example poses an apt parallel, where the accomplishment of an internal, harmonious balance in the patient's constitution (or the body politic) affords resilience against external threat. Rather like the achievement of dental fitness prior to cardiac surgery, extracorporeal contaminants are drawn out from the body in anticipation of an impending threat to the body's structural integrity.

In northwest Tanzania, a comparable ritual of removing teeth from infants and young children (*ebiino* or 'plastic teeth') emerged in the Haya community in the late twentieth century, temporally associated with the introduction of human immunodeficiency virus (HIV) and Western capitalist economies (Weiss, 1992). Like infective endocarditis, *ebiino* is believed to be life-threatening to the child and is also thought to have an exogenous origin, supposedly in the form of a living worm (*kijoka*) that may have been imported inadvertently via migrants from Uganda or Rwanda. Weiss argues that the metaphorical description of these 'plastic' teeth among the Haya signifies their understanding of plastic goods as a commodity form, underscoring the recognition of 'plastic' teeth as a foreign object that embodies and represents the turbulence of modern sociocultural transformation in the Haya community. As an anthropological case study, *ebiino* proves a strong resemblance to the Western phenomenon of infective foci: a dormant threat once localised to the afflicted teeth which then begins to disseminate throughout the body, impinging on the vital organs with capricious, and sometimes deadly, consequences (Mogensen, 2000).

In this chapter, I set out to trace the conceptual development of the metaphor 'dental fitness' in relation to cardiac surgery, beginning with its historical origins in focal infection theory. From this vantage point, I describe how the military language of dental fitness became affixed to the vestiges of focal infection theory, supplanting the connotations of cardiac surgery with those of warfare. I then undertake a critical analysis of dental fitness as the diagnostic manifestation of a societal norm, and consequently make a preliminary sketch towards a theory of iatronormativity.[3] Without clinical guidelines for achieving dental fitness, I argue, these normative judgements will continue to be enacted and sustained by an informal surveillance network of tacit and codified practices.

## A body under siege

In 1891, the American dentist and microbiologist Willoughby Dayton Miller published an essay in the periodical *Dental Cosmos* entitled 'The Human Mouth as a Focus of Infection'. He claimed that in recent years 'the conviction has grown continually stronger, among physicians as well as dentists, that the human mouth ... performs a significant role in the production of varied disorders of the body', and went on to speculate that 'if many diseases whose origin is enveloped in mystery could be traced to their source, they would be found to have originated in the oral cavity' (Miller, 1891, p. 689). This enduring and all-encompassing hypothesis was soon to be recognised more widely in the field of medicine as 'focal infection theory'.[4] Stemming from the germ theory of disease espoused by microbiologist and physician Robert Koch, the theory of focal infections was typical of contemporaneous efforts to ascribe each and every human disease to a specific microbial aetiology (Carstairs, this volume). In the context of dentistry, this theory held that the human mouth, situated along the border delineating interior from exterior, could act as a portal of entry to the body for pathogenic microbes; from oral infections, principally in the guise of dental and periodontal abscesses, bacteria could then disseminate throughout the bloodstream (or lymphatic network) and contribute to an array of distant pathologies. By way of evidence, Miller compiled an extensive catalogue of case studies, ranging from a seven-year-old boy with carious teeth who subsequently died from a brain abscess to a 33-year-old woman with a fistula on her breast that reportedly healed after the offending tooth had been extracted.

With additional case reports and series being published in the United States (Billings, 1912, 1914), across the Atlantic, a number of British doctors were beginning to take notice. One of these physicians, the prolific William Hunter became, in turn, a forceful advocate for the theory of focal infections. Announcing in 1900 the discovery of 'oral sepsis' as a prominent source of disseminated infections, inter alia, the distant cause of meningitis, gastritis and osteomyelitis, he criticised the apparent hypocrisy of his contemporaries:

> No physician or surgeon would tolerate for a moment that a patient with a foul septic ulcer, say in his forearm, should from time to time apply his lips to the ulcer to clean it. Yet this is – pathologically – precisely what happens in the case of patients with necrosed teeth and stomatitis. (1900, p. 215)

No doubt he would have felt vindicated in the following decade by experimental results published at the Mayo Clinic in Rochester, Minnesota, in which animal subjects were injected intravenously with bacterial cultures obtained from human dental infections (Rosenow, 1919). In 1921, he expanded upon these claims and decried the ignorance of many dentists in valuing the technical expertise of traditional dental surgery over the biological foundations underlying their craft (Hunter, 1921). Such a criticism tapped into existing desires to advance the professionalisation of dentistry beyond a mere technical apprenticeship; in the same year, the Dentists Act of 1921 had mandated the compulsory registration of practising dental surgeons with a newly created Dental Board of the United Kingdom (Gelbier, 2005).

One year later, in 1922, the writer Virginia Woolf experienced the consequences of focal infection theory first-hand, undergoing a series of tooth extractions to alleviate a bout of 'influenza' that left her bed-ridden for several days. She detailed the rationale behind this decision to her friend Janet Case:

> The dr. now thinks that my influenza germs may have collected at the roots of three teeth. So I'm having them out, and preparing for the escape of microbes by having 65 million dead ones injected into my arm daily. It sounds to me too vague to be very hopeful – but one must, I suppose, do as they say. (Nicolson and Trautmann, 1976, p. 529)

Shortly after the procedure (and subsequent 'vaccination'), she returned to London having made a brief stay of recuperation at her country home in Rodmell, Sussex. On arrival she wrote in her diary: 'The depression of a return from Rodmell is always acute. Perhaps this continued temperature – I lost three teeth in vain the other day – may be some sort of cause for my ups & downs' (Bell and McNeillie, 1978, p. 176). The recognition that these teeth were extracted 'in vain' is key here, implying as it does her view that the prescribed treatment was taken unnecessarily and, furthermore, seemingly with fruitless effect.

Woolf's raised temperature and heart 'murmur' gave few signs of abating in the days that followed, and she outpoured this frustration through her letters: 'I'm so cross. Three teeth pulled out that might have lasted a lifetime, and temperature still up. Next they'll cut out my tonsils, and then I suppose adenoids, and then appendix, and then – what comes next?' (p. 531). Unfortunately, there is an underlying truth in this morbid parody of modern medicine. Rosenow outlines the truly circular reasoning of many physicians in their belief that 'if improvement does not follow the removal of a given focus, it is considered presumptive evidence that the particular operation was not properly performed or that other foci exist' (1919, pp. 205–6). In another letter, Woolf compares the continued regularity of her influenza to 'a very respectable grandfather's clock', regretting the loss of teeth she could 'ill spare' with 'so far no result' (p. 532). Whether or not this therapy was ever prescribed for her mental health is left unsaid; however, her former psychiatrist George Savage was renowned for his commitment to focal infection theory (Lee, 1996). In his efforts to spearhead the movement in Britain, Hunter similarly believed that 'oral sepsis' could, on occasion, be responsible for nervous or mental disorders in a phenomenon he referred to as 'toxic neuritis' (Hunter, 1901; Hunter and Moynihan, 1927).

Back in the United States, a psychiatrist and medical director of the New Jersey State Hospital, Henry Cotton was enthusiastically championing tooth extraction as a means to resolve mental illness (Cotton, 1919). With nineteenth-century innovations in antisepsis, analgesia, and anaesthesia, surgical intervention had begun to emerge as a modish panacea for the more troublingly evasive illnesses, popularising the colectomy, appendicectomy and tonsillectomy (Porter, 1997). Hysterectomies were increasingly performed for the 'hysterical' woman, mirroring an ancient belief in the 'wandering womb' – an errant uterus intent on provoking emotional maladies. 'Another fashionable inter-war diagnosis', Porter notes, 'was focal sepsis: the notion that pockets of pus were lurking in the sickly body, causing infections and requiring surgical extraction. It thus became routine to extract teeth, often *all* the teeth of patients in psychiatric hospitals' (1997, p. 601). No longer content with damage limitation alone, Cotton proceeded to treat his patients prophylactically, extracting relatively healthy teeth as a precaution against the insidious surfacing of focal infections concealed within the mouth (Scull, 2005). In these prophylactic measures, the nascent roots of dental fitness as a means to circumvent the risk of infective endocarditis become increasingly evident.

Focal infection theory remained influential until the 1940s, by which time the underlying scientific argument was falling into disrepute and losing its adherents (Reimann and Havens, 1940). As methods for the analysis of mortality statistics in psychiatric institutions were being steadily refined, the frequent deaths from 'surgical bacteriology' began to outweigh any anecdotal benefits and led to its swift, unequivocal demise. Yet, a few remnants of this theory have survived, most exceptionally with regard to dental health and the infectious complications resulting from cardiac surgery. Diseased teeth are still thought to behave like infective foci, shedding bacteria into the bloodstream in what is known as a 'transient bacteraemia'. And still more, patients scheduled for cardiac surgery are routinely referred to dental surgeons for prophylactic extraction of their teeth, purportedly as a measure against the risk of transient bacteraemia. Towards the latter half of the twentieth century, a subtle change occurred in the way that dental surgeons and cardiologists spoke with one another on the subject of dental health: no longer in terms of 'focal infection', 'oral sepsis' or 'surgical bacteriology', but, instead, of 'dental fitness'. Thenceforth, the military language of dental fitness became affixed to the vestiges of focal infection theory, supplanting the connotations of cardiac surgery with those of warfare. In so doing, the conflict of heart surgery gradually became an embodied surrogate for the conflict of war.

Dental fitness first emerged in the context of military conflict, the implication being that teeth are fit for a certain purpose such as warfare. In the early phase of the Boer War, poor dental health had been recognised as a major contributing factor to military recruits being deemed unfit for service (Strong, this volume). Among nearly 70,000 men who had been examined, as many as 4,400 were rejected for having decayed teeth (Gelbier and Randall, 1982) and, moreover, roughly 3,000 men were invalided home from South Africa for the sequelae of dental caries (Welshman, 1998). Establishing the dental fitness of military recruits has since become a routine procedure; for instance, the North Atlantic Treaty Organization (NATO) uses a military classification of dental fitness for risk assessment of its personnel prior to their deployment. As Richardson (2005) explains in more detail, the NATO classification extends from 'category 1, fully dentally fit' to 'category 4, dental examination is overdue', with corresponding remedial action to be taken as appropriate. The precise definitions of these categories, however, vary between the member states of NATO.

By contrast, the first mention of dental fitness in a non-military context seems to have taken place in the latter half of the twentieth century. The late 1980s saw the terminology of dental fitness being co-opted by the oil and gas industry as an indication of whether employees' dental health was considered suitable for commencing work on offshore installations (Ballantine et al., 1990). Furthermore, it was around this time that dental fitness was adopted as a metaphor for the pre-surgical preparations that anticipated the impending conflict of cardiac surgery (Rogers, 1989). This gradual transformation in the semantic associations attached to cardiac surgery's risk of infective endocarditis is not entirely unexpected, however. Indeed, military metaphors are rife in the medical world. In her essay *Illness as Metaphor*, Susan Sontag observes how 'the controlling metaphors in descriptions of cancer are, in fact, drawn … from the language of warfare', lamenting that 'every physician and every attentive patient is familiar with, if perhaps inured to, this military terminology' (Sontag, 1978, p. 65). The so-called war on cancer, instigated by U.S. President Richard Nixon in 1971, formed the apogée of efforts to peddle military metaphors on illness, re-establishing norms in public sentiment and behaviour towards cancer patients (Sontag, 1978). As such, the metaphorical language affixed to concepts of dental health is similarly able to instil societal norms and thereby regulate the health behaviour of individuals.

In the concluding section, I undertake a critical analysis of dental fitness as the diagnostic manifestation of a societal norm. Having traced the conceptual development of this metaphor, I go on to explore how the semantic associations formerly attached to military fitness now impact on the dental health of cardiac surgery patients. In doing so, I elaborate the philosopher of medicine Georges Canguilhem's theory that health and disease are independently normative concepts which do not simply correspond to normal and abnormal states of being. I then proceed to make a preliminary sketch towards a theory of iatronormativity, exploring how normative judgements are enacted and sustained by an informal surveillance network of tacit and codified practices.

## The iatronormative

Should one say that it is *normal* for our teeth to be healthy? Or are these adjectives – *normal* teeth and *healthy* teeth – precisely one and the same? Is dental disease merely an abnormality; a divergence from what is considered biologically normal for the human mouth? Ever since the golden years of physiology in the nineteenth century, a recurring assumption has posited health to be the state of biological normality, in necessary contrast to the (relatively) abnormal state of disease. In accordance with this line of thought, it follows that dental disease should be defined in opposition to, and as a deviation from, the norm of dental health. Further, it is possible that dental fitness could then be regarded as a subset *within* the norm of dental health; a subset that tolerates only limited deviation from the optimal standard; a much slender definition of peak health. But is this fundamental assumption – the belief that pathology is strictly a deviation from biological normality – a reasonable one? To propose a counter-example, if orthodontic therapies for dental malocclusion were to be withheld, then 'crooked' teeth would occur quite as often as 'straight' teeth (Wickström, 2016). But, then again, is it true that a lack of geometric alignment in itself counts as disease? Or that the norm is what we find most commonly in nature? This case stresses a marked discontinuity between received notions of ubiquity and the norm, health and normality.

One of the pivotal figures in the philosophy of medicine, Georges Canguilhem discards the persistent claim that health is a biological norm, and disease the deviation from that norm. 'Disease is still a norm of life', he argues, 'but it is an inferior norm in the sense that it tolerates no deviation from the conditions in which it is valid' (Canguilhem, 1991 [1943] p. 183). Such a viewpoint is especially relevant to dental health, where diseases of the mouth are considered phenomenologically atypical due to their ubiquity and hyper-monitorability (Rakhra, 2019). Canguilhem clarifies this point by adding that 'the sick living being is normalized in well-defined conditions of existence and has lost his normative capacity, the capacity to establish other norms in other conditions'.[5] Indeed, Canguilhem's reasoning would indicate that a person's dental health can be described more accurately as a capacity of his/her mouth to normalise; that is, a capacity that enables the mouth to establish new biological norms relative to its fluctuating physical and social environment. In other words, 'The sick man is not abnormal because of the absence of a norm but because of his incapacity to be normative' (p. 186). Hence, a person can only be considered truly 'sick' or diseased in relation to their individual circumstances, not simply in relation to the biological characteristics typical of a population to which they belong. Of course, this is not to say that the existence of dental disease is relative to a person's unique inner perspective but that the dental health of an individual must be judged in consideration of their material and social environment in the widest sense.

Canguilhem goes on to contend that while illness may appear to differ from the biological norm of health solely on a quantitative or statistical scale (e.g. high blood pressure), the threshold bridging health and illness is at least partly qualitative in nature and therefore derives substantially from value-based judgements. Further, he argues that the normal is a polysemous term that compounds both statistical and moral conceptions under a single umbrella: (i) what is most *frequently* the case (or that which constitutes a statistical average), and (ii) what *ought* to be the case (i.e., a value-based, moral understanding). In this way, the normal state designates both the 'habitual' and the 'ideal' (p. 126). The philosopher Eva Kittay delineates these two kinds of normal as 'a descriptive sense and a prescriptive sense' (2006, p. 93), taking this latter sense one step further by postulating the desire for normality as a possible tautology: a desire for what is desirable. Clearly, it is the moral or prescriptive sense of normality that would apply most readily to the condition of dental fitness; rather than addressing the typical or representative state of dental health, it focuses on what is thought desirable under the present circumstances. The degree of dental health that might be considered *normal* for a cardiac surgery candidate would therefore depend to some extent upon the perceived values and moral judgements of the responsible clinician.

A fundamental distinction separating the example of dental fitness from Canguilhem's biological normativity, however, is the clinician's exclusive privilege in setting these new norms, in what might be termed iatronormativity. This concept derives from Freidson's (1970) claim that medical diseases can be addressed as socially constructed phenomena rather than simple biological facts and that, therefore, it is the clinician who is, to a certain extent, responsible for the 'creation' of disease. However, in contrast to Freidson's social construction of disease and Illich's (1975) equally influential concept of social iatrogenesis (i.e., the overmedicalisation of society), the enactment of iatronormativity would necessitate the creation of new norms, not diseases. The undisputed authority of the clinician to attribute dental fitness to certain individuals, embedded in particular circumstances, can be seen as an example of the normative judgements that are routinely undertaken in medical practice. Once a declaration of dental fitness has been made, the clinician creates a new norm corresponding to an alternate modality of health. Thus, the achievement of dental fitness is ultimately both normalising and normative: it measures patients against an imagined norm and, in so doing, reinforces this ideal as the new normal. This normative tendency is even more remarkable when one acknowledges the dearth of clinical guidance on which criteria ought to establish dental fitness, and to what extent interventions should be undertaken to achieve it. Without clinical guidelines for achieving dental fitness, these normative judgements are enacted and sustained by an informal surveillance network of tacit and codified practices.

Contemporary usage of the metaphor 'dental fitness' across the cardiac-dental care boundary contributes towards an illusion of dental fitness assuming a merely descriptive or statistical role. However, through extension of Canguilhem's theory that health and disease are independently normative concepts which do not simply correspond to normal and abnormal states of being, dental fitness may instead be considered a value-laden term rather than a descriptive subset of dental health. Indeed, tooth extraction with the intent to achieve dental fitness can therefore be seen to assume the role of a dramaturgical act: a performance that functions symbolically as a ritual of purification and anticipates the embodied conflict of cardiac surgery. The passage towards candidacy for cardiac surgery involves the dental surgeon inventing a new norm; one that sustains a restricted capacity for varying from idealised dental health. Now that the patient is being considered for cardiac surgery, the outcome of a previous dental check-up is no longer held to be valid. And, of course, whether the patient considers his/her existing state of dental health to be normal for himself/herself is quickly discarded as irrelevant.

In Alasdair Gray's dystopian and surrealist novel *Lanark*, the eponymous protagonist takes refuge from the morbid city of Unthank by descending through a gaping human mouth. Clinging tightly to an incisor, he clambers down into the subterranean Institute – an authoritarian clinic where recalcitrant patients are discreetly processed into canteen cuisine. Lanark's visceral passage exemplifies how casually the human mouth is symbolised as a gateway to the body; a metaphor reflected in the *mouths* of rivers and caves, the *lips* of cups and pots. My exploration of the metaphor 'dental fitness' set out to articulate and explicate this metaphor, challenging how it is currently wielded across the cardiac-dental care boundary. Dental fitness is interpreted by dental surgeons on an ad hoc basis, gathering together both explicit forms of professional knowledge and a tacitly shared, collective meaning behind the term. Whilst proffering the semblance of scientific objectivity – despite the absence of explicit criteria with which to judge dental fitness – the expression conceals and obscures its largely social function. This involves the accomplishment of dental fitness through establishment of a new norm set by the clinician's authority: an instance of iatronormativity. Rather, the removal of teeth as a means to achieve dental fitness operates as a ritual of purification, the consummate extraction of extra-corporeal contaminants, an act that aims to restore the body's integrity in readiness for the external threat of cardiac surgery. Those individuals thought to be particularly susceptible are evaluated against a new norm; a norm set by the clinician that tolerates a much narrower definition of health.

## Notes

1 From Woolf's essay *Gas*, published in Clarke (p. 452, 2011).
2 See Gibson and Exley (2013) for a historical overview of the symbolic significance attached to the human mouth in Western and non-Western societies.
3 The meaning and derivation of this term will be outlined more precisely in the final section of the chapter.
4 In contrast to Nettleton's (1988) assertion that the mouth became 'separated' from the body as a distinct corpus of medical knowledge during the nineteenth century, the emergence of focal infection theory seems to indicate resistance to this line of thought. It is perhaps a notable exception that (as in the case of physiologist May Mellanby's support for the nutritional deficiency theory of dental caries) efforts to reunite dental

health and general health continued well into the twentieth century (Nicolson and Taylor, 2009).

5  Building upon this interpretation, Mol (1998) considers the multiplicity of norms that ensues and asks how the many norms of medicine might relate. She proposes, taking the case of diabetes, that social and laboratory norms may be interdependent and 'hang together' or may instead contradict one another and coexist in tension. The normative practices of medicine thus constitute a societal discourse of perpetual conflict and compromise.

# References

Ballantine, B. N., Costigan, F. and Anderson, R. J. (1990) 'A survey of the dental health of the workers on two groups of offshore installations', *Journal of the Society of Occupational Medicine*, 40, pp. 143–148.

Bell, A. O. and McNeillie, A. eds. (1978) *The Diary of Virginia Woolf, Volume II: 1920–1924*. London: The Hogarth Press.

Billings, F. (1912) 'Chronic focal infections and their etiologic relations to arthritis and nephritis', *Archives of Internal Medicine*, 9, pp. 484–498.

Billings, F. (1914) 'Focal infection: its broader application in the etiology of general disease', *Journal of the American Medical Association*, 63, pp. 899–903.

Canguilhem, G. (1991 [1943]) *The normal and the pathological*. New York: Zone Books.

Clarke, S. N. ed. (2011) *The essays of Virginia Woolf: volume VI, 1933–1941, and additional essays, 1906–1924*. London: The Hogarth Press.

Cotton, H. A. (1919) 'The relation of oral infection to mental diseases', *Journal of Dental Research*, 1, pp. 269–313.

Freidson, E. (1970) *Profession of medicine: a study of the sociology of applied knowledge*. Chicago: University of Chicago Press.

Gelbier, S. and Randall, S. (1982) 'Charles Edward Wallis and the rise of London's School Dental Service', *Medical History*, 26, pp. 395–404.

Gelbier, S. (2005) '125 years of developments in dentistry, 1880–2005. Part 2: Law and the dental profession', *British Dental Journal*, 199, pp. 470–473.

Gibson, B. and Exley, C. (2013) 'The mouth and society', *Social Science and Dentistry*, 2, pp. 50–57.

Gray, A. (1981) *Lanark: a life in four books*. Edinburgh: Canongate Books.

Hunter, W. (1900) 'Oral sepsis as a cause of disease', *British Medical Journal*, 2065, pp. 215–216.

Hunter, W. (1901) *Oral sepsis as a cause of 'septic gastritis', 'toxic neuritis', and other septic conditions*. London: Cassell & Co.

Hunter, W. (1921) 'The coming of age of oral sepsis', *British Medical Journal*, 3154, p. 859.

Hunter, W. and Moynihan, B. (1927) 'Chronic sepsis as a cause of mental disorder', *British Medical Journal*, 3487, pp. 811–818.

Illich, I. (1975) *Medical nemesis: the expropriation of health*. London: Calder & Boyars.

Isaac, R. E., Hayes, J. and Ashraf, S. (2017) 'Are cardiac valve patients 'dentally fit' and can oral and maxillofacial surgery provide a means of optimising patient outcome?', *Journal of Oral and Maxillofacial Surgery*, 46, pp. 109.

Kittay, E. F. (2006) 'Thoughts on the desire for normality', in: Parens, E. (ed.) *Surgically shaping children: technology, ethics, and the pursuit of normality*. Baltimore: John Hopkins University Press.

Lee, H. (1996) *Virginia Woolf*. London: Chatto & Windus.

Miller, W. D. (1891) 'The human mouth as a focus of infection', *Dental Cosmos*, 33, pp. 689–713.

Mogensen, H. O. (2000) 'False teeth and real suffering: the social course of 'germectomy' in Eastern Uganda',*Culture, Medicine and Psychiatry*, 24, pp. 331–351.

Mol, A. (1998) 'Lived reality and the multiplicity of norms: a critical tribute to Georges Canguilhem', *Economy and Society*, 27, pp. 274–284.

Nettleton, S. (1988) 'Protecting a vulnerable margin: towards an analysis of how the mouth came to be separated from the body', *Sociology of Health and Illness*, 10, pp. 156–169.

Nicolson, M. and Taylor, G. S. (2009) 'Scientific knowledge and clinical authority in dentistry: James Sim Wallace and dental caries', *Journal of the Royal College of Physicians of Edinburgh*, 39, pp. 64–72.

Nicolson, N. and Trautmann, J. eds. (1976) *The Letters of Virginia Woolf: Volume II, 1912–1922*. London: The Hogarth Press.

Pantiora, A. (2017) 'OMFS: Dental fitness prior to cardiac surgery', *British Dental Journal*, 222, pp. 643–644.

Porter, R. (1997) *The greatest benefit to mankind: a medical history of humanity from antiquity to the Present*. London: Harper Press.

Rakhra, D. (2019) 'The dental anomaly: how and why dental caries and periodontitis are phenomenologically atypical', *Philosophy, Ethics, and Humanities in Medicine*, 14(15), pp. 1–7.

Reimann, H. A. and Havens, W. P. (1940) 'Focal infection and systemic disease: a critical appraisal – the case against indiscriminate removal of teeth and tonsils', *Journal of the American Medical Association*, 114, pp. 1.

Richardson, P. S. (2005) 'Dental risk assessment for military personnel', *Military Medicine*, 170, pp. 542–545.

Rogers, S. (1989) 'A study of the dental health of patients undergoing heart valve surgery', *Postgraduate Medical Journal*, 65, pp. 453–455.

Rosenow, E. C. (1919) 'Studies on elective localization: focal infection with special reference to oral sepsis', *Journal of Dental Research*, 1, pp. 205–267.

Scull, A. (2005) *Madhouse: a tragic tale of megalomania and modern medicine*. London: Yale University Press.

Sontag, S. (1978) *Illness as metaphor*. New York: Farrar, Straus & Giroux.

Turner, V. (1967) 'A Ndembu doctor in practice', in: *The forest of symbols: aspects of Ndembu ritual*. London: Cornell University Press.

Weiss, B.(1992) 'Plastic teeth extraction: the iconography of Haya gastro-sexual affliction', *American Ethnologist*, 19, pp. 538–552.

Welshman, J. (1998) 'Dental health as a neglected issue in medical history: the School Dental Service in England and Wales, 1900–40', *Medical History*, 42, pp. 306–327.

Wickström, A. (2016) 'I hope I get movie-star teeth': doing the exceptional normal in orthodontic practice for young people', *Medical Anthropology Quarterly*, 30, pp. 285–302.

Woolf, V. (2012 [1926]) *On being ill*. Ashfield, MA: Paris Press.

# 7 'DO AS YOUR DENTIST TELLS YOU'[1]: mouthwash advertising in interwar America

*Alexander C. L. Holden*

## Introduction

The association of oral hygiene with the prevention of dental disease has led to a long connection between those engaged in the practice of dentistry, and those who sell oral hygiene products. This chapter is concerned with the depiction of dentists within an advertising campaign for Lavoris mouthwash featuring in the *Saturday Evening Post* during the years 1929 and 1930. Lavoris is one of the largest manufacturing chemists in the industry and a well-known brand of mouthwash in the United States where it is been sold since 1903. Lavoris has long been associated with the dental profession. As an example, the report of the Fourth Annual Meeting of the Southwestern Society of Orthodontists in January 1924 documents that as an exhibitor, Lavoris donated a box of golf balls as prizes for the golf tournament held at the meeting (Fisher, 1924). The firm's initial association with the profession during the interwar period is important because it was during this period that Americans began to routinely visit the dentist for examinations and treatment. It is also during this period that the work of the profession became firmly rooted within a scientific evidence base, giving the work of dentists legitimacy and creating distance between dentists deemed to be of good standing within the profession and those considered to be 'empirics'.

To build on interwar consumer demand for dental services, Lavoris published its first advertisement from the 'Lavoris Reciprocation Program' in 1929 (Figure 7.1; Table 7.1, advert reference 1).

Lavoris' campaign, and its first advertisement 'tendered to the American Dentist in appreciation of more than 25 years' acceptance and good will', is particularly significant for demonstrating the firm's primary purpose: to champion professional dentists. The promotion of Lavoris mouthwash to the wider public appears as a secondary purpose. Despite this, the advertising of dentists as men of science and good character, coupled with the overt linkage of Lavoris as a key partner to the profession, should be acknowledged as allowing the adverts to also simultaneously build the scientific credibility and legitimacy of the Lavoris mouthwash brand.

DOI: 10.4324/9781003047674-9

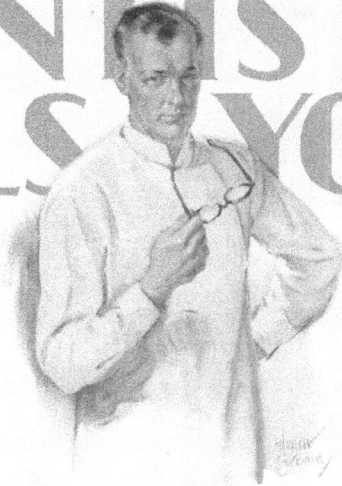

THE SATURDAY EVENING POST    63

*Figure 7.1* 'Do As Your Dentist Tells You'.

Source: Retro AdArchives/Alamy Stock Photo.

The importance of historic dental advertising has been recognised by previous analyses (Miskell, 2004; Grumsen, 2009; 2012; Hujoel, 2019), as well as within this collection by Catherine Carstairs, who critically analyses toothpaste and toothbrush advertising within the interwar period. Grumsen (2009) notes that advertising has both shaped and been shaped by the actions and reactions of the dental profession. The advertising campaign being examined in this chapter gives us a sense of the portrayal of the dental profession and the dentist–patient

*Table 7.1* Description of Lavoris advertisements within the series

| Advert reference | Main caption of advert | Overview of advert illustration |
| --- | --- | --- |
| 1 | DO AS YOUR DENTIST TELLS YOU | A dentist, with glasses in his hand and wearing a stern facial expression, stands in front of the main caption. This is written in all-capitals and in a bold, red font (Figure 7.1). |
| 2 | Who Stole This Dentist's Hour? | A dentist stands looking at a clock on the surgery wall with his hands on his hips. A dental assistant makes notes (Figure 7.2). |
| 3 | Three Years Old, so to the Dentist We Will Go! | A dentist, on bended knee, introduces himself to a smiling young girl in the dental surgery. She is accompanied by her mother (Figure 7.3). |
| 4 | Is Your Name Among the Missing? | A dentist sits at his desk at night, the empty surgery in the background. He is examining papers. |
| 5 | D is for Dentist – do as he says! | The dentist in the illustration is surrounded by children who are being taught about oral hygiene. |
| 6 | Don't Expect Your Dentist to Perform Miracles | A charlatan performs dentistry as a crowd watch on. He is accompanied by a minstrel wearing "blackface" makeup. |
| 7 | Your Dentist rates a Salute, too | Two US military servicemen stand at attention. The Army and Navy Dental Corps insignia feature below them. |
| 8 | Suggestion for A New Year's Resolution | A male patient who is wearing a suit swears an oath, his right arm raised, as the dentist watches. His hands are on his hips. |
| 9 | YEARS OF LIFE FOR SALE HERE | The scene of a dentist and assistant at work in surgery features. On the surgery door, a sign with the main caption features. |

relationship of almost ninety years ago. The advertisements capture the profession at a time of fragility; dentists were still emerging as professionals, striving to differentiate their legitimate practice from those they described as charlatans, while at the same time also solidifying the nature of oral health as an essential component of wellbeing within the zeitgeist. The advertisements also express to the reader the expectations of the dental profession of how patients should interact and perceive their dentist. But the campaign is also worthy of consideration today and provides an understanding of the contemporary nature of professionalism. Understanding the historic social cues of professional consolidation illuminates how these expectations may have evolved or have been preserved through to the present day.

To develop insights into the presentation of the profession and the dentist's relationship with his or her patients within the illustrations of the advertisements, Kress' and van Leeuwen's (2006) framework for analysing the grammar of visual design is employed. This, coupled with discourse analysis of the language within the written advertisements, allow an in-depth assessment of the depiction of the dentist, professional identity and the dentist–patient relationship. Discourse is an important concept within social semiotics. Kress and van Leeuwen (2001, p. 21) define discourse to be

> socially situated forms of knowledge about (aspects of reality). This includes knowledge of events constituting that reality (who is involved, what takes place, where and when it takes place, and so on) as well as a set of related evaluations, purposes, interpretations and legitimations.

In the context of dentistry, dental discourse encompasses the language of the profession, the knowledge produced and the professional institutions and social spaces that it occupies (Nead, 1988). All three of these elements to dental discourse are explored within this analysis in order to develop greater insight into what this advert series might give into the nature of dental professionalism.

Kress and van Leeuwen's method for examining visual grammar is derived from Halliday's (1978) definitions of different types of semiotic 'work', termed metafunctions. In assessing visual media, Kress and van Leeuwen describe three metafunctions: representation, interaction and composition. These metafunctions are described within the analysis as they are encountered. Kress and van Leeuven's methodology for semiotic analysis provides a framework for descriptive analysis, but alone it does not give the full depth of insight allowing for detailed interpretation (Jewitt and Oyama, 2001). It is important to draw upon knowledge of the history and context of the time period from where these advertisements were originally situated to provide direction to the application of this analytical approach: in this case, these advertisements must be seen in the context of the interwar period, when American dentistry was gaining professional and scientific legitimacy.

This analysis is limited to nine advertisements, being a study of a particular programme run by Lavoris that is unique in its direction and purpose as a limited series and the most blatant representations of the firm's aim to help legitimise the dental profession in the eyes of the public. The nine advertisements have a common layout; they feature an illustration with irregular borders, with text beneath the visual component. A brief summary of the adverts is featured in Table 7.1.

Lavoris continued to advertise following the release of the reciprocation programme, but these later advertisements were more concerned with highlighting and selling Lavoris mouthwash as a product rather than showcasing the dental profession, thus demonstrating further change in the dentists–company–patient relationship.

It is also worth noting that the legitimacy of the science of dentistry was a major feature of this period in the dental profession's development.

Carstairs (2015) notes that in interwar United States, dental schools revised their curricula and extended the training time required to qualify. The dental profession also sought to gain legitimacy through its adoption and promotion of the theory of focal sepsis (Dussault and Sheiham, 1982). The profession's keen adoption of the focal sepsis theory in the 1910s and 1920s where oral infection led to systemic infections or chronic diseases may explain the advertisements' expansion of the dentist's role to 'a staunch ally of Nature and Medicine'. Yet, despite the importance of science in dentistry's journey towards professional legitimacy, the series almost exclusively focuses on the character and professionalism of dentists.

## The reader: who do the adverts speak to?

The *Saturday Evening Post* grew its readership to two million between the years of 1908–1937, and predominantly appealed to white, middle-class Americans, mainly men, promoting traditional values of family and business life (Cohn, 1989). Where they appear, the dental patients depicted in the advertisements, who are representative of the readership, often hold less salience within the series than the dentists they appear alongside. Like other advertising of the period within the newspaper, the actors are all white. The discourse within the advertisements aligns with the readership of the magazine, the messaging being tailored to readers from a higher socioeconomic and affluent background. For example, the text refers to the reader 'as a tax-payer, as a good citizen' and makes repeated references to the reader as an employer: 'protect others, your acquaintances or employees, from the menace of quackery' and 'Go to him for regular examination as frequently as he suggests. Encourage your family, your employees to this custom too'. Also, one of the advertisements presents a fictional oath for a patient to give to their dentist: 'I will encourage employees or business associates to give more attention to oral health'.

The implication of this repeated reference to the patient as a businessman or employer (both roles are given masculine gender) is that the dentist, whilst presented as an altruistic professional, is not a universally accessible service available to all. This is compounded by the portrayal of the 'quack' dentist within one of the advertisements, performing dentistry for the masses. Those dentists who advertised their services as being affordable or discounted in some way were believed by the profession to 'attract a less desirable class of people' (Noyes, 1915). When the studied advertising campaign commenced in 1929, the average annual income in the United States was reported to be $692 (U.S. Department of Commerce, Bureau of Economic Analysis, 1989) with dentists reported to have an average net salary of $4,267 (Weinfeld, 1950). The majority of pre–World War Two dental care was funded by patients themselves, rather than through any government funding or insurance arrangements (Weinfeld, 1950). It was therefore financially beneficial for Lavoris and dentists more broadly to attract wealthier patients by advertising in the *Saturday Evening Post*.

# Legitimising the professional status of the dentist

## *Male and Pale*

In order to legitimise the dentist in the eyes of the typical *Saturday Evening Post* reader, the representation of the dentist (where portrayed) is a white man, wearing a white clinical coat and is frequently bespectacled. When not pictured, the dentist is still referred to with male pronouns within the advert text. The whiteness of the dentist's coat achieves salience through its contrast with the other objects, figures and environmental settings featured in the colour advertising illustrations. The white clinical coat is a representative semiotic resource used to signify the characteristics of the dentists featured in the advertising, linking this depiction of dentists also to the portrayal of medical doctors and scientists of the time. Within Kress and van Leeuwen's framework, conceptual structures of representation relate to the essence or static qualities of actors or objects (circumstances); in this series of advertisements, the dentist provides a clear representation of professional power and status. The clearly gendered and racially homogenous nature of the portrayal of the dentist presented (and indeed the advertisement reader) has been noted in assessments of other dental advertising from the same period. Grumsen (2009, p. 77) notes that female dentists and African American dentists have been present in America since 1866 and 1869, respectively, yet have no presence in this advertising series nor any series of this period. Nye (1997) discusses how the masculine-dominant nature of professional cultures in medicine persisted after the inclusion of female practitioners due to the existence of 'honour-codes' and this may help to explain the lack of gender or racial diversity within the adverts. But here, it is significant that the majority of readers of the newspaper in which the advertisement appeared were wealthy males.

## *Professional authority and good dental citizenship*

The advertisements all extol and promote the professional virtues of the dentist as men of skill, as well as presenting the dentist as an authority, both in respect to professional knowledge and as a figure to be obeyed. In the first advertisement in the series (Figure 7.1 and Table 7.1, reference 1), the image of the dentist appears front and centre-right of the advert illustration. He appears in front of the lower part of large text, written in red, which states 'DO AS YOUR DENTIST TELLS YOU'. He wears a stern expression and holds a pair of glasses in his right hand. He looks straight at the reader, making eye contact as male readers of the newspaper might do if they met the dentist in person. Jewitt and Oyama (2001) refer to this as a demand image; the dentist in the advert is demanding that readers heed the advertisement's command to being deferent to the orders of a dentist. Semiotically, the dentist within the advertisement makes direct contact with the reader, compelling action as instructed. The image text is written in red, block letters and takes up the entire top half of the advert. This large red lettering and the direct eye contact from a representation of authority demand obeyance.

The legitimacy of the dentist's authority is reinforced by the advertisements' text, the discourse focusing on the dentist's role as an expert in life and as a trained professional: 'Know your dentist and so know more about yourself' and 'For your dentist is more than a repairman'. The dentist's expertise is also expanded beyond the oral cavity: 'He wants to safeguard you from needless suffering, protect you from troublesome systemic disorders – rheumatism, arthritis, afflictions of heart or kidneys – that can arise for oral defects'. One of the advertisements starkly illustrates the true impact of the dentist's role in health; a dental surgery sign states: 'YEARS OF LIFE FOR SALE HERE' (Table 7.1., advert reference 9). The advertisement is quick to point out 'Actually, you will never find such a sign as this', suggesting that the ethical dentist would find advertising in such a manner to be unprofessional, but that this represents the reality of undergoing regular dental examinations and oral care.

The dentist is described by Nettleton (1994, p. 82) as a 'tooth judge.' Within the Lavoris campaign, we see the visual embodiment of this in the advertisement 'Suggestion for A New Year's Resolution'. In this advertisement, a patient stood with their right arm raised, making an oath stating their commitment to oral health and dental treatment, whilst a dentist looks on in a stance of disciplinary authority. The wording of the oath fits within the discourses found within the other advertisements of the campaigns. Deference to the professional dentist is evident as one of the prevailing discourses within the oath: 'I will abide by his decisions, for he knows best' and 'I will return promptly and regularly until this work is completed. I will do my best to cooperate with him'. The narrative representation of this image reinforces the dentist's power and legitimacy to pass judgement upon the public for their commitment to oral health.

The advertisements depict the dentist as stern. In three of the advertisements, the dentist is depicted with at least one hand on his hips either in a position of dominance, or in frustration. In the advert titled 'Who Stole This Dentist's Hour?' (Figure 7.2.; Table 7.1, advert reference 2), the dentist is shown, facing away from the reader, with the narrative of his attention being connoted by a vector connecting his gaze with the clock on the wall. The dental assistant in the illustration with the dentist faces towards the reader, but away from the dentist who, with the familiar stance of hands-on hips, is implied to be irritated and having his time wasted, or as the title suggests, stolen. The dental assistant, a woman wearing a white gown and a nurse's cap, looks down, her head seeming to be bowed in deference to the dentist. The text chastises those who miss appointments or attend late: 'There are men and women who consider it their privilege to break an appointment with the dentist for little or no reason. Many are habitually late'. This advertisement also embodies a theme that is common to the campaign: the discourse that the dentist works hard has trained extensively and has a right to earn a living and social status matching this. Here, dentistry is again described as 'arduous'

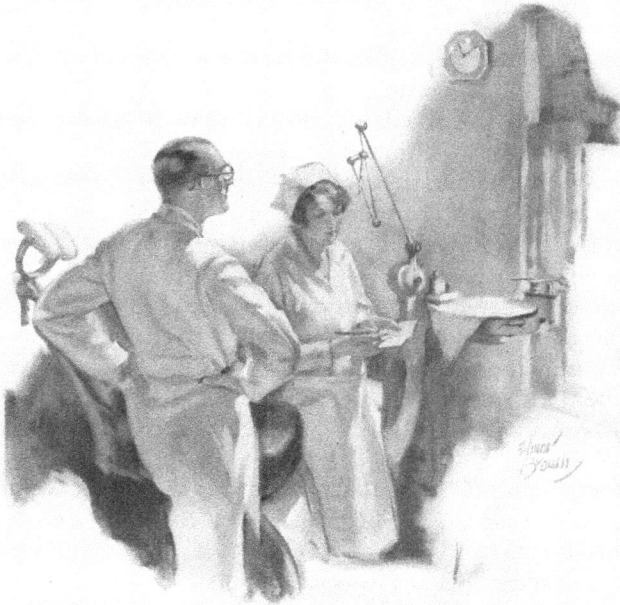

Figure 7.2 'Who Stole This Dentist's Hour?'
Source: Retro AdArchives/Alamy Stock Photo.

and it is also suggested that the patient who misses their appointment contributes to an inequity that prevents the dentist from earning a fair living: 'Increasing costs of overhead and assistance, improved standards of cleanliness and equipment all combine to make it difficult for the dentist to earn a fair profit, a living commensurate with his education and value to society'. This discourse interacts with a similar discourse within the advertisements that presents the dentist as simply wanting an opportunity to perform his duty, to help and to heal: 'Your dentist wants an opportunity to serve you. Visit him regularly – as often as he suggests. Don't rely too much on ordinary brushing. Let this man who has trained himself for just this duty keep constant vigil over your mouth' and 'Give him opportunity to rend you and your family the valuable service for which he is fitted'. The patient who is late or absent is presented has having breached an assumed contract existing between the profession and the public. Within the campaign, there are overt references to the obligations of the public and the individual patient. The relevance of oral and dental health and the notion of being a good 'dental' citizen has been described in relation to oral health being linked to status (Horton and Barker, 2010; Gibson and Exley, 2013). This advertising campaign demonstrates that the rhetoric of 'dental citizenship' (also discussed at length by Scott, in this volume in the context of 'dental fitness'), embodied by regular attendance for examination and compliance with professional advice, has been promulgated by the profession from its origins, supporting the assertion that dentistry was born from public health, rather as a purely clinical discipline (Nettleton, 1994).

In the advertisement 'Three Years Old, so to the Dentist We Will Go!' (Figure 7.3, Table 7.1, advert reference 3), the dentist is portrayed as friendly; the dentist kneeling down to be at the child's level. The text does not address children but encourages parents to take children to the dentist regularly: 'Parents! Your youngsters deserve the opportunity to form early habits of oral hygiene'. Whilst neither this advertisement, nor the other advertisement featuring representations of children (Table 7.1, advert reference 5), shows the dentist visually to be authoritative, the text is nevertheless commanding and demands the same deference to professional advice. The other advertisement follows this same pattern, a feature which is clearly discernible from the title: 'D is for Dentist – do as he says!' The representation here is of the dentist as an educator, a 'teacher in a white coat'. The dentist here is presented as someone seeking to help: 'Your dentist wants an opportunity to serve you' and this is blended with an appeal to a 'civic responsibility' in delivering oral health education to children. This notion of public service and altruism is reinforced: 'Let this man who has trained himself for just this duty keep constant vigil over your mouth'. The dentist here is presented as a professional with a strong sense of public service and duty. This reference to service further reinforces the close links between the notion of altruistic service being integral to an identity as a health professional. The use of the term 'vigil' suggests a higher or spiritual component of the professional role and indicates that the dentist's duty is related to far more than a commercial interaction.

The dentist's role as educator is further enhanced by two of the advertisements titled 'Who Stole This Dentist's Hour?' (Table 7.1., advert reference 2) and 'Is Your Name Among the Missing?' (Table 7.1., advert reference 4). These advertisements use the word 'truant' to describe patients who do not attend for regular examinations and comply with the dentist's professional advice. Another advertisement 'Is Your Name Among the Missing?' (Table 7.1., advert

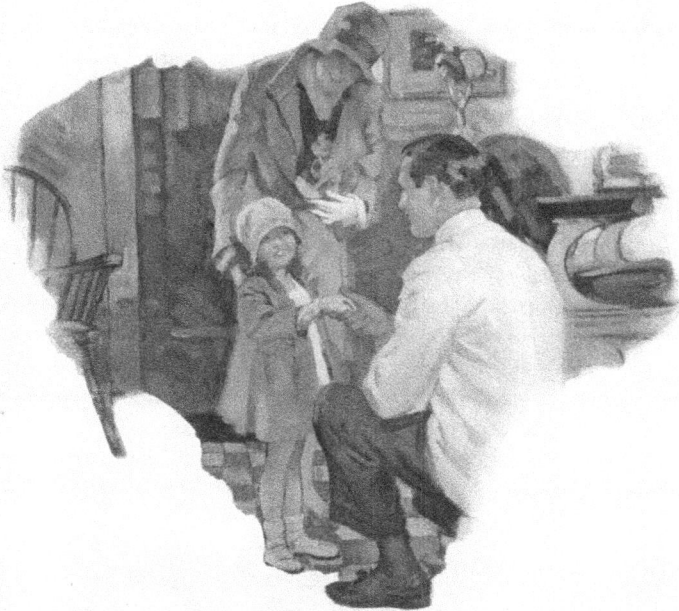

148      THE SATURDAY EVENING POST      *October 5, 1929*

## Three Years Old, so to the Dentist We Will Go!

Here is a room all bright and clean, and full of such wonderful things to see. A nice man, too, who is glad to meet 3-year-old people. Lots of children, he says, never go to the dentist. They get toothache, and are cross, and never have good sound teeth.

*Parents!* Your youngsters deserve the opportunity to form early habits of oral hygiene. Take them at three, or soon thereafter, to the dentist. Give your

dentist opportunity to do all within the power of modern science to help the child enjoy the advantages of oral health. First teeth require attention to protect the permanent teeth. Keep your dentist on guard over your child's future. Your dentist is trained for this important work. You will do him and the youngster a favor if you start the habit of regular dental examination early. Young children learn easily to use

a gargle, or mouthwash. Set a good example for them; they are enthusiastic mimics.

And grown-ups, too, must remember that oral health is closely related to body health. See your dentist regularly. Toothbrush, and mouthwash, every day—of course—but just as important for young and for old is to "Do As Your Dentist Tells You."

LAVORIS CHEMICAL COMPANY
Minneapolis, Minn. · Toronto, Ont.

This page is a part of the Lavoris Reciprocation Program tendered the American Dentist in recognition of more than 25 years' acceptance and good will

*Children like the pleasant taste of Lavoris solution. Teach them early the habit of a mouthwash at every brushing. Lavoris is safe and refreshing.*

*Refuse imitations—ask for Lavoris by name. Large and small bottles at drug counters everywhere.*

*Figure 7.3* Three Years Old, so to the Dentist We Will Go!'
Source: Retro AdArchives/Alamy Stock Photo.

reference 4) also uses the term 'delinquent' to describe those who deviate from prescribed treatment plans. The advertisement features an illustration of a dentist, sat in a darkened room adjacent to the surgery (we see the chair, empty, situated behind the dentist) looking through a collection of patient record cards.

The implication is that he knows each one and recognises those who has been absent from his care for too long. The only source of light in this scene is the lamp on the dentist's desk, the suggestion to the reader is that this is a scene set at night, which implies that this is a professional who cares so much, they are kept up at night worrying about those who have not attended. The dentist is large in the frame of this advertisement, the only other advertisement where the dentist appears as large is the first in the series titled 'DO AS YOUR DENTIST TELLS YOU' (Figure 7.1.; Table 7.1., advert reference 1). The size of the figure within the frame is important in relation to the sense of intimacy that this creates. Here, the reader is encouraged to relate to the dentist, to sympathise with him and see him as being invested in the care of his patients. This is reinforced by the words of the text which suggest that he feels 'pity' for those who do not come, thus drawing on the emotions of the reader. The text also reinforces his professional superiority: 'Do not expect your dentist to implore you to accept his services. Go to him voluntarily'. The text also describes how the professionalisation of dentists prevents the dentist from advertising or so-liciting for the public to take up services: 'The very same code that protects you from dental quackery restrains the reputable and ethical dentist from soliciting your appearance or return'.

### The Dentist as military man

The dentist's virtue, character and social status are reinforced by the series through military symbolism. The advertisement titled 'Your dentist rates a sa-lute, too' (Table 7.1., advert reference 7) features two officers from the US military stood at attention. The advertisement highlights that dentists in the military receive high rank and status and are 'respected and obeyed' and builds on the call for obedience and respect of other advertisements in the campaign by suggesting that civilian patients should accord their dentist the same respect they might give to a military officer (Sweet, in this volume, also demonstrates how military dress and status imbue powerful influence in Chapter 5). Its social semiotics support the fact that this is the primary mode of action of this ad-vertisement. The two depicted dentists do not wear white coats in this re-presentation, but military uniform. The only suggestion that these characters are dentists is the inclusion of the insignia of the US Dental and Navy Corps, respectively, beside each figure from that service. Whilst these men represent dentists, they primarily represent commissioned officers. Many of the readers of the advertisement will have likely seen military service, either directly or through the participation of loved ones, thus, the advertisement has a particular emotional appeal to the reader. It implores the reader to be 'a good soldier', as well as using rhetoric chosen to inspire civil and military duty: 'Volunteer your co-operation in keeping your mouth in good condition of repair' and 'Give him opportunity to lead you to oral health. For you, no less than the soldier or sailor, need regular dental service to keep you present for duty – active, comfortable and efficient'. The text also presents the dentist as having 'enlisted' in a profession and undergone 'long and arduous training' which further encourages the parallel between the vocational nature of both dentistry and a military career.

### Excluding the charlatan

The one advertisement that does not fit with the other depictions of dentists is titled 'Don't Expect Your Dentist to Perform Miracles' (Table 7.1., advert reference 6). Its illustration focuses upon the historic dental practitioner, performing alongside minstrels and operating on stage, portraying him to be a charlatan: 'The itinerant charlatan who dispensed minstrelsy and "painless" malpractice has fled before the law and public opinion. Yet there remains the Quack – the dentist who claims to be able to do what the reputable, ethical dentist will not'. The scene shows the charlatan performing on stage, clutching extraction forceps behind his back. The scene is marked in its difference from the other social environments found in the advertising campaign. The charlatan also does not wear the white clinical garb of the other practitioners portrayed in the series. This noticeable distinction acts to separate this individual and asserts that he does not belong within the dental profession. The patient in the chair being treated is shown screaming in agony. The scene is dark (being set at night) and chaotic; a crowd gathers around the stage, watching the dentist at work, whilst a minstrel wearing 'black-face' make-up performs music. Fire from torches burns behind the stage, adding to the perception of chaos, with the scene appearing almost sinister. In the forefront, a man clutching his face is shown walking from the stage. His position at the front of the scene gives him marked salience and importance. The reader is invited to identify this figure as having just undergone painful and unpleasant treatment at the hands of this dentist. Both this character and the unfortunate individual undergoing care wear drab and shabby clothing, suggesting a lower social status compared to the patient presented as wearing a suit and smart clothing in the advertisement 'Suggestion for A New Year's Resolution' (Table 7.1., advert reference 8). The implication is that this is dentistry for the poor and the vulnerable, the opposite of the intended target readership of this advertising campaign. Despite this charlatan dentist being the focus of the advertisement visually, the written text focuses upon the contemporary dentist (in 1929) who engages in misleading advertising. The advertisement aims to separate the ethical dentist, whose practice is based on merit, from the dentist who makes exaggerated claims and promises that cannot be delivered. For the reader, the advertisement's message is that these unscrupulous dentists are not part of the dental profession, despite potentially having professional training.

The Lavoris campaign stresses the selfless nature of the professional dentist as being the reason for the public to submit to professional discipline and justifies the establishment of a professional monopoly. The inclusion of the example of the 'quack' dentist in the advertisement 'Don't Expect Your Dentist to Perform Miracles' (Table 7.1., advert reference 6) suggests that the dental profession of this era in America was still struggling to assert a professional identity, with the need to differentiate the role of the professional dentist from that of the un-trained charlatan who mixed dental treatment with circus tricks. The adver-tisement embodies the rhetoric of historic figure, Pierre Fauchard. As an eighteenth-century Parisian dentist, Fauchard separated himself from the gau-diness, showmanship and inflated claims of many tooth-drawers of the time, by being one of the first to align the practice of dentistry with the medical pro-fession. Part of Fauchard's success in his endeavour of legitimising dental practice is due to his recognition of the increasing desire of the Parisian public to improve their dental appearance, rather than just have teeth 'pulled' (Jones, 2014). A contemporary dentist to the period of this campaign who was often accused of being a charlatan was Dr Edgar Parker, better known as 'Painless Parker' who operated the 'Parker Dental Circus'. Despite having received a formal dental education, Parker was a showman:

> The first 'patient' extraction was usually a sham in that the patient was a member of the Parker troupe, a tooth was palmed, and the extraction was 'performed' and announced with the tooth held high in the forceps, with the patient testifying there was no pain at all … and the crowd cheered (Behrents, 2015, p. 522)

Parker's activities continued well into the 1930s. The profession's unease with Painless Parker and his ilk of dentist can be summarised well by Parker's own words: 'I like being a dentist and a salesman at the same time' (Garant, 2013, p. 403). The question of whether these two identities can harmoniously exist still perplexes the profession into the twenty-first century (Holden, 2018; Holden, Lee and Thomson, 2020).

## Conclusion

The collection of advertisements under study in this chapter was published at a time when the dental profession, both in the United States and other countries, was seeking to gain professional legitimacy through building associations with the interwar authority of science and medicine. It is of note that while the advertisements reference the dentists to be a 'staunch ally of science and medicine', there is little within the advertisements to suggest that science is the underlying base of dentistry. Rather, the focus of the multimodal texts is the expression of a strong professional identity and notion of appropriate conduct in relation to practice as a dentist. Through analysis of the advertisements, it is clear to see importance being placed upon issues such as how dentists should and should not advertise or solicit business, the notion of professional duty and service and a commitment to professionally sanctioned modes of practice. Whilst some of these principles remain valued today, many do not; for example, advertising in dentistry in the United States is now largely de-regulated (Jerrold and Karkhanehchi, 2000). The profession's position towards advertising has much in common with the status quo before the establishment of organised dentistry and monopolisation (Holden et al., 2021). The dental profession, along with other health professional groups, have been forced to accept that society desires a more equal relationship with those that provide them with care. Despite this, the health professions still enjoy professional respect, trust and prestige.

This case study portrays dentists in United States at a key point in the development of dentistry as a legitimate health profession, a point where the professional status of dentistry existed in a fragile state. Within the advertisements, alongside the commitment shown by the profession to public service and duty, is a palpable anxiety for the profession to compete against the less scrupulous elements of dental practice: advertising and commercialised practice. Contemporary narratives in private dental practice demonstrate similar concerns of how ethical practitioners might compete against dentists who value commercial profits over patient interests and care (Holden, Lee and Thomson, 2020).

This series of advertisements portrays the dental profession as being bound to an obligation to promote good oral health and serve the public and being proud of this commitment. Contemporary members of the dental profession may also reflect upon the concept of fragile professionalism, whereby the monopoly of professionalised practice is inhibited by an uncertainty within society as to whether this is needed and warranted. Dentists in the twenty-first century may perceive a similar need to differentiate their services from non-dental professionals seeking to provide services that were once firmly within the purview of regulated dentists, such as orthodontics using aligners and teeth whitening (see Lala in this volume for cosmetic dentistry). The rise of modern non-professional providers of dentistry, aided by technology, may elicit similar demonstrations and announcements of professional status and legitimacy to those seen within this analysis. Maintaining an overt commitment to the profession's obligations to society is still as essential and relevant as it was during professional consolidation in the interwar period.

## Note

1 This quotation is taken from the advert in Figure 7.1.

## References

American Board of Internal Medicine., (2002) 'Medical professionalism in the new millennium: a physician charter', *Annals of Internal Medicine*, 136(3), pp. 243–246.

Anderson, N. A. (2003) *Discursive analytical strategies: understanding Foucault, Koselleck, Laclau, Luhmann*. Bristol: Policy Press.

Behrents, R. G. (2015) 'Dr Edgar R. R. Parker: his time and now', *American Journal of Orthodontics and Dentofacial Orthopedics*, 148(4), pp. 521–524.

Carstairs, C. (2015) Debating water fluoridation before Dr. Strangelove, *American Journal of Public Health*, 105(8), 1559–1569.

Cohn, J. (1989) *Creating America: George Horace Lorimer and the 'Saturday Evening Post'*. Pittsburgh: University of Pittsburgh Press.

Dussault, G. and Sheiham, A. (1982) 'Medical theories and professional development: the theory of focal sepsis and dentistry in early twentieth century Britain', *Social Science and Medicine*, 16(15), pp. 1405–1412.

Fisher, C. (1924) 'Fourth annual meeting of the Southwestern Society of Orthodontists', *International Journal of Orthodontia, Oral Surgery and Radiography*, 10(2), pp. 120–126.

Garant, P. R. (2013) *The long climb: from Barber-surgeons to doctors of dental surgery*. Hanover Park, IL: Quintessence Publishing.

Gibson, B. J. and Exley, C. (2013) 'The mouth and society', *Social Science and Dentistry*, 2(2), pp. 50–57.

Grumsen, S. (2009) 'The era of whiter teeth: advertising in American dentistry 1910-1950', *Journal of the History of Dentistry*, 57(2), pp. 75–84.

Grumsen, S. S. (2012) 'Zeal of acceptance: balancing image and business in early twentieth-century American dentistry', *Medicine Studies*, 3, pp. 197–214.

Halliday, M. A. K. (1978) *Language as a social semiotic*. London: Edward Arnold.

Holden, A. C. L. (2018) 'Consumer-driven and commercialised practice in dentistry: an ethical and professional problem?', *Journal of Medicine, Healthcare and Philosophy*, 21(4), pp. 583–589.

Holden, A. C. L., Lee, A. and Thomson, W. M. (2020) [Forthcoming] 'Dentists' perspectives on commercial practices in private dentistry', *JDR Clinical & Translational Research* [online]. [Viewed 15 September 2021]. Available from: 10.1177/2380084420 0975700

Holden, A. C. L., Nanayakkara, S., Skinner, J. Spallek, H. and Sohn, W. (2021) 'What do Australian health consumers believe about commercial advertisements and testimonials? a survey on health service advertising', *BMC Public Health* [online], 21, pp. 74. [Viewed 15 September 2021]. Available from: 10.1186/s12889-020-10078-9

Horton, S. and Barker, J. C. (2010) 'Stigmatized biologies: examining the cumulative effects of oral health disparities for Mexican American farmworker children', *Medical Anthropology Quarterly*, 24(2), pp. 199–219.

Hujoel, P. P. (2019) 'Historical perspectives on advertising and the meme that personal oral hygiene prevents dental caries', *Gerodontology*, 36, pp. 36–44.

Jerrold, L. and Karkhanehchi, H. (2000) 'Advertising, commercialism, and professionalism: a history of the ethics of advertising in dentistry', *The Journal of the American College of Dentists*, 67(4), pp. 39–44.

Jewitt, C. and Oyama, R. (2001) 'Visual meaning: a social semiotic approach',in: van Leeuwen, T. and Jewitt, C. (eds.) *The handbook of visual analysis*. London: Sage, pp. 183–204.

Jones, C. (2014) *The smile revolution*. Oxford: Oxford University Press.

Kress, G. and van Leeuwen, T. (2001) *Multimodal discourse: the modes and media of contemporary communication*. London: Bloomsbury Academic.

Kress, G. and van Leeuwen, T. (2006) *Reading images: the grammar of visual design*. 2nd ed. London: Routledge.

Miskell, P. (2004) 'Cavity protection or cosmetic perfection? Innovation and marketing of toothpaste brands in the United States and Western Europe, 1955–1985', *Business History Review*, 78(1), pp. 29–60.

Nead, L. (1988) *Myths of sexuality: representations of women in Victorian Britain*. Oxford: Blackwell.

Nettleton, S. (1994) 'Inventing mouths: disciplinary power and dentistry', in: Jones, C., and Porter, R. (eds.) *Reassessing oucault: power, medicine and the body*. London; New York: Routledge, pp. 73–90.

Noyes, E. (1915) *Ethics and jurisprudence for dentists*. Chicago: Tucker-Kenworthy.

Nye, R. A. (1997) 'Medicine and science as masculine 'fields of honor', *Osiris*, 12, pp. 100–120.

U.S. Department of Commerce, Bureau of Economic Analysis. (1989) *State personal income: 1929–87: estimates and a statement of sources and methods*. Washington DC: U.S. Department of Commerce, Bureau of Economic Analysis.

Weinfeld, W. (1950) 'Income of dentists, 1929–1948', in: Sawyer, C. and Meehan, M. J. (eds.) *Survey of current business*. Washington DC: U.S. Department of Commerce, Bureau of Economic Analysis, pp. 8–16.

# 8 Science, beauty and health: the explosion of toothpaste and toothbrush advertising in interwar America

*Catherine Carstairs*

## Introduction

In the interwar years, Americans learned about how to care for their mouths and teeth in school, from their dentists, and perhaps most importantly, from advertisers of oral hygiene products. During these years, a thriving market for toothpastes and toothbrushes developed, part of the mass marketing of consumer care products such as soap that developed at the turn of the century. This chapter will undertake a content analysis of toothpaste and toothbrush advertisements in the *Ladies Home Journal* and *Good Housekeeping*. With prices generally ranging from 25 cents to a few dollars, toothpaste and toothbrushes were inexpensive items that a large section of the population could afford to buy. Like the soap advertisements that exploded in the early years of the twentieth century, toothpaste advertisements promised beauty, romance and success. These advertisements also stressed the marvels of science. As Roland Marchand (1986) described in *Advertising the American Dream*, advertisers were 'Apostles of Modernity' who instructed people how to live and how to consume in a modern world. Toothpaste advertising created new expectations for what the teeth should look like (straight, white and 'glistening'); they told people (especially women) how often to smile and what their breath should smell like. While dentists emphasized that toothbrushing would help keep the mouth clean and prevent decay, there was no evidence that toothpaste had any health benefits in the years before fluoridated toothpaste and dentists were sceptical of the value of toothpaste advertising. Even so, toothpastes were much more heavily advertised than toothbrushes. This chapter will briefly explore how toothpaste and toothbrush advertisements drew on the dental science of the day. Advertisements stressed the importance of hygiene to twentieth-century life and suggested how the problems of modernity could be solved through science and consumption. It will also address how dentists responded to these advertisements and question if these advertisements had an impact on the practice of toothbrushing.

There is a small literature on the history of toothpaste advertising. Danish historian Stine Grumsen examined how dentists appeared in American advertisements for toothpastes and toothbrushes, using the on-line database available

DOI: 10.4324/9781003047674-10

through the John W. Hartman Centre at Duke University. She argues that advertisements played an important role in creating a new culture of oral hygiene in the United States. Yet, because the Hartman Centre only draws on the records of a few advertising firms, her analysis focuses on S.S. White Toothpaste, Sanitol, Dr. West's and Pepsodent, thereby missing some of the most important players in the field (Grumsen, 2009, pp 75–84). Segrave (2010), the author of more than forty books on topics ranging from policewomen to tipping, wrote *America Brushes Up: The Use and Marketing of Toothpaste and Toothpaste in the Twentieth Century*, using the contemporary periodical literature. *America Brushes Up* is a useful romp through the history of oral hygiene, although Segrave tends to treat her sources rather uncritically. Business historian Peter Miskell (2004) has written a superb article on toothpaste advertising, although he focuses on a later time period when therapeutic toothpastes, including fluoridated toothpastes, transformed the market. In Chapter 7 of this volume, Alex C. L. Holden examines Lavoris mouthwash advertising in the *Saturday Evening Post*, demonstrating dentists' commitment to being represented as being in service to the public. In contrast to previous work, this chapter provides a thorough review of the advertisements that appeared in two of the leading women's magazines in the United States: *Good Housekeeping* and the *Ladies Home Journal* during the interwar years when many Americans started purchasing toothpaste. It looks more at the popular culture of oral health care than at the history of dentistry, and argues that it was advertising, more than dentists, that made regular toothbrushing part of the practices of hygienic modernity.

## Methodology

Women's magazines were chosen because women made the vast majority of purchasing decisions in the United States at the time, especially for smaller items such as toothpaste (Ewan, 1976, p. 167). *Ladies Home Journal* first appeared in 1883 and became an immediate success. By the turn of the century, it was considered to be the 'monthly bible of the American home' (Wood, 1956, p. 113). In the interwar years, it had the largest circulation of any women's magazine in the United States, just under three million printings per issue (Fox, 1990, p. 28; Hammill, 2020). *Good Housekeeping* was established in 1895. The magazine became particularly well-known for its 'Good Housekeeping Institute' which tested household appliances, cleaning agents and household products and gave the best of these the 'Good Housekeeping Seal of Approval' (Wood, 1956, p. 121). *Good Housekeeping*'s readers were women from small- and mid-sized towns (Chuppa-Cornell, 2005, p. 456). Both of these magazines were rich with advertisements. As advertising historians Stuart Ewen, Marchand and others have shown, advertising exploded in the interwar years (Ewen, 1976, p. 32; Marchand, 1986, p. 6). In the 1910s, toothpaste advertisements were usually small, black and white advertisements. By the 1920s, full-page coloured advertisements were common, especially for the leading brands, and the number of advertisements skyrocketed, demonstrating toothpaste's growing significance in the market.

For both of these magazines, I examined all of the advertisements related to toothpaste and mouth hygiene in four issues per year. For the *Ladies Home Journal*, the most important brands were: Colgate's Ribbon Dental Cream, which advertised in nearly every issue; Ipana, which became a major advertiser in 1925 and usually had an advertisement in every issue thereafter; Pepsodent, which was a heavy advertiser from 1920–1935; Pebeco, which advertised heavily in the late 1920s; and Listerine Toothpaste, which became a major advertiser in the 1930s. Squibb's advertised more irregularly, but its advertisements were usually full-page and in colour, making them quite striking. Dr. Lyon's Tooth Powder was the only other significant player. Toothbrush manufacturers Dr. West's and Pro-phy-lac-tic also made regular appearances. The brands were similar in *Good Housekeeping*: Ipana had advertisements every year after 1920 while Colgate's Ribbon Toothpaste and Pepsodent all advertised regularly, although Pepsodent appeared less frequently in the late 1930s. Squibb's also advertised on occasion. The most frequent toothbrush advertisers were Dr. West's and Pro-phy-lac-tic. Both magazines had occasional advertisements from a range of other products including Kolynos, Calox, Iodent, Forhan's and Arm & Hammer Baking Soda. In short, there was little difference between the two magazines in terms of the products advertised and not surprisingly, the same advertisements appeared in both publications. As a result, I will focus my analysis on Colgate's Ribbon Toothpaste, Ipana, Pebeco, Listerine, Pepsodent and Squibb's. I will also briefly discuss the toothbrush brands: Dr. West's and Pro-phy-lac-tic. Most of these were large advertisements with prominent images as well as considerable text. My analysis takes into account the images used to illustrate the advertisements, as well as the text, using a semiotic approach that examines how the advertisement might have been interpreted or understood in the culture of the day (Barthes, 1972).

## Dental science and 'mouth hygiene'

Like the vitamin advertisements studied by Rima Apple (1988, pp. 65–83), toothpaste advertisements frequently drew on science to support their claims, so it is important to understand the changes that were underway in the field of dentistry at the time. When the so-called father of modern dentistry, Pierre Fauchard, published *Le chirugien dentiste* in 1723, he focused on mechanical reparation. He argued for the importance of mouth cleanliness, but this would remain secondary to the mechanical business of 'fixing teeth' (Ring, 1993, p. 166; Hoffman-Axthelm, 1981, pp. 196–207). From the 1830s onwards, some dentists argued that caries were caused by acids that were the result of the decomposition of foods (Black, 1917, pp. 62-5). Even so, dentistry would remain primarily focused on mechanical repair until 1890 when W. D. Miller, an American dentist inspired by the bacteriologist Robert Koch, published *Micro-Organisms of the Human Mouth*, which argued that tooth decay was a two-part process. In the first stage, acid left by food residues dissolved the tooth enamel. Then, microorganisms were able to attack the inner layers of the tooth. Miller's work helped inspired a 'mouth hygiene' movement that urged people to brush their teeth (Ring, 2002, pp. 34–7). A National Mouth Hygiene Association was founded to do educational work in the early twentieth century, showing films and giving lectures across the country (Jones, 1915, pp. 405–9). This was similar to other hygienic campaigns at the turn of the century in the United States and Europe that encouraged people, especially the poor, to keep their homes and bodies clean to prevent disease (Ward, 2019). Dentists also educated people on the importance of diet to oral health. The work of James Sim Wallace, who emphasized the importance of eating 'detergent foods' that encouraged mastication and avoiding sweets, was particularly influential (Wallace, 1912; Johnson, 1923; Nicholson and Taylor, 2009). Wallace was sceptical about the value of toothbrushing, but most of the leading dental texts believed in the importance of both diet and toothbrushing (Black, 1917; Johnson, 1923).

The campaign for prevention and mouth hygiene was further aided by the theory of focal infection. (Dussalt and Sheiham, 1982, pp. 1405–12; Herschfeld, 1981, pp. 34–5; Kumar, 2017, p. 467; Beeson, 1992, pp. 13–23. See also chapter 6 by Scott in this volume). It had long been claimed that infections in the mouth could lead to illness elsewhere in the body. Hippocrates claimed to cure a case of arthritis through removing a tooth, as did the famed American physician Benjamin Rush (Kumar, 2017, p. 467; Kersley, 1949, p. 151). But the theory was re-invigorated by the British surgeon William Hunter. In 1900, Hunter published an article in the *British Medical Journal* claiming that 'the constant swallowing of pus' was 'a most potent and prevalent cause of gastric trouble'. He claimed that oral sepsis was also a cause of tonsillitis, ulcerative endocarditis, meningitis, osteomyelitis and other conditions. He recommended that all dead teeth be removed, that all tooth plates be vigorously sterilized daily and that dentists refrain from 'conservative dentistry' such as bridges which could not be kept sterile (Hunter, 1900, pp. 215–6). At a lecture at McGill in 1910, subsequently published in *The Lancet*, he asserted that he admired the 'sheer ingenuity and mechanical skill' of the dental surgeon, but that their work created 'ghastly tragedies'. He claimed that the 'worst cases of anaemia, gastritis, colitis … nervous disturbances of all kinds … chronic rheumatic affections' and kidney disease were caused by building 'a veritable mausoleum of gold fillings, crowns and bridges over a mass of sepsis' (Hunter, 1911, pp. 79–86). As the theory of focal infection gained support from physicians, dentists and the public, dentists increasingly focused on the prevention of dental disease through toothbrushing and diet (Black, 1917, p. xvi; Fones, 1921; Hunt, 1911, pp. 7–9).

Miller's theory of cavity formation and the theory of focal infection were promoted by dentists and public health advocates, but they also met a ready audience among the producers of oral hygiene products. As historian Nancy Tomes has detailed in *Gospel of Germs*, germ theory was not just promoted by bacteriologists. The manufacturers of household products such as soap, toilets and vacuum cleaners also embraced germ theory to sell their goods (Tomes, 1998). She argues that germ theory was being sidelined by the 'new public health' by the 1920s, which put more focus on individual health be-haviours, but advertisers of products such as Kleenex, Kotex, paper cups and cellophane only intensified their focus on the sanitary benefits of their pro-ducts in the interwar years. Certainly, this was true in the field of toothpaste and toothbrush advertising, where advertisers took advantage of the theory of focal infection and the still relatively new mouth hygiene movement. As B. J. Gibson and O. V. Boiko have argued elsewhere, health communication is polyphonic, coming from health professionals, family members and in this case, advertisers (2012).

## Advertising toothpaste and toothbrushes: removing the film and preventing pink toothbrush

Each toothpaste and toothbrush had a tag or a slogan that differentiated it. Pepsodent touted that it would 'remove the film' that allowed germs to breed. Pebeco claimed to stimulate the 'mouth glands to protect the teeth'. Colgate's promised that its foam 'penetrates into every tiny crevice' where 'it softens and dislodges the decaying impurities, washing them away in a detergent wave'. Ipana warned about 'pink toothbrush' and promised that its special ingredient Ziratol would heal the gums. Squibb's warned about 'The Danger Line' where the gums met the teeth and where food would linger, ferment and cause decay. Listerine traded on the reputation it already had for antisepsis and emphasised that it was a quality toothpaste at a reasonable price. Dr. West's promoted its 'health curve' that allowed it to reach spots that were hard to get at with other toothbrushes. Pro-phy-lac-tic promised that its large end tuft would allow you to reach 'every tooth'. Many of the advertisements used highly scientific language to describe how their special ingredients or special shape in the case of tooth-brushes would improve the care of the teeth. So, for example, Colgate's pro-mised that it contained no 'harsh grit' or other dangerous substances. It described its 'double action' – 'the fine precipitated chalk loosens deposits upon the teeth. At the same time, the pure vegetable-oil soap washes away the loo-sened particles' (Colgate's, 1921, p. 176). Similarly, Pepsodent claimed that it was 'based on pepsin, the digestant of albumin. The film is albuminous matter. The object of Pepsodent is to dissolve it, then to day by day combat it' (Pepsodent, 1920, p. 107). In *Captains of Consciousness*, Stuart Ewen argues that this 'mystification' was an inherent part of consumer culture in the interwar years, encouraging people to put their faith in corporate solutions (Ewen, 1976, pp. 107–8). But it also spoke to the faith that existed in science and medicine at a time of significant advances in halting infectious diseases (Burnham, 1982, pp. 1474–9). Toothpaste advertisements advised prospective customers to visit their dentist regularly, and several claimed that dentists recommended their brand most frequently (Colgate's, 1921, p. 176).

In the 1920s, toothpaste advertisements often provided detailed instruction on how to brush the teeth and why one should do so. In 1921, an advertisement for Colgate's told prospective buyers: 'For the sake of your health, take care of your teeth'. The advertisement instructed people to brush their teeth twice a day: once in the morning and once at night before going to bed, explaining that the upper teeth should be brushed downwards and the lower teeth upwards (Colgate's, 1921, p. 176). Pro-phy-lac-tic toothbrush ran advertisements with half set of teeth and a toothbrush demonstrating the correct toothbrushing motion (Pro-phy-lac-tic, 1924a, p. 163). Dr. West's admonished people to spend four minutes a day brushing their teeth – two in the morning and two at night (Dr. West's, 1927, p. 143). Colgate's drew on the theory of focal infection to claim that 'bad teeth endanger the health, often being responsible for rheumatism, indigestion, heart troubles, impairment of sight, etc'. They suggested that in addition to brushing that people visit their dentist twice a year. A 1925 Colgate's advertisement (Figure 8.1) went even further – beside the photo of a beautiful young woman in the bathroom admiring herself in the mirror, there was an insert of a young woman in bed, a doctor taking her pulse. It pronounced: 'Bad Teeth May Lead to Years of Agony: Tooth Decay Can Cause Diseases Which Result in Complete Breakdown of Health'. In the text, Colgate's claimed that 'scientific research traces rheumatism, heart disease, kidney trouble, even insanity and death, to bad teeth' (Colgate's, 1925, p. 48). Pepsodent explained that 'germs by the millions' bred in the film that Pepsodent promised to remove 'and they, with tartar, are the chief cause of pyorrhea and most gum disorders' (Pepsodent, 1927, 112).

While many toothpaste advertisements stressed the health benefits of brushing the teeth, the beauty benefits were perhaps even greater. This was a period of increased attention to beauty and cosmetics. As Kathy Peiss (1998, p. 97) has shown, the number of perfume and cosmetic manufacturers nearly doubled in the United States from 1909–1929 and the factory value of their products increased by ten. Many advertisements for Pepsodent and Colgate's featured young white women looking in the mirror. In *Captains of Consciousness*, Ewen (1976, p. 177) argues that this was a common trope in advertising in the era – as he put it 'women were reminded that it was their appearance more than their organizational capacities which ensure fidelity in particular and home security in general'. Marchand (1986, p. 149) argues that photographs only began to dominate over drawings in magazine advertisements in the late 1920s, but photography was common in toothpaste advertisements earlier than this, showing the importance of demonstrating what the toothpaste could accomplish in terms of improving a woman's looks. In the late 1920s and early 1930s, Colgate's (1930, p. 85) ran advertisements featuring a series of close-up photographs of a woman's mouth, showing how closely women should be inspecting their mouths and teeth.

Toothpaste advertisements regularly reminded women that love could be gained or lost through their choice of toothpaste. One Pepsodent advertisement featured a seated young woman looking in the mirror, with her beau admiringly looking at her (Pepsodent, 1921, p. 67). Another featured a young woman in a ball dress, presumably waiting for a suitor to ask her dance – the advertisement headlined 'a delightful test' referencing the ten-day trial tube on offer but possibly also suggesting

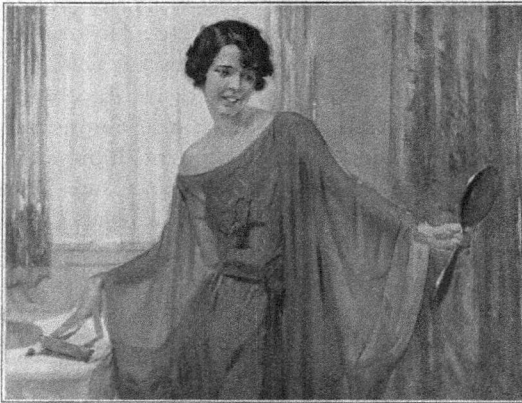
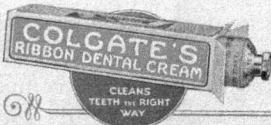
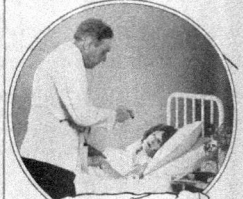
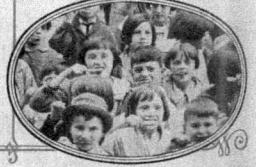

*Figure 8.1* Colgate advertisement.

Source: Ladies Home Journal, August 1925, p. 48.

that the real test was whether or not she would be asked to dance (Pepsodent, 1922, p. 47). Similarly, Pebeco advertisements usually featured white couples: sometimes at the swimming pool, sometimes at the opera, sometimes enjoying nature, always with broad smiles and straight teeth (Pebco, LEHN & FINK, Inc, 1924, p. 94; Pebco, LEHN & FINK, Inc, 1925a, p. 79; Pebco, LEHN & FINK 1925b, p. 201). The idea that norms around teeth and smiling were changing (and why it was important to keep up) was a frequent feature in Pepsodent advertisements. One asked: 'Why Women Smile As they never did before: Teeth are prettier today – Millions combat film' (Pepsodent, 1924, p. 131). Similarly, Dr Lyon's claimed that it was the 'dentifrice that made fine teeth fashionable' (Dr. Lyon's, 1921, p. 104). It is important to note that this message was always directed towards a white audience. While these magazines were read by a broad array of Americans, they usually portrayed a fairly bourgeois existence, one that would have been out-of-reach for many consumers. Typical for advertising in the period, no African-Americans or Asians appeared in any toothpaste or toothbrush advertising in these two magazines (Chambers, 2008).

## The parables of toothpaste advertising

In *Advertising the American Dream*, Marchand argues that certain parables were repeated regularly in advertising in the interwar years. These were: the parable of the first impression, the parable of the democracy of goods, the parable of civilization redeemed and the parable of the captivated child. Surprisingly, the last of these appeared infrequently in toothbrush and toothpaste advertising, although advertisements did occasionally suggest that children liked the taste of a particular toothpaste (Listerine, 1934, p. 97), but the others were ubiquitous. The parable of the first impression was the idea that young people would miss out on love or employment through failing to make a good first impression. Listerine antiseptic which had invented the ailment of halitosis had long been a leader in so-called shame advertisements. They featured attractive girls who could not figure out why their boyfriends had left them for another, or why they could not get a date, until a kindly friend suggested that that they had halitosis. Listerine quickly solved the problem and weddings ensued (Marchand, 1986, p. 218–20). Not surprisingly, the firm adopted this marketing for their toothpaste as well. One Listerine advertisement heralded: 'Many a first impression has been ruined by some seemingly little thing'. It warned that people 'quite unconsciously' look at people's teeth when they are talking. If they are 'unclean' or 'improperly kept', the 'fastidious' person will automatically keep their distance (Listerine, 1924, p. 162). In the late 1930s, Colgate (the brand dropped the apostrophe in the mid-30s) began using cartoon advertisements, a trend that was then sweeping the advertising world. In one, Janey's father catches her writing a letter to 'Lonely Hearts'. He exclaimed that the town was full of nice young people – there was no need for her to be lonely. She retorted that she just wasn't able to keep friends. He suggested that perhaps it was her breath. Her dentist recommended Colgate and soon the phone was ringing off the hook (Colgate, 1938, p. 41). In the late 1930s, Ipana ran a series of advertisements featuring beautiful young women with their mouths firmly closed. The headlines screamed that the young women were 'a perfect partner', 'a beau-catching beauty' and 'So young – so Lovely' until they smiled (Ipana, 1938, p. 1; Ipana, 1939a, p. 1; Ipana 1939b, p. 1). In the 1930s, it was not just romance that could be lost, it was jobs as well. One Colgate advertisement featured a secretary who had been laid off because of her bad breath while a Listerine advertisement suggested that 'career girls could overcome the greatest handicap to success' by improving their breath (Colgate, 1937, p. 54; Listerine, 1937, p. 7).

The parable of civilization redeemed was the dominant motif in Ipana advertisements. This parable suggested that fast modern life had dangers, but that these could be overcome by the use of the advertised product. Ipana advertisements featured wealthy Americans, often in the process of dining on the rich foods that Ipana claimed could cause the dreaded 'pink toothbrush'. One 1925 advertisement featured two women and on man sitting around a dining room table, a maid in the background. There were fresh flowers and candles – the man was wearing a suit and the women were wearing sheer fashions with bobbed hair. The advertisement promised that you could 'Ward off "pink toothbrush" with Ipana'. It warned that the 'soft foods' deprived the gums of the stimulation they needed. An insert included quotations from 'professional papers' emphasizing the dangers of eating soft foods and failing to exercise the jaws (Ipana, 1925, p. 246). A similar advertisement from 1927 warned that 'to change the culinary habits of our households is a task too radical to attempt. Servants would leave. Guests might not enjoy it' (Ipana, 1927, p. 266). In the mid-1930s, Ipana began running an innovative campaign, prominently featured on the inside cover of *Good Housekeeping* (Figure 8.2). It featured young attractive women chomping on huge pieces of food: a T-bone, a head of celery and a drumstick. '"BARB-AROUS!" *Says* Good Housekeeping Beauty Editor "INTELLIGENT" *Says* your own dentist'. The advertisement warned that eating like this could be 'social suicide' even if it exercised the gums in the way that dentists thought was necessary. Instead, it suggested, try Ipana (Ipana, 1935, p. 1; Ipana, 1936a, p. 1; Ipana, 1936b, p. 1). Similarly, Pro-phy-lac-tic ran advertisements featuring a pre-historical man who had never had a toothache and Dr. West's claimed that in the time of the Sphinx, toothaches were rare (Pro-phy-lac-tic, 1924b, p. 92; Dr. West's, 1924, p. 63). Modern times, by contrast, required the regular use of the toothbrush.

The parable of the democracy of goods was also used by toothpaste and toothbrush manufacturers. This was the idea that everyone could enjoy the same pleasures or conveniences as the rich. Ipana's luxurious surroundings suggested that it was a toothpaste for the wealthy, but like other toothpastes, it offered a free trial tube to anyone who requested it. In the early 1930s, Ipana ran an advertisement with a young woman on a horse and a young man driving a truck – despite their class differences, they both used Ipana to avoid pink toothbrush (Ipana, 1933a, p. 1). In the early 1930s, Listerine insisted that the elite used Listerine toothpaste because they knew that it was a quality toothpaste even though it was cheap compared to other toothpastes. One such

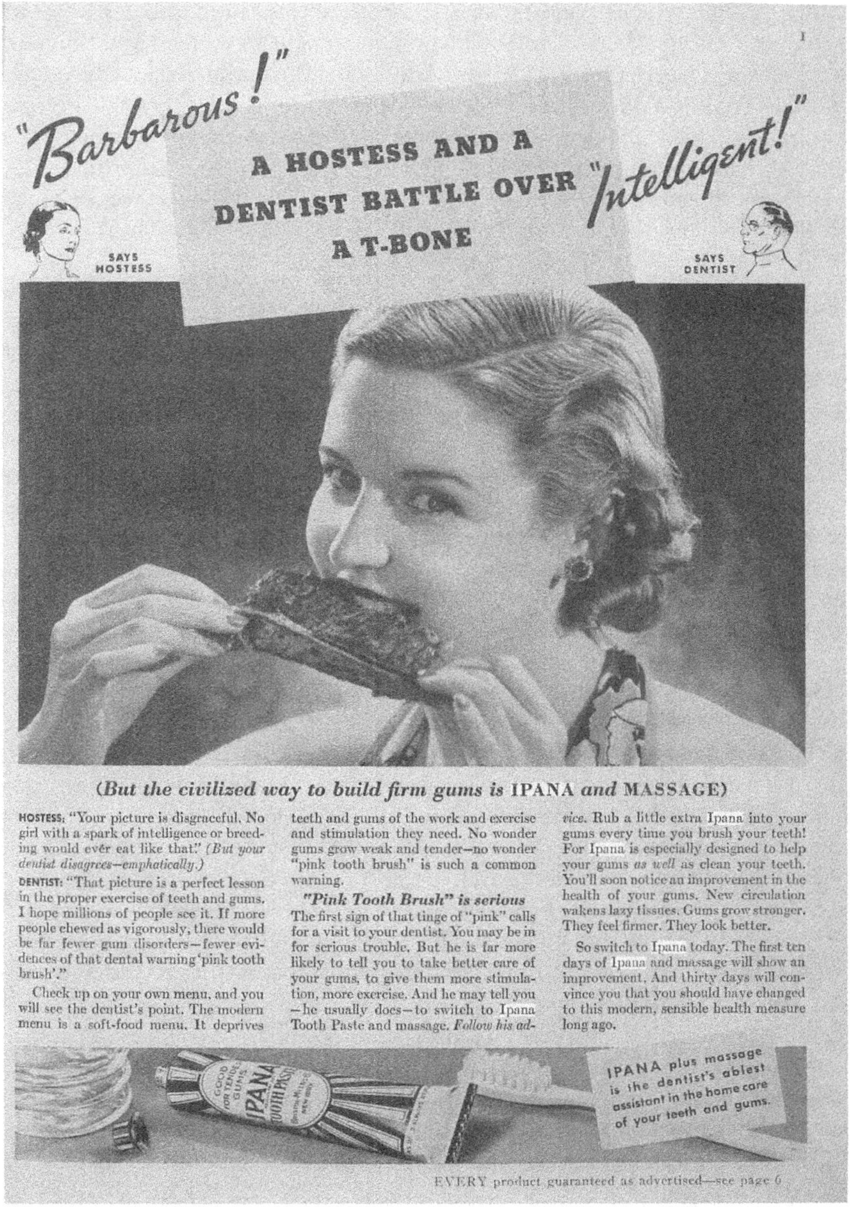




*Figure* 8.2 Ipana advertisement.

advertisement featured people out on a yacht and the claim 'Odd that Listerine toothpaste seems most popular with those who least need the $3 it saves' (Listerine, 1933, p. 43). Indeed, saving money become an increasingly common theme during the Depression. In the late 1920s, Listerine began advertising what you could do with all of the money that you saved by buying Listerine toothpaste – they included having a facial, buying dainty handkerchiefs and starting a bank account for your child (Listerine, 1928, p. 142; Listerine, 1929, p. 103). By the early 1930s, these became more practical – 30 loaves of bread and new bath towels (Listerine, 1931, p. 107; Listerine, 1930, p. 125).

## Dentists and toothpaste advertising

While these toothpaste advertisements encouraged the daily practice of toothbrushing, they appalled dentists, who were concerned about their in-accuracies. Before the introduction of fluoridated toothpastes, there was no evidence that any brand of toothpaste had any beneficial effect other than freshening the breath, and perhaps encouraging the act of tooth brushing. The advantages of toothbrushing entirely lay with the act of brushing. In 1929, the American Dental Association formed the Council on Dental Therapeutics to research the claims of commercial dental products, which many dentists felt were false and misleading. To gain acceptance as a 'dental remedy', manu-facturers needed to provide a full list of the ingredients and needed to truthfully advertise their products (Palmer, 1935, pp. 245–51).

The opposition to false toothpaste advertising was part of a larger consumer movement. A series of books in the late 1920s and 1930s, including *100,000,000 Guinea Pigs, Your Money's Worth* and *Eat, Drink and Be Merry*, ignited a much broader consumer movement that argued that ignorant con-sumers needed to be protected from unscrupulous manufacturers and adver-tisers (Glickman, 2009, pp. 194–5). *100,000,000 Guinea Pigs*, the best-selling book of the decade, included an entire section on toothpastes, excoriating Pebeco because its principal ingredient was poisonous, Pepsodent because it contained an abrasive that could damage tooth enamel and Kolynos because it contained too much soap. It declared that 'probably no other commodity has been responsible for so much downright and expensive lying by the re-spectable advertising agencies' (Kallet and Schlink, 1933, p. 62). *Your Money's Worth* lambasted tooth brush advertising as well, saying that no toothbrush could be made to conform itself to the dental arch; that most tooth brushes in the market were too large and that bristles tended to buckle and did not penetrate between the teeth (Chase and Schlink, 1936, 20). In 1935, dentist Bissell Palmer, who had played an important role in the creation of the ADA's Council on Dental Therapeutics, published *Paying Through the Teeth*, a scathing account of the claims of toothpaste manufacturers. He worried that toothpastes that promised that they could cure 'pink toothbrush' or clean between the crevices of the teeth misled consumers into believing that they could care for their teeth properly without going to the dentist.

Even so, the vast majority of consumers likely knew little about the false claims of toothpaste manufacturers and began purchasing toothpaste (and toothbrushes) in the hopes of attaining a brighter smile.

## Advertising and the rise of toothbrushing

It is impossible to know whether the ubiquitous advertising for toothpastes and toothbrushes in the interwar years increased the practice of tooth-brushing, but some evidence suggests that toothbrushing was becoming a daily habit for more and more Americans. In 1935, the managing editor for the advertising periodical *Printer's Ink* claimed: 'Colgate and Pro-phy-lac-tic performed a tremendous health service to the country by their teaching of oral hygiene … these advertisers taught the public not only to keep its teeth clean but also to visit the dentist with reasonable frequency' (Larrabee, 1935, p. 68). *Printer's Ink* was hardly an unbiased source – advertisers wanted to believe that they were contributing to the common good, but dentist C. J. Hollister, writing for the *Journal of the American Dental Association*, agreed that Americans were becoming more 'tooth-conscious', a result of 'commercial advertising' (Hollister, 1930, p. 742). At the beginning of the time period examined here, dentist Sidney Rauh estimated, based on toothbrush sales, that less than 20 per cent of Americans even owned a toothbrush (Rauh, 1926, p. 1439). By the late 1930s, the vice-president and general manager of Pepsodent claimed that the market for toothpaste had stabilized 'some years ago'. It was impossible to get Americans to buy more toothpaste – the only option was to get them to switch brands (Luckman, 1939, p. 16). A 'cupboard inventory' of thousands of homes in the United States in 1938 found that 65 per cent had toothpaste (Miskell, 2004, p. 39). A few years later, *Time* confidently proclaimed 'all good Americans brush their teeth' (*Time* 1945). During the interwar years, it seems, many Americans, especially those in the middle and upper classes, became convinced that daily toothbrushing was necessary to achieve beauty, health and success in a modern society.

Ironically, as Americans adopted the toothbrushing habit, some dentists began to question it. As previously mentioned, they were irritated by what they regarded as the false claims of toothpaste advertising. But they were also influenced by new scientific developments. Dentists had always believed that diet was important in preventing tooth decay, but the interwar developments in nutrition intensified the focus on diet. The work of May Mellanby on Vitamin D was particularly influential (Mellanby and Pattison, 1928, pp. 1079–82; Mellanby, 1928). Some dentists, such as Weston Price, who was then doing research on diets and dentition around the world, began to question the value of tooth brushing altogether (Campbell, 1936, pp. 105–10). Russell Bunting, a prominent dental researcher at the University of Michigan, argued that refined sugars were the most important factor in tooth decay and that mouth cleanliness 'except when carried to an extreme and impractical degree' did not provide 'much protection' (Bunting, 1933, p. 29; Bunting, 1962, p. 29). William Brady, a physician who wrote a syndicated column on nutrition that was reprinted in many American newspapers, was one of the toothbrushing doubters. Although very few dentists questioned the merits of toothbrushing, they started to acknowledge that 'a surgically clean tooth is an impossibility in the normal mouth' (Davis, 1949, p. 16). While public health dentists never rescinded their advice to brush their teeth, they acknowledged that the problem of tooth decay was more complicated than 'mouth hygiene'. The search for new solutions would bring them to fluoride and usher in a whole new era of toothpastes.

## Acknowledgements

Thanks to Trina Gale for her excellent research assistance. Thank you to the Social Science and Humanities Research Council of Canada and to AMS Healthcare for funding this research. Thank you to McGill-Queen's University Press for allowing me to republish a few sections of my book *The Smile Gap: a History of Oral Health and Social Inequality* (2022).

## References

Anon (1962) 'Russell Bunting', *New York Times*, 23 November. pp. 29.

Anon (1945) 'So you brush your teeth', *Time Magazine* [online], 45(4). [Viewed 15 September 2021]. Available from: http://content.time.com/time/subscriber/article/0,33009,791929,00.html

Apple, R. (1988) 'They need it now': science, advertising and vitamins, 1925–1940, *Journal of Popular Culture* [online], 22(3), pp. 65–83. [Viewed 15 September 2021]. Available from: doi: 10.1111/j.0022-3840.1988.2203_65.x

Beeson, P. (1992) 'Fashions in pathogenetic concepts during the present century: autointoxication, focal infection, psychosomatic disease and autoimmunity', *Perspectives in Biology and Medicine* [online], 36(1), 13–23. [Viewed 15 September 2021]. Available from: doi: 10.1353/pbm.1993.0014

Barthes, R. (1972) *Mythologies*. Trans Annette Lavers New York: Hill and Wang.

Black, G. V. (1917) *A work on operative dentistry*. 3rd edn. Chicago: Medico-dental Publishing Company.

Burnham, J. (1982) 'American medicine's golden age: what happened to it', *Science* [online], 215(4539), pp. 1474–1479. [Viewed 15 September 2021]. Available from: doi: 10.1126/science.7038876

Bunting, R. W. (1962) 'Recent developments in the study of dental caries', *Science* [online], 78(2028), pp. 419–424. [Viewed 15 September 2021]. Available from: doi: 10.1126/science.78.2028.419

Chambers, J. (2008) *Madison avenue and the colour line*. Philadelphia: University of Pennsylvania Press.

Campbell, J. M. (1936) 'Is the 'local theory' impermeable', *Journal of the Canadian Dental Association*, 2(3), pp. 105–110.

Chase, S. and Schlink, F. J. (1936) *Your money's worth*. New York: Macmillan.

Chuppa-Cornell, K. (2005) 'Filling a vacuum: women's health information in *Good Housekeeping's* articles and advertisements, 1920–1965', *Historian*, 67(3), pp. 454.

Colgate's (1921) 'For the sake of your health', *Ladies Home Journal*, 38(10), pp. 176.

Colgate's (1925) 'For the sake of beauty and health', *Ladies Home Journal*, 42(2), pp. 248.

Colgate's (1930) 'You need this penetrating dentifrice', *Ladies Home Journal*, 47(8), pp. 85.

Colgate (1938) 'Dear lonely hearts', *Ladies Home Journal*, 55(8), pp. 41.

Colgate (1937) 'Stranded until her dentist told her why', *Ladies Home Journal*, 54(10), pp. 54.

Davis, W. A. (1949) 'Dentistry and the public health movement', in: Pelton, W. J. and Wisan, J. M. (eds.) *Dentistry in public health*. Philadelphia: W.B. Saunders Company, pp. 14–23.

Dr. Lyon's (1921) 'You can't be too careful of your teeth', *Ladies Home Journal*, 38(10), pp. 104.

Dr. West's (1924) 'The secret revealed', *Ladies Home Journal*, 41(4), pp. 63.

Dr. West's (1927) 'When BEAUTY depends solely on your SMILE', *Good Housekeeping*, 85(1), pp. 143.

Dussalt, G. and Sheiham, A. (1982) 'Medical theories and professional development', *Social Science Medicine* [online], 16, pp. 1405–1412. [Viewed 15 September 2021]. Available from: doi: 10.1016/0277-9536(82)90135-6

Ewen, S. (1976) *Captains of consciousness: advertising and the social roots of the consumer culture*. 1st edn. New York: McGraw-Hill.

Fones, A. (1921) *Mouth hygiene: a text-book for dental hygienists*. 2nd ed. Pennsylvania: Lea and Febiger.

Fox, B. (1990) 'Selling the mechanized household: 70 years of ads in *Ladies Home Journal*', *Gender and Society*, 4(1), pp. 25–40.

Gibson, B. J. and Boiko, O. V. (2012) 'The experience of health and illness: poly-contextural meaning and accounts of illness', *Social Theory & Health* [online]. pp. 1–32. [Viewed 15 September 2021]. Available from: doi: 10.1057/sth.2011.22

Glickman, L. B. (2009) *Buying power: a history of consumer activism in America*. 1st edn. Chicago: University of Chicago Press.

Grumsen, S. (2009) 'The era of whiter teeth: advertising in American dentistry, 1910–1950', *Journal of the History of Dentistry*, 57(2), pp. 75–84.

Hammill, F. (2020) *Circulating American magazines: visualization tools for U.S. magazine history*. 25 March. [Viewed 15 September 2021]. Available from: https://sites.lib.jmu.edu/circulating/2020/03/25/what-is-a-mass-circulation-magazineby-faye-hammill/

Herschfeld, J. (1981) 'William Hunter and the role of 'oral sepsis' in American dentistry', *Bulletin of the History of Dentistry*, 33(1), pp. 35–45.

Hoffman-Axthelm, W. (1981) *History of dentistry*. 1st edn. Chicago: Quintessence.

Hollister, C. J. (1930) 'Dental health week', *Journal of The American Dental Association*, 17(4), pp. 742–744.

Hunt, G. E. (1911) 'What is the best way?', *Oral Hygiene: A Journal for Dentists*, 1(1), pp. 7–9.

Hunter, W. (1900) 'Oral sepsis as a cause of disease', *British Medical Journal* [online], 2(2056), pp. 215–216. [Viewed 15 September 2021]. Available from: doi: 10.1136/bmj.2.2065.215

Hunter, W. (1911) 'The role of sepsis and antisepsis in medicine', *The Lancet* [online], 177(4559), pp. 79–86. [Viewed 15 September 2021]. Available from: doi: 10.1016/S0140-6736(01)60080-1

Ipana (1925) 'Ward off 'pink toothbrush' with Ipana', *Ladies Home Journal*, 42(4), pp. 246.

Ipana (1927) 'Pink 'tooth brush' is a protest from over-coddled gums', *Ladies Home Journal*, 44(4), pp. 266.

Ipana (1933) 'Neither wealth nor health', *Ladies Home Journal*, 50(4), pp. 1.

Ipana (1933a) 'Pink toothbrush' threatens them both', *Good Housekeeping*, 96(2), pp. 1.

Ipana (1935) 'Savage', *Good Housekeeping*, 100 (5), pp. 1.

Ipana (1935) 'Shocking!' Says editor of Vogue, *Ladies Home Journal*, 52(1), pp. 1.

Ipana (1936a) 'Barbarous!: a hostess and a dentist battle over a T-bone', *Good Housekeeping*, 103(1), pp. 1.

Ipana (1936b) 'Shocking', *Good Housekeeping*, 102(1), pp. 1.

Ipana (1938) 'So young – so lovely', *Ladies Home Journal*, 55(8), pp. 1.

Ipana (1939a) 'Beau catching beauty', *Ladies Home Journal*, 56(8), pp. 1.

Ipana (1939b) 'A perfect partner', *Ladies Home Journal*, 56(10), pp. 1.

Johnson, C. N. (1923) *A textbook of operative dentistry*. 4th ed. Philadelphia: P. Blakiston's Son & Co.

Jones, J. (1915) 'Popular education in mouth hygiene through organized publicity', *American Journal of Public Health* [online], 5(5). pp. 405–409. [Viewed 15 September 2021]. Available from: doi: 10.2105/ajph.5.5.405

Kallet, A. and Schlink, F. J. (1933) *100,000,000 guinea pigs*. 1st edn. New York: Vanguard Press.

Kumar, P. S. (2017) 'From focal sepsis to periodontal medicine: a century of exploring the role of the oral microbiome in systemic disease', *Journal of Physiology* [online], 595(2), pp. 465–476. [Viewed 15 September 2021]. Available from: doi: 10.1113/ JP272427

Kersley S. (1949) 'Dental sepis and chronic rheumatism', *Proceedings of the Royal Society of Medicine*, 42(3), pp. 151–3.

Larrabee C. B. (1935) 'Dentists and advertising', *Printer's Ink*, 172, pp. 68–70.

Listerine (1924) 'Ruined', *Good Housekeeping*, 78(4), pp. 162.

Listerine (1928) 'Have a facial', *Good Housekeeping*, 87(1), pp. 142.

Listerine (1929) 'Tooth paste starts baby's bank account', *Good Housekeeping*, 88(1), pp. 103.

Listerine (1930) 'Teach her the secret of healthy teeth and economy', *Good Housekeeping*, 90(6), pp. 125.

Listerine (1931) 'Millions acclaim quality results of a new thrift dentifrice'. *Good Housekeeping*, 92(1), pp. 107.

Listerine (1933) 'Odd that Listerine tooth paste seems most popular with those who least need the $3 it saves', *Good Housekeeping*, 97(5), pp. 103.

Listerine (1934) 'It tastes swell', *Good Housekeeping*, 98(1), pp. 97.

Listerine (1937) 'How career girls overcome the greatest handicap to success', *Ladies Home Journal*, 54(1), pp. 7.

Luckman, C. (1939) 'Pepsodent's 7 points', *Printer's Ink*, 186, pp. 15–18.

Marchand, R. (1986) *Advertising the American dream: making way for modernity*. 1st edn. Berkeley: University of California Press.

Mellanby, M. and Pattison, C. L. (1928) 'The action of vitamin D in preventing the spread and promoting the arrest of caries in children', *British Medical Journal* [online], 2(3545), pp. 1079–1082. [Viewed 15 September 2021]. Available from: doi: 10.1136/ bmj.2.3545.1079

Mellanby, M. (1928) 'The influence of diet on the structure of teeth', *Physiological Reviews* [online], 8(4), pp. 545–577. [Viewed 15 September 2021]. Available from: doi: 10.1152/physrev.1928.8.4.545

Miskell, P. (2004) 'Cavity protection or cosmetic perfection: innovation and marketing of toothpaste in the United States and Western Europe, 1955-1985', *The Business History Review* [online], 78(1), pp. 28–60. [Viewed 15 September 2021]. Available from: doi: 10.2307/25096828

Nicholson, M. and Taylor, G. S. (2009) 'Scientific knowledge and clinical authority in dentistry: James Sim Wallace and dental caries', *Journal of the Royal College of Physicians of Edinburgh*, 39(1), pp. 64–72.

Palmer, B. (1935) *Paying through the teeth.* 1st edn. Michigan: The Vanguard Press.

Peiss, K. (1998) *Hope in a jar: the making of America's beauty culture*, 1st edn. New York: Metropolitan Books.

Pebco, LEHN & FINK, Inc., (1924) 'The harmful mouth condition you must overcome', *Ladies Home Journal*, 41(10), pp. 94.

Pebco, LEHN & FINK, Inc., (1925a) 'Your white teeth – do you know how to keep them safe', *Ladies Home Journal*, 42(2), pp. 79.

Pebco, LEHN & FINK, Inc., (1925b) 'Teeth stay white and safe', *Ladies Home Journal*, 42(6), pp. 201.

Pepsodent (1920) 'Glistening teeth are Seen everywhere now – this is why', *Ladies Home Journal*, 37(4), pp. 107.

Pepsodent (1921) 'Twice daily: teeth need these five effects', *Ladies Home Journal*, 38(10), pp. 67.

Pepsodent (1922) 'A delightful test', *Ladies Home Journal*, 39(4), pp. 47.

Pepsodent (1924) 'Why women smile', *Good Housekeeping*, 78(4), pp. 131.

Pepsodent (1927) 'Cleanse teeth of dingy film', *Good Housekeeping*, 84(5), pp. 112.

Pro-phy-lac-tic (1924a) 'Fight tartar', *Good Housekeeping*, 78(4), pp. 163.

Pro-phy-lac-tic (1924b) 'A 400,000-year-old head that never had a toothache', *Ladies Home Journal*, 41(1), pp. 92.

Rauh, S. J. (1926) 'The teaching of oral hygiene in schools', *Journal of the American Dental Association*, 13(10), pp. 1439.

Ring, M. E. (1993) *An illustrated history of dentistry.* 1st edn. New York: Abradale Press.

Ring, M. E. (2002) 'W. D. Miller: the pioneer who laid the foundation for modern dental research', *New York State Dental Journal*, 68(2), pp. 35–37.

Segrave, K. (2010) *America brushes up: the use and marketing of toothpaste and toothbrushes in the twentieth century.* 1st edn. Jefferson: McFarlane & Company.

Tomes, N. (1998) *Gospel of germs: men, women, and the microbe in American life.* 1st edn. Cambridge: Harvard University Press.

Wallace, J. S. (1912). The Prevention of Dental Caries. London: Published at the Office of The Dental Record.

Ward, P. (2019) *The clean body: a modern history.* Montreal and Kingston: McGill-Queen's University Press.

Wood, J. (1956) *Magazines in the United States.* New York: The Ronald Press.

# Part III
# The patient's perspective

# 9 Tommy's teeth: trench mouth, dentures and dental health among British army recruits in World War One

*Helen Strong*

During World War One, British army medical officers medically examined and rejected potential army recruits due to their poor oral condition. Yet, many men slipped through the recruitment process with bad teeth. It was not long after their dispatch to war that these otherwise fit young men began to suffer. The existing level of poor oral health of the voluntary recruit was compounded by the appalling conditions in the trenches and the lack of dental hygiene behaviours – this soon led to a dental problem in the field. From August to December 1914, one of the chief causes of military hospital admissions for non-battle casualties was disease of the teeth and gums, which accounted for 2,495 cases, a ratio per 1,000 ration strength of 13.1 of the fighting force (Mitchell and Smith, 1931).

Many of these men were suffering from Vincent's gingivostomatitis, or trench mouth. The symptoms of this disease include severe pain and bleeding of the gingiva caused by excessive pathogenic activity of bacteria normally present in the oral cavity, owing to several predisposing factors including stress, smoking and a poor diet (Chaubal and Bapat, 2017). Trench mouth reached epidemic proportions in combatants during World War One as pathogenic bacteria was easily spread through the unhygienic cooking pots and shared eating utensils used by mobile canteens (Woods, 1926).

Although trench mouth was widespread among soldiers during the war, the historiography on oral disease and dentistry in the military is limited (Grant, 2012; Woods, 1938). Rather than seeing poor oral health of recruits as the result of a complex set of underlying inequalities which gave rise to a chronic dental problem for the army, the current literature on dental matters in military situations draws heavily on the role of the dental profession, particularly during the Boer War (Gelbier, 2005). This is because the history of dentistry has been largely written by, and about, dental professionals.[1] The 'top down' rather than a 'history from below' or 'people's history' approach thus limits historical understanding of the social, political and economic antecedents of oral disease, particularly in relation to the lived experience of the working-class (Samuel, 2000). Moreover, focus on the professional view often leads to scholarly neglect of the emotional impact of dental pain in the fighting force. Uncovering the effects of

DOI: 10.4324/9781003047674-12

dental pain on the body and mind in the trenches is important for understanding more about the soldiers' experience.

Poor oral health, including trench mouth, impacted on a soldier's everyday life in more fundamental ways than historians have recognised. Hitherto neglected oral histories and written memoirs show that many soldiers reported on their tooth troubles in letters home to family, or recounted their experience in later life. By uncovering more about the soldier's experience of dental health and how they suffered unduly as a consequence of broader societal oral health inequalities, this chapter offers a new perspective on the morbidity of British soldiers who served during World War One and by extension, provides a broader picture of oral health among the British population in this period than hitherto exists. By providing the first study on trench mouth, this chapter also builds on recent scholarship that has focussed on combatant's physical and psychological experience of trench warfare (Anderson, 2014; Dyde, 2011; Humphries, 2014; Goodman, 2014; Conroy, 2018), and trench diseases, such as trench fever (Atenstaedt, 2006, 2011). The chapter also challenges the current view that concern towards the oral health of soldiers began in earnest during the Boer War (Gelbier, 2005). As we will see, oral health was a more pressing and debilitating medical issue than the authorities were willing to acknowledge and prepare for at the beginning of the war. Rather, concern towards the problem of soldiers' oral health was not fully appreciated by the state until after the Great War – when the Army Dental Corps (ADC) was established in 1921. The problem of Tommy's teeth was a matter left to the charitable sector on the Home Front which funded and developed a spontaneous dental treatment service for soldiers in the theatres of war.

This chapter is presented in three sections. Firstly, it will outline the history of dentistry in the British army and relate how dental malaise was perceived by military medical officers in the years leading up to and during World War One. It will then discuss how recruits from 1914 onwards enlisted despite their poor oral health, and the ways in which they coped with their dental health situation in the battlefields. The final section will discuss how charity provided dental treatment for the serving soldier.

## Dentistry in the British army: a historical overview

By 1914, only four Medical Officers had completed a dental module as part of their training for the entire fighting force. Such a limited number of trained dental personnel available to the whole army indicates that the oral health of soldiers was simply not a priority of the authorities at the time. Between the seventeenth and nineteenth centuries, army dentistry was undertaken by the infantry's surgeon (Woods, 1938). This situation changed when Mr Newland Pedley became the first of five civilian registered dentists, permitted by the War Office, to treat soldiers in the field during the second Boer War (1899–1902) (Woods, 1938; Gelbier, 2005). Dental sick-wastage during this war was a serious issue; dental caries and septic conditions affected nearly 7,000 men, a third of whom were invalided back to the UK unfit for service (Great Britain, 1904). However, the War Office did not seem to appreciate the severity of the dental issues among its men in South Africa, nor how the same problem could affect troops in a European war. Had this government department taken the dental problem more seriously, more effort would have been made to increase the numbers of dentists in the army.

But the roots of dental issues among the military were located at home. As chapter 12 in this volume by Claire Jones has shown, in the late Victorian and Edwardian periods, oral disease was quite the norm across the British population. Furthermore, the draining effect of oral health problems on workforces was a matter much overlooked by many employers unless they were shamed into providing dental welfarism or wished to increase productivity. In this respect, serving troops can be seen as the national defence labour force and a similarly neglected group.

The widespread oral malaise was caused by several factors. Perhaps most notable was the considerable increase in the nation's annual sugar consumption over the nineteenth century which contributed to the incidence of dental caries (Ross, 1994, p. 234). Dental treatment was widely available for the average working-class man, but most 'dentistry' was not preventive – nature took its course until the pain could be borne no more. Who extracted the tooth was dictated by what could be afforded, perhaps the local chemist, a non-registered dentist, or itinerant quack (Beier, 2008, pp. 90–1).

In terms of dental hygiene behaviours used to prevent oral disease, it is difficult to establish and quantify the routine use of toothbrushes in the adult British population in the early decades of the twentieth century. But it is likely that their use among the young male working-class population was low. Although toothbrushes were issued to soldiers from 1901 onwards, early reports suggested that young soldiers were ignorant about how to use them, though education and weekly inspections apparently increased the number of those who 'put down for a toothbrush' (Allport, 1904). Little changed in the oral health practices of the Tommy as a Dental Officer reported at the end of the war that 'the percentage of men who show evidence of a daily use of a toothbrush is very small, numbers frankly stating that they have never used a toothbrush in their lives' (Coe, 1915–9). It is not surprising, perhaps, that young recruits were lacking in knowledge about oral hygiene. The lack of toothbrush ownership and use by working-class schoolchildren was noted by the Medical Officer of Health for the London School Board Dr James Kerr. In 1905, he and his assistant carried out a dental inspection on the pupils of a South London elementary school to find that only 3 of the 245 children had toothbrushes and used them regularly (Wallis, 1908, p. 4).

The experience of the South African war did little to develop a dedicated army dental service. Rather, the military's understanding of dental fitness of young men was based on their own official statistics at the beginning of the twentieth century, which claimed that the rate of rejection for potential recruits with bad teeth had been relatively low. However, such statistics were not a reliable measure considering there was no definitive 'dental standard' until after the war when the Army Dental Corps was established. Before the ADC, medical officers relied on their interpretation of a series of regulations and orders, as they inspected the mouth of the recruit and made a subjective decision on what constituted 'adequate dentition'. The loss of several teeth was common, but a strong, able-bodied man could be passed fit and enlisted even if he could only masticate with his front teeth and stumps of decayed molars (Westcott, 1907).

## Enlisting soldiers with bad teeth during World War One

On 6 August 1914, the new Secretary of State for War, Lord Kitchener, began the expansion of the British army (Simkins, 1988, p. 39). Amid heightened levels of patriotism, the army recruitment service struggled to cope with the boom of volunteers, particularly in London (Silbey, 2005, pp. 22–6). Although additional recruiting centres were quickly opened to ease the load, civilian doctors, who were not *au fait* with the physical requirements of the army, were called to inspect the vast numbers of new recruits, often over 200 men a day each (Winter, 1980). One working-class soldier recounted his medical examination as a swift affair, his hair was clipped off, then he was given a shilling and sworn in, after which he was marched to the dentist for extractions (Silbey, 2005, pp. 24–5). During the recruitment boom of 1914, any perceived 'dental standard' certainly slipped; a bad mouth could have easily been overlooked, deliberately or otherwise (MacPherson, 1921, p. 134; Robinson, 2016). Inspections were carried out in little time, under poor lighting conditions in temporary recruitment stations and the civilian doctors drafted in were initially paid a fee for each man passed, but nothing for those rejected.

The exact numbers of rejections on the grounds of defective teeth in World War One is impossible to know. Firstly, the recruitment process meant that many men were rejected immediately by the recruitment officer. Secondly, some men made a number of unsuccessful attempts before being accepted as war progressed, particularly during the conscription months (Clarke, 2015). But by November 1914, it was realised that many men enlisted had with poor teeth. To cope with this issue, the War Office announced that no man should be discharged if they required dental treatment but were otherwise fit (MacPherson, 1921, p. 134). Given the lack of dental personnel at their disposal, it was left to members of the British and Scottish Dental Associations who had offered to treat new recruits for free and see them fit for service. By February 1915, recruits could be 'subject to dental treatment' (MacPherson, 1921, p. 135).

Shortcomings in the lax 'dental standard' of early recruitment and enlistment process soon led to dental problems in the field as one of the chief causes of sick wastage.

Table 9.1 shows that by 1915, disease of the teeth and gums is one of the principal causes of hospital admissions, 24,703 men with a ratio (per 1,000 ration strength) of 41.8. The records for 1915, represented by Table 9.1, relate

*Table 9.1* Causes of overseas hospital admissions, 1915

| Cause of hospital admission | Number of admissions | Invalided home | Deaths |
| --- | --- | --- | --- |
| Diseases of the digestive system | 67,663 | 461 | 506 |
| Influenza | 44,392 | 30 | 23 |
| Diseases of the respiratory system | 31,141 | 632 | 94 |
| Scabies | 25,242 | 7 | 2 |
| Diseases of the teeth and gums | 24,703 | 42 | 6 |
| Frostbite | 16,256 | 227 | 19 |
| Trench foot | 6,462 | 40 | 6 |

solely to the British Expeditionary Force (BEF) – those who were sent to war on the continent, and considered the most complete, thus the best representation available of the morbidity of the force on the Western Front. The British Expeditionary Force consisted of ten sections of the British army sent to the Western Front, a total average ration strength of 662,342. Whilst most men returned to duty, forty-two cases are invalided home, and there were six recorded deaths. Unlike any civilian death attributed to oral disease (e.g. those from phossy jaw discussed in Chapter 12) which had capacity to ignite political unrest in the workforce, these deaths were not sufficient to warrant the army's attention to the oral health of the soldier.

Socially inferior Tommy was simply lucky to be alive. Indeed, this data represents men who were suffering so badly that they were admitted to hospital but does not account for those suffering in the trenches. Army medical services in the field were under so much pressure that diseases of the teeth and mouth were responsible for relatively few men being sent home or deaths compared to other causes of non-casualty admissions, so teeth were obviously not the most pressing issue for the army medics. Furthermore, a soldier could decide to literally keep his mouth shut and carry on despite the dental pain he was in. It was normal for men to put up with toothache, coupled with an awareness that their fellow soldiers were losing their lives not only to enemy fire, but to other diseases which prevailed during the cold, wet and foggy first winter of the war, such as influenza, respiratory disease and frostbite (Mitchell and Smith, 1931, p. 135). These diseases were less easy to conceal from others than toothache; a man suffering with flu or frostbite would be unable to walk or fight the enemy. It was up to Tommy to cope with his own dental problems in the field.

## Tommy's teeth in the trenches

This section outlines some of the lived experiences of officers and soldiers using oral and written memoirs and reports of the medical officers and dentists who treated them. Oral history can be a reliable source which enlightens how people – particularly the working-classes – coped with a situation at the time, and their reflections thereafter (Portelli, 2006). Furthermore, archived oral history, especially interviews collected by the 'life-history' method, is considered to be more spontaneous and richer in nature compared to a structured interview, and potentially more valid (Gallwey, 2013, p. 47).

The Imperial War Museum Sound Archive (https://www.iwm.org.uk/collections/sound), from which these testimonies are drawn, is the largest of its kind in the world. The Museum's oral history collection forms the bulk of this archive, the majority of which has been digitised. This important historical resource is invaluable for historians, as the oral histories have been collected from both service personnel and non-combatants, men and women.

As we have seen, it was not long into the war before many thousands of soldiers were hospitalised on account of oral health problems. Even those who enlisted with a healthy mouth would have struggled against the onslaught of poor rations, particularly lacking in vitamin C, supplemented with parcels of sweets, jam and tobacco from home.

One way some men coped with their poor oral health (and in particular, their lack of dentition) was by wearing false teeth. In 1917, a report on the examination of 10,000 Scottish recruits claimed that 928 had dentures, a figure that was likely to be conservative (Galloway, 1920). Dentures had both positive and negative connotations about men who wore them, as suggested in this volume by Sweet. However, here evidence shows that Medical Officers viewed those who enlisted with false teeth positively; dentures signalled a 'clean and healthy' mouth, with no risk of septic conditions, added to which well-fitting dentures provided good mastication (Helliwell, 1928). This attitude to dentures was the prevailing social norm; whereas natural teeth were considered unreliable. Such beliefs led to the widespread practice of edentulism or 'full clearances' of teeth, replaced with dentures, often in early adulthood.[2] Men who were 'lucky' enough to have false teeth could sign up for service, be quickly attested, trained and sent onto the Western Front, at which point the reality of war set in.

Accounts of some denture wearing soldiers expressed adversity, whilst others used their situation to their advantage – they took back some control into their lives. One of the key problems was eating the rations, because dentures were easily broken: 'I had a full set of dentures when I was seventeen' recalled Edwin Bigwood, a British private from Bristol who served with 7th Battalion Worcestershire Regiment on the Western Front from 1916 to 1917. When describing hard tack,[3] he recalled: 'these biscuits they snapped off all those teeth … [interviewer: they were very hard?] … yes, like dog biscuits today'. Edwin visited the medical officer, who suggested he soaked the biscuits, but fortunately soft bread was sent from home (Smith, 1988, Reel 1, 24:45). The tasteless biscuits did not go to waste despite being so hard (Haines and Beck, 1994, p. 251). They were used as cooking fuel instead of kindling (which was scarce) to boil up water in their dixies for their sickly sweet ration tea (Graves, 1960, p. 82).

Aside from the damage from hard tack, dentures were easily lost – sometimes deliberately. Soldiers concocted all manner of stories to tell the medical officer, who had little option but to send the soldier back to base, which often meant being put on 'light' duties until the new set was ready. Stories of 'lead swinging' included a man who claimed he had accidentally lost his dentures as he vomited overboard the sea vessel in Bay of Biscay, whilst another claimed a jackal stole them in the middle of the night from the glass of water next to his bed. On both occasions, it was suggested the 'lost' dentures were often 'hidden' quite safe in the bottom of the kit bag (Roe, 2004).

The official military statistics, as seen in Table 9.1., do not unfortunately break down the proportions of men hospitalised specifically for trench mouth. However, there was certainly an acknowledgement that there was a dental health problem given the availability of dental treatment for soldiers in the BEF which increased as the war progressed. More dentists were enlisted, but the standard of facilities and equipment varied in the theatres of war. This was owing to the fact that the dental treatment of British soldiers in the field was a matter left to the efforts of St John and the British Red Cross who collaborated to form the Joint War Committee in October 1914.

The St John Ambulance Brigade Hospital in Etaples, near Boulogne, northern France, was the largest medical facility to serve the BEF and renowned for being well-equipped (Museum of the Order of St John 2016). It opened on 1st September 1915, with a dedicated dental department, under the Chief Dental Officer W.E Coe, who wrote: 'No expense was spared in fitting the surgery with the most modern appliances, so as to facilitate the work in every way' (Coe, 1915–9). One such piece of modern apparatus was a dental X-ray machine, whilst a separate dental workshop, staffed by Lance Corporal McConway, attended to the denture cases.

Coe kept detailed monthly statistics on patient numbers and types of treatment carried out in the department. From September 1915 to January 1919, a total of 9,099 patients received dental treatment these included: 3,608 fillings, 1,981 extractions, 510 dentures, and 2,589 other procedures such as root canal treatment. In the first four months, eleven fractured jaws were attended to, but from the beginning of 1916, these cases were sent directly to a special centre for facial injuries, at a hospital in Wimereaux, along the northern French coast. As Gelbier (2005) has noted, the development of maxillo-facial surgery came in response to modern warfare in World War One. However, it was categorised as trauma of the face/mouth rather than disease.

Treating both inpatients and outpatients, officers and other ranks, Coe was well experienced by the end of his time in Etaples. His final handwritten report is notable for reflecting a class-based attitude towards oral health inequalities and blaming the soldier for his own poor dental condition:

> The general condition of the teeth of patients was deplorably bad ... the proportion presenting with active and wholly neglected caries was extremely high. So long as there is no pain from these conditions men are unwilling to have their teeth attended to. There is a marked want of appreciation of the importance to health of the maintaining of efficient masticat[ion] by conservative treatment...there is almost an entire absence

of previous dental treatment, other than extraction of the teeth for the relief of pain … From the point of view of Public Health, most of the men would require dental treatment (Museum of the Order of St John 2016).

As we have seen, dental sick-wastage in the field can be attributed to a combination of compounding factors including existing poor oral health, sugar-laden rations and dirty canteens. Yet for poor Tommy, trench life brought more pressing issues to the fore; keeping warm and dry was far more important than a clean mouth and preventive dental treatment. Even men with good teeth and gums would have struggled to maintain a daily oral hygiene regime. Soldiers were issued with a toothbrush and a tin of toothpowder (Tilbury and Co toothbrush and Kropp, Sheffield razor, 1918). Compared to their civilian counterparts, these items could be difficult to replenish.

Octavius Moore Haines was nineteen when he passed his medical school entrance exam in March 1914. He signed-up for the army in January 1915 and undertook his basic training in the Royal Army Medical Corps. He served in a military hospital in Cairo and later a field station in Salonica, Greece, where he set up an army dental surgery and laboratory (Haines and Beck, 1994, p. 5). His letters home to his family asked for replacement 'comforts' not being supplied by the army or in short supply locally, he wrote:

> 30.4.16 … Things are awfully expensive, I will get you to send me some soap, writing material, toothpowder & **brush**. (216)

> 12.6.16 … Thanks also for the toilet requisites…the toothbrush too was most welcome … what luxuries. (225)

Such letters point out that despite Haines's upper-class background and position as a dental officer in training, like Tommy, he too struggled to obtain the kit for basic oral hygiene because they were seen as comforts by the military authorities. The dental health of serving men was not prioritised, despite the high sick wastage from dental disease and the problem of trench mouth.

## On the home front

The plight of poor Tommy dealing with toothache in the trenches and dentures in the dug outs prompted sympathy on the Home Front. Voluntary action raised funds for dental equipment to treat soldiers near to enemy lines. Philanthropy during World War One was phenomenal. Between 1916 to 1920, just under 18,000 new charities were registered under the War Charities Act 1916 (Grant, 2014, p. 135). Men, women and children were inspired to 'do their bit' – they boosted morale as they raised money (Haines and Beck, 1994). Existing large national charity organisations pooled resources during the war.

Such resources allowed the Army to improve its dental services as the war went on. As we have seen, the Joint War Committee provided much-needed medical care for servicemen (Meyer, 2015). Field stations and hospitals, such as that mentioned in Etaples, were opened in each theatre of war, often some distance from the front line. Ambulances and other vehicles would bring the sick and injured to the hospital. The mobilisation of medical units, and more specifically mobile dental units, brought dentistry services to those serving nearer enemy lines. By the end of the war, there were six mobile dental vehicles in the field, together with mobile x-ray and dental laboratories. Dentures could be mended in a few hours, compared to losing a man for up to a month if sent to a hospital (Museum of the Order of St John [c. 1915]).

The first dental unit was inspected by the King and Queen at Buckingham Palace on 7th October 1916 and funded by the Civil Service Federation. Dentist Mr E. Curtice was in charge of the vehicle, which was well-appointed with two dental chairs, gas cylinders and sterilisation apparatus for clinical work, as well as equipment to make dentures (Anon, 1916). The fifth mobile vehicle of the fleet was presented by the 'Silver Thimble Fund' on 4th May 1918. The Fund was started by Miss H. E. Hope-Clarke of Wimbledon who found a hole in the thimble she was using and decided to put an advertisement in *The Times* on 8 July 1915, asking people to donate worn out silver thimbles to buy a motor ambulance. Between 1915 and 1920, about 65,000 thimbles and many other silver trinkets were donated, and sold by auction or melted down for scrap raising over £60,000 (Museum of the Order of St John [c. 1915]).[4]

The appeal spread internationally. In New Zealand, *The Wanganui Chronicle* reported that whilst the local branch of the Silver Thimble had collected a good amount of old silver, folks were encouraged to donate 'clumsy and hideous early Victorian jewellery' and sacrifice sentimental trinkets to help those who have made supreme sacrifices (Anon, 1917). The reaction of the public to this charity demonstrated a collective social consciousness to the dental needs and pain which Tommy endured in the trenches. Without mobile dental units or the philanthropically funded hospital dental departments, such as Coe's in Etaples, more soldiers would have suffered with their teeth.

## Conclusion

This chapter has argued that the poor dental health of soldiers in World War One, particularly the debilitating and prevalent disease of trench mouth, has been overlooked by historians because other non-battle illnesses contributed to higher mortality statistics. Nevertheless, this chapter has shown that otherwise fit men suffered from trench mouth, dental pain from caries, and coped with problems associated with dentures – all of which had a detrimental impact on their everyday life in the trenches. Letters home and oral histories bring to life the significance of their experience, both then and now. However, the ignorance of the military authorities to the potential of oral health problems in the trenches, despite the shortcomings of the Boer war, was symptomatic of the wider inequalities in public dental health. Teeth affected soldiers' everyday life, both at war and at home.

## Notes

1 For example, Gelbier, 'Part 7: War and the Dental Profession', considers the 'dental health problem' as a matter addressed by the dental profession and military during the Boer war, when actually the army officials did little to learn by this experience. The number of dentists drafted in during the Great War was pitiful given the widespread problem.
2 For more details on the sociological aspects of edentulism, see: Gibson et al. (2017) and Sussex Thomson and Fitzgerald (2010). These studies showed that in Scotland and later in New Zealand, edentulism was a decision which was social in nature; a response to the perceived unreliability of natural teeth, particularly by the working-class. The practice of edentulism and wearing of dentures offered a 'status passage' – a socially accepted solution to the inevitability of tooth loss and of benefit to the individual during life transitions.
3 Hard tack was a type of ship biscuit – very hard, cheap to produce, very long-lasting and tasteless – designed to provide calories in the rations. In Britain, they were made by the biscuit manufacturers Huntley and Palmer.
4 This amount of £60,000 is equivalent to at least £3.5 million today.

## Reference List

Allport, H. K. (1904) 'Training soldiers in personal hygiene', *Journal of the Royal Army Medical Corps*, 3(6), pp. 621–623.

Anderson, J. (2014) 'Rehabilitation and restoration: orthopaedics and disabled soldiers in Germany and Britain in the First World War', *Medicine, Conflict and Survival*, 30(4), pp. 227–251.

Anon (1916) 'Care of the wounded', *The British Journal of Nursing*, 57, (14 October), pp. 307.

Anon (1917) 'Silver Thimble Fund', *Wanganui Chronicle*, LX, (10 February).

Atenstaedt, R. (2011) *The medical response to the trench diseases in World War One*. Newcastle upon Tyne: Cambridge Scholars Publishing.

Atenstaedt, R. L. (2006) 'Trench fever: the British medical response in the Great War', *Journal of the Royal Society of Medicine*, 99(11), pp. 564–568.

Beier, L. M. (2008) *For their own good: the transformation of English working-class health culture, 1880–1970*. Columbus: Ohio State University Press.

Chaubal, T., and Bapat, R. (2017) 'Trench mouth', *The American Journal of Medicine*, 130(11), pp. 493–494.

Clarke, N. (2015) *Unwanted warriors: the rejected volunteers of the Canadian Expeditionary Force, Studies in Canadian military history*. Vancouver: UBC Press.

Coe, W. E. (1915–9) Report on the Dental Dept St John's Ambulance Hospital Étapes. [unpublished]. At: Museum of the Order of St John, OSJ/1/2/1/1/11.

Conroy, K. (2018) 'Hearing loss in the trenches – a hidden morbidity of World War I', *The Journal of Laryngology & Otology*, 132(11), pp. 952–955.

Dyde, S. (2011) 'The chief seat of mischief: soldier's heart in the First World War', *Journal of the History of Medicine and Allied Sciences*, 66(2), 216–248.

Galloway, J. S. (1920) *Report upon the physical examination of men of military age by National service medical boards from November 1st, 1917 - October 31st, 1918. Vol.1.* [S.l.]: H.M.S.O.

Gallwey, A. (2013) 'The rewards of using archived oral histories in research: the case of the Millennium Memory Bank', *The Journal of the Oral History Society*, 41(1), pp. 37–50.

Gelbier, S. (2005) '125 years of developments in dentistry, 1880–2005. Part 7: war and the dental profession', *Br Dent J*. 199, 12(24), pp. 794–798.

Gibson, B. J., Sussex, P. V., Fitzgerald, R. P. and Thomson, W. M. (2017) 'Complete tooth loss as status passage', *Sociology of Health and Illness*, 39(3), pp. 412–427.

Goodman, M. (2014) 'The other side of the poison cloud: Canadian soldiers as English patients after the first gas attacks', in: Barkhof, S. and Smithm, A. (eds.) *War and displacement in the twentieth century: global conflicts*. London: Routledge, pp. 53–69.

Grant, E. J. (2012) *The toothwrights' tale: a history of dentistry in the Royal Navy, 1964-1995*. Gosport: Chaplin.

Grant, P. (2014) *Philanthropy and voluntary action in the First World War:mobilizing charity*. London: Routledge.

Graves, R. (1960) *Goodbye to all that*. Harmondsworth: Penguin Books.

Great Britain. (1904) *Appendix to the Report of the Inter-Departmental Committee on Physical Deterioration*. Parl. Papers, 1904 [Cd 2186]. London: The Stationary Office.

Haines, O. C. M. and Beck, B. (1994) *My dearest Mamma and Papa: 1914-1918 war letters*. Cowbridge: D. Brown and Sons Ltd.

Helliwell, J. (1928) 'The dental standard of the recruit', *Journal of the Royal Army Medical Corps*, 50(3), pp. 163–174.

Humphries, M. (2014) 'Wilfully and with intent: self-inflicted wounds and the negotiation of power in the trenches', *Histoire sociale / Social History*, 47(94), pp. 369–397.

MacPherson, W. G. (1921) *Medical services: general history*. London: HMSO.

Meyer, J. (2015) 'Neutral caregivers or military support? The British Red Cross, the Friends' Ambulance Unit, and the problems of voluntary medical aid in wartime', *War & Society*, 34(2), pp. 105–120.

Mitchell, T. J., and Smith, G. (1931) *Medical services: casualties and medical statistics of the Great War*. London: HMSO.

Museum of the Order of St John [c. 1915]. Newspaper articles - Silver Thimble Fund. OSJ/1/13/2/1.

Museum of the Order of St. John. (2016) 'St John in the First World War'. [online], *Museum of St John*. [Viewed 29 October 2021]. Available from: http://museumstjohn. org.uk/research/projects/st-john-first-world-war/

Portelli, A. (2006) 'What makes oral history different?'. in: Robert, R. P. and Thomson, A. (eds.) *The oral history reader*. London: Routledge.

Robinson, M. (2016) 'Broken soldiers: the chaos of enlistment in the British Army in the early months of the Great War', *History Ireland*, 24(2). [Viewed 27 October 2021]. Available from: https://www.historyireland.com/wwi/broken-soldiers-the-chaos-of-enlistment-in-the-british-army-in-the-early-months-of-the-great-war/

Roe, E. P. (2004) *Diary of an old contemptible: Private Edward Roe, East Lancashire Regiment, from Mons to Baghdad, 1914-1919*. Barnsley: Pen & Sword Military.

Ross, R. (1994) *The development of dentistry: a Scottish perspective circa 1800-1921*. Ph.D. thesis, University of Glasgow.

Samuel, R. (2000) 'People's history', in: Tosh, J. (ed.) *Historians on history: an anthology*. Harlow: Pearson Education.

Silbey, D. (2005) *The British working class and enthusiasm for war, 1914-1916*. London; New York: Frank Cass.

Simkins, P. (1988) *Kitchener's army: the raising of the new armies, 1914-16*. Manchester: Manchester University Press.

Smith, L. E. (1988) Interview with Edwin Charles Bigwood. At: Imperial War Museum Sound Archive, 10115.

Sussex, P. V., Thomson, W. M. and Fitzgerald, R. P. (2010) 'Understanding the 'epidemic' of complete tooth loss among older New Zealanders', *Gerodontology*, 27, pp. 85–95.

Tilbury, W. R. and Co (toothbrush) and Kropp, Sheffield (razor) (1918) Holdall, toiletry equipment. At: London: Imperial War Museum, EQU 2556. [Viewed 27 October 2021]. Available from: http://www.iwm.org.uk/collections/item/object/30013732

Wallis, C. E. (1908) *The care of the teeth in public elementary schools; with special reference to what is being done in Germany.* London: J&A Churchill.

Westcott, S. (1907) 'The teeth of the soldier', *Journal of the Royal Army Medical Corps*, 8(2), pp. 141–150.

Winter, J. (1980) 'Military fitness and civilian health in Britain during the First World War', *Journal of Contemporary History*, 15(2), pp. 211–244.

Woods, S. H. (1938) 'An outline of dentistry in the British Army, 1626-1938: (Section of the History of Medicine)', *Proceedings of the Royal Society of Medicine*, 32(2), pp. 99–112.

Woods, S. H. (1926) 'Post-war acute ulcerative gingivitis', *Journal of the Royal Army Medical Corps*, 47(4), pp. 241–251.

# 10 The mouth as the gateway to the leaky body: the visibility of internal bleeding in the mouths of people with haemophilia

*Alison Dougall, Blánaid Daly, and Sasha Scambler*

## Introduction

Haemophilia is an X-linked bleeding disorder that prolongs clotting times. At its most severe, this can cause spontaneous life-threatening bleeding into organs, muscles and joints and in its milder form classically manifests with increased bleeding following trauma or surgery. Due to advances in medical care and the availability of factor replacement therapy, most younger people living with Haemophilia in Ireland are now able to control bleeding through digitalised risk based programmes that match factor requirements with activities and allow people to pre-plan and manage their activities to avoid the risks of internal bleeding. The activities matched for factor requirement affect many areas of the body but there are no specific risk factors associated with the mouth (aside from receiving dental treatment itself). This effectively removes the mouth from the risk of self-management undertaken for other parts of the body and is the first indicator of the separation of the mouth and the body. For those that still experience bleeds these are largely seen through signs such as bruising, swelling and associated intense and familiar pain rather than encounters with blood directly. With the exception of the increased rate of deaths observed during the 1980s and 1990s due to blood-borne viral infections in factor replacement therapy, the lifespan of people with haemophilia now approaches that of the general population. There currently remains no cure, however, and access to the most effective treatment, factor replacement therapy, varies geographically according to economic viability, local custom and practice, and individual patient doctor preferences (Colvin et al., 2008; O'Mahony et al., 2013; Srivastava et al., 2013; Gringeri et al., 2014).

Despite huge improvements in the general health of people with haemophilia, there is some evidence that adults and children living with the condition have poorer oral health status and poorer oral health-related quality of life than the general population. People with haemophilia may have difficulty in accessing general dental care by virtue of their medical condition and many avoid dental care due to dental anxiety related to a family history of bleeding

DOI: 10.4324/9781003047674-13

following previous dental treatment. The World Federation of Haemophilia (WFH) suggest that this impacts on their members' physical and psychosocial wellbeing and that dental services should be available as part of the comprehensive care of people with haemophilia worldwide in order to enhance their quality of life. This reflects the fact that dental services are not routinely incorporated as part of the comprehensive care of people with haemophilia in many parts of the world, and even where they are, as in the example of Ireland, the mouth is treated differently, largely outside factor self-management regimes, and with many people feeling safe only when accessing specialist dental care. Despite this call for better integration then, the mouth remains largely separated out from the body, both in haemophilia care and in the attitudes and experiences of people with haemophilia towards their bodies.

Whilst there is relatively little sociological research focusing specifically on the mouth, one notable exception is the work of Nettleton (1992) who describes the development of dentistry and the separation of the mouth from the body. Nettleton charts the growth of the dental profession and the deliberate separation of medicine focused on the mouth from medicine focused on the body. This has resulted in the routine, unthinking, exclusion of oral health care from packages of care focused on the body and reflects the position within haemophilia care as well as in many other areas, including dementia care and palliative care. She suggests, further, that the mouth can be seen as the boundary between the internal and external bodies and as such becomes associated with regulation and social control of the body. This is the starting point for our analysis of the mouth as a leaky boundary in people with haemophilia.

Drawing on empirical data from a study exploring the lived experience of bleeding from the mouth for people with haemophilia, this chapter highlights the significance of the mouth uniquely within the body as the boundary through which the body leaks and the internal becomes external (Shildrick, 2015). Even in countries with excellent support and healthcare regimes in place for people with haemophilia, such as Ireland, the mouth is experienced differently from other parts of the body. Bleeding from the mouth is common and impacts significantly on daily life. This contributes to high levels of dental fear and avoidance of dentists and dental treatment. In this context, the mouth is the site where the immediate, visceral reality of a condition which remains largely enclosed within the material body becomes visible. Focusing on difference, separation and the mouth as a leaky breach in the boundary of the body, this chapter starts with a brief sociological take on existing research on the mouth and oral health for people with haemophilia, drawing on relevant work on the social construction of the body, deviance, bodily boundaries and fluid, leaky bodies. Experiences of bleeding from the mouth are then explored drawing on data from an in-depth qualitative study of people with haemophilia in Ireland and the wider impacts of the separation of the mouth and the body are explored.

## A sociological take on haemophilia and the mouth

The risk of oral disease for people with haemophilia is the same as for the general population, and the risk factors of oral disease are well known and can be modified or prevented (Gregory and Fenton, 2014). Despite this, extensive or prolonged bleeding from the mouth due to poor oral health, as a consequence of a dental intervention, or through trauma to the mouth, is cited as both a perceived and experienced problem for people with haemophilia (Brewer, 2008; Hewson et al., 2011; Srivastava et al., 2013). Extensive or prolonged bleeding from the mouth, alongside higher levels of periodontal disease, gingivitis and poor oral hygiene all potentially impact on the body as a social entity in interactions with others. Sociologists have long argued that the body is not just a biological entity but a social one, we live our lives through and within our bodies and our engagement with the world around us is embodied. In this way, 'bodies are not just individual entities; they link us to other humans and to the world around us' (Fox, 2018, p. 265). This is reflected in Goffman's (1968) concept of 'body idiom' and the way in which we use the body in human interaction as a non-verbal tool to communicate social position. 'Body idiom' is used to back up what people say and do in social interactions and involves the wearing of appropriate clothes, the way hair is styled and the use of gestures and expressions. Those with shared culture are then enabled to read unspoken cues and label and grade those around them. This is a continual process which shapes both self and social identities. If the body that we are expressing ourselves through is deemed unsanitary, or unsightly this then has the potential to impact on both self and social identity. This is not a new phenomenon; however, in their work on aids for deaf people in Victorian Britain, Gooday and Sayer (2017) highlight aids marketed specifically to be 'invisible' thus working to hide the wearer's impairment. An advert by A. A. Marks published in 1888 (cited in Sweet, 2017) shows prosthetic legs designed specifically to render invisible the 'unsightly' single limbed body. As Sweet explains, the ongoing attempts to develop invisible prosthesis 'validate attempts to eradicate disability via a medical model, which sees physical loss as a potentially fixable issue' (Sweet ibid, p. 132).

Building on this, Goffman (1968) looked at the impact of being labelled as deviant or abnormal on those with what he termed 'abominations of the body'. This included those living with a long-term condition or disability and, within the context of this chapter, would include people diagnosed with haemophilia. These people, Goffman suggested, were living in bodies that may not be able to engage in 'body idiom' and conform to cultural expectations and so were forced to undertake information management to combat the negative perceptions or stigma surrounding their label. People with conditions that were immediately visible on interaction were 'discredited' and focused on managing the tension of the reactions of 'normals', whilst people with conditions that were not immediately apparent (often termed 'invisible disabilities') focused on managing information and disclosure/non-disclosure of the diagnosis. In this case, haemophilia managed through an effective treatment regimen could largely be considered invisible with the majority of symptoms unseen, except through the mouth where visible bleeding might precipitate disclosure of the condition and exposure as deviant.

Social constructionists highlight the increased importance of the 'body' in a consumer culture, the emphasis on looking good and the implications of this for the non-normative body, be that through disease, impairment or age:

> A body that does not function 'normally' or appear 'normal', that is confined to a wheelchair or bed, is both visually and conceptually out-of-place, as evidenced by the lack of public facilities for people with disabilities or the elderly.
>
> (Lupton, 1994, p. 38)

At the same time the body, now required to be perfect, is provided with all kinds of opportunities for improvement from medical technology to diet and fitness regimes. Implicit throughout this literature is the idea that weak, ill, unattractive or disabled bodies are to be rejected or avoided as distasteful. Healthy, 'able' bodies are seen as morally superior (Elias, 1978). Building on this, the work of Mathieson and Stam (1995) identifies the effect that the onset of illness has on body consciousness and the awareness that the body is not functioning in the way that is expected of it. This again highlights the impact of visible difference and is illustrated in our empirical findings through normalised, everyday bleeding from the mouth as well as through dramatic bleeds.

This difference is also immediate and obvious when people with haemophilia require dental care. Excessive bleeding following dental procedures remains one of the most frequent complications occurring in people with haemophilia (Franchini et al., 2005) and one-third of all surgical admissions amongst people with haemophilia in New Zealand were for elective or emergency dental procedures (Park et al., 1999). A study carried out in the UK in 2012 found that 20 per cent of those surveyed had been refused treatment by a local dentist because of their bleeding disorder and a further 45 per cent did not have confidence that their local dentists could treat their condition appropriately despite available guidelines (Kalsi et al., 2012). The World Federation of Haemophilia (WFH) suggest that lack of access to safe appropriate care impacts on the physical and psycho-social well-being of their members and can adversely affect their oral health related quality of life (OHrQoL) (Srivastava et al., 2013; World Federation of Haemophilia, 2006). In these studies, visible difference impacts not just on psycho-social wellbeing but the ability to access services needed to control symptoms.

In relation to oral health specifically, very little is known about people with haemophilia's experiences of the mouth and research undertaken tends to be limited to small cross-sectional studies which measure caries experience (Boyd and Kinirons, 1997; Ziebolz et al., 2011), periodontal disease

(Ziebolz et al., 2011) or anxiety (Dogan et al., 2013) using a variety of measures. The few qualitative studies available report high levels of dental anxiety, avoidance behaviours and trust issues (Kalsi et al., 2012) which is perhaps unsurprising given experiences of trying to access, and of receiving, dental care. In addition, people with haemophilia were found to be less likely to practice good oral hygiene measures (Azhar et al., 2006), brush their teeth (Alpkilic Baskirt et al., 2009), use a toothbrush and toothpaste (Kabil et al., 2007) or use floss (Hitchings, 2012). Potential reasons for this are explored in the following section. Oral problems are cumulative and progressive (Shtereva, 2006) yet there is no robust literature describing the oral health of people with haemophilia as they age, how they manage and access dental care or their understanding of oral health while living with a chronic condition. Further, Hitchings (2012) suggested that people with haemophilia 'often experienced dental pain or gingival bleeding but had not recognised it as a need to seek treatment'. They frequently attributed bleeding from their mouth to their haemophilia rather than oral health but recognised the negative impact it had on their quality of life.

Bleeding from the mouth, whether excessive and prolonged, or routine and normalised, emphasises the importance of seeing bodies not just as social but also as material entities. Longhurst (2000) suggests we need to under-stand bodies as material entities that exist in space and interact with that space, bodies that are fluid and leaky. This idea of leaky bodies stems from McDowell's (1993) work on feminism and space, arguing that women's embodied experiences challenge bodily boundaries and the assumed bound-aries between the internal body and the social world, between 'self and other'. Through menstruation, lactation and childbirth, the boundary of the body becomes permeable and the internal body leaks into the external social world. Thus, she argues, 'The feminine construction of self is an existence centred within a complex relational nexus, compared to the masculine construction of self as separate, distinct and unconnected' (McDowell, 1993, p. 306). Building on this, Longhurst (2000) highlights the links made be-tween leaky, irrational female bodies and solid, rational male bodies. She states that bodies that leak (in this case, female bodies) are not seen as appropriate or trusted in public spaces. This can be seen in the debates on the morality of breastfeeding in public places and in the social isolation and shame associated with the impact of period poverty on girls and women, preventing them from social interaction with their leaky bodies potentially on display. Conversely male, bodies with secure boundaries, can be trusted in public spaces to act in a rational, controlled way. Longhurst suggests that these conceptualisations have little do with the biological body but are powerful in 'constructing relationships to space'. This raises interesting questions about the role of the mouth in relation to the body, and parti-cularly about the role of the mouth as a leaky boundary in the male bodies of people living with haemophilia.

## Experiences of bleeding from the mouth

What we have thus far is a long-term condition which involves internal bleeding throughout the body, has no cure but is well managed through a complex, self-managed factor replacement programme. The exception to this seems to centre around the mouth, exacerbated by the epistemological and geographical separation of the mouth from the body. Whilst other activities and parts of the body can be, and are, managed with reference to the factor/activity lists provided by the Irish Haemophilia Society, the mouth is largely absent from this and activities and treatments related to the mouth are located in specialist centres of expertise in the main cities.

The data presented here come from a qualitative study exploring the relationship between the mouth and the body for people living with haemophilia in Ireland. Face-to-face semi-structured interviews were conducted with 29 adults with haemophilia, or diagnosed as carriers of haemophilia across the four provinces of Ireland. Participants were purposively sampled across five groups: men under and over 40 with mild haemophilia, men under and over 40 with moderate or severe haemophilia; women diagnosed with haemophilia or as carriers. In addition, a mix of people living in urban and rural areas were recruited to reflect the particularities of the Irish context. Interviews were audio recorded, transcribed verbatim and a five-stage thematic analysis was undertaken (Ritchie et al., 2013). Informed, written consent was obtained from all participants and ethical approval for the study was obtained from Kings College London and Trinity College, Dublin Ref. BDM/12/13–121.

The results of the analysis are presented here with a specific focus on the mouth as a gateway to the leaky body and the site where bleeding, and with it deviance or difference, becomes visible. To set the scene we start with an outline of the limited visibility of bleeding in other parts of the body for people living with haemophilia and then move on to focus on the mouth. Bleeding from the mouth can then be seen to have a range of impacts, from the more obvious trauma and pain associated with severe bleeding through acting as a trigger for diagnosis through to the impact on others, fear, stigma and labelling. Each of these areas is explored and illustrated with quotes from the interviews. Each quote is identified through the pseudonym of the participant, the severity of their diagnosis (S = moderate to severe, M = mild) and whether they are under or over 40.

## Internal bleeding, invisible blood

Haemophilia is characterised by internal bleeding, as Eóin explained:

> My haemophilia is not about external bleeding it's about internal bleeding and so I don't really have the external bleeding you see … and so I get bleeding into my kidneys and my head and that sort of thing – my joints are not really an issue or the bruising. (Eóin Sv<40)

Whilst the bleeding occurs and has an impact on the body and life of the participant, the blood itself is visibly missing. This concept of bleeding without visible blood was described in many of the interviews. Participants talked about pain or heat, limited movement, or the need for injections of factor.

> You wouldn't be able to put pressure on it, it would be really really hot ... That's how you know it's a bleed, it's really really hot. (Finn S<40)

Niall talked about the fact that there were no visible signs of the haemophilia, aside from the severe pain he experienced.

> I got worse when I was about 10 ... like my arms locking up and just agony ... I couldn't do nothing. (Niall S<40)

Others, such as Patrick, talked about visible bruising as the only obvious external sign of internal bleeding.

> well 'J' senior ... we were out for a meal there the other day ... and he was at the table and he was all black and blue everywhere and I don't think people like looking at him because you can see he's got the severe form. (Patrick M>40)

In these examples, the body is not leaky and the results of the haemophilia, the bleeding, is contained. Even where the bleeding can be seen it is contained within the skin of the body.

## Visible blood

What makes the mouth particularly interesting is that it is one of the only sites of the body where the blood becomes visible, where the body leaks and the bleeding is no longer contained, it can be tasted, its temperature experienced and it leaves its mark on clothes, sheets and skin. This leads to the mouth taking on a more significant role in the embodied lives of people with haemophilia. The mouth in this situation is both internal and external, the breach through which the internal can be seen. As Eóin explained:

> Mmm I think it's to do with, I know my mouth is internal, I didn't for a long time but then when I had to start getting procedures done, like getting a tooth out then my mum said to me that I'd have to get factor and I'd have to get this and realise my mouth is internal, they don't just mean under my skin inside my body when they say internal ... I would have considered my mouth not to be internal bleeding because it's not under my skin it's something I can see, so. (Eóin Sv<40)

The mouth was almost always the first site where the visceral reality of a bleed was experienced. For some this was a dramatic bleeding experience, as vividly described by Patrick.

> It was when we got a tooth out, the dentist came to the school and I was maybe 14 ... but my mother then came into the room the next morning and she looked at me and the plug [tooth pack] was out by then and I was stuck to the pillow and with congealed blood and of course she panicked. (Patrick M>40)

Outside of dental care this kind of dramatic bleed was only seen in cases where traumatic injury occurred as Ciaran highlighted, recounting his treatment following a car accident.

> Because I bleed out ... I remember them telling me it was like a war zone going on in A&E, they were putting the blood in but ... [It was just coming out]. (Ciaran M>40)

Whilst this kind of bleeding is dramatic and often linked to dental trauma or treatment, sometimes visible blood was more insidious. Aidan recalled the story he was told about his first bleed from the mouth aged two.

> I cut the connection there between the lip and the gum: and mmm that would set off, and every time I fed it would just start bleeding again ... it just kept bleeding, from the mouth, every time I had a bottle it would just. (Aidan S<40)

All of these stories highlight the impact that visible blood has for people with an oftentimes contained internal bleeding disorder. It also highlights the role the mouth plays in making the internal externally visible. The descriptors 'stuck to the pillow with congealed blood' and 'like a war zone' highlight the immediacy and impact of having internal bleeding become visible. This can be a signifier of deviance, of having this unusual leakiness of the body becoming apparent, whether dramatic or insidious in presentation.

## Blood and dentists

Often major bleeding episodes were linked to dentists and dental treatment. For many of the participants this was the only invasive medical treatment they had received and thus the only situation where a bleed was caused by something other than an accident. This effectively separates out the mouth and dental care from the rest of the body and other forms of healthcare. In these cases, the bleeding from the mouth could act as a trigger for diagnosing the haemophilia:

Well me and my brother were diagnosed the same day … it was my fecking teeth again – … well we had always been bleeders in those days they called them bleeders of course – but anyway we went to the dentist at the school and we both had a load of teeth out – anyway – I was oozing for days afterwards – and actually me brother was far worse than me cos I think I only had a couple of teeth out but he had had a whole bunch and in the end my ma had to take us both to the hospital and they couldn't even stop it there so anyway they kept packing it with stuff … but it wouldn't stop and I think me brother was in the hospital for a good few days – but I wasn't bad enough for that – but anyway in the end we went up to Dublin and they told us we were haemophiliacs and we had it from my mother's side … no one had ever mentioned it before as we were just typical bleeders and not haemophiliacs. (Tomas M>40)

What is interesting here is that the label 'haemophiliac' was gained through formal diagnosis following dental treatment. Prior to this there was a lay understanding that the boys were 'bleeders' and that this ran in their families. This label of 'bleeders' was very common amongst our sample, a multi-generational identity as a family of 'bleeders'. Whilst this led to an informal acceptance of the need to avoid some activities and warn healthcare workers of potential problems with uncontrolled bleeding, access to an effective treatment regime was not in place until a formal diagnosis was received, often following a trauma and significant bleed.

Teeth the first time we'd been in Our Lady's [Children's Hospital] in the 1970s and my big stay in hospital was after me dentist … I went to me dentist in around 72/73 and I ended up in hospital about 3 days after … He took a tooth out and it kept bleeding … 3 days bleeding away to my heart's content, giving me nothing … They put the gauze on it and eventually it stopped. (Hugh M>40)

In these examples, prior to the dental treatment, there was no diagnosis and no treatment was being received. This was the case even where the identity as a 'bleeder' was common knowledge in the family, and often in the wider community. The dental clinic then becomes the site of change, of acquiring a new label, and potentially an altered identity, as well as the site of access to treatment.

Even where the diagnosis was known, dental treatment was often the cause of significant bleeds and led to visceral descriptions of the feel, taste and sight of blood in the mouth.

I got knocked down a few years ago and had to get root canal treatment and the bleeding, I swallowed so much blood I got sick on blood. (Finn S<40)

This, unsurprisingly, often led to significant and long lasting dental fear.

> I am petrified of dentists, it comes from my childhood ... every milk tooth that came out was a least a week to 3 weeks in hospital for every tooth, every tooth had to be taken out surgically it was an absolute nightmare, I hated the dentist, I came to hate them very early in life and I still have this fear. (Sean S>40)

Frequently this fear was linked to experiences in childhood and to historical treatments prior to an understanding of either the haemophilia itself or prior to the development of effective factor-based treatment.

> They were scared to give you injections for fillings and that ... to freeze it up in case it caused a bleed ... and if you had a tooth out you couldn't have it stitched so you just had to be laid up afterwards on the wards and they would keep plugging the hole for days until it stopped ... and you weren't supposed to eat anything. (Joe S>40)

Sometimes it was also linked to the reactions and experiences of others within the family, again highlighting the mouth as a site of deviance and of difference/ deviance becoming visible. Tomas describes his memories of the experiences of family members who also had haemophilia:

> Well she (his mother) was blaming the dentist of course and I can remember her screaming at him and shouting at them but of course they couldn't do anything. They held down my brother to stitch his gums up to try and stop the bleeding but anyway – there was no going back to the dentist after that for the rest of us. (Tomas M>40)

Even where factor was available and bleeding was controlled, dental treatment could be traumatic. A number of the participants in this study had contracted HIV or Hepatitis C through contaminated blood products in the 1980s. Tomas described how he contracted HIV and how he found out.

> Well – I only had the factor a couple of times in my teens and my twenties and both times was my teeth - because I needed teeth out ... I needed a filling done and I got factor for it – like you had to in them days – and – well – that was the time – it was in the early eighties – well I know it was exactly it was march the 13th 1984 at 10.30 in the morning and anyway – yes that's when I got the blood with the HIV and then later hit with the hepatitis too and anyway – yes – you can imagine that I hated the dentist –I wished nothing had been done with the tooth – and I had left it in and put up with the pain – but. (Tomas M>40).

In this example the mouth becomes more than the breach in the body where the internal bleeding becomes external, and it becomes the cause, if not the site, of the breach where the external infection gets in.

## A daily bloody mouth

Many of the descriptions of bleeding from the mouth given by participants in this study were dramatic and traumatic for the participants, and often for their families too. Many more of the descriptions, however, were mundane and ordinary. For most participants, the feel and taste of blood in the mouth was simply a daily experience, often as part of the usual routine of keeping the mouth clean.

> Yeah just gums and stuff bleed a lot easier than just a normal person, I'm just so used to seeing blood now, it doesn't even bother me like, constantly you see blood and I'm just used to it. (Niall S<40)

This was seen as frustrating but not overly worrying, routine oral hygiene practices simply cause bleeding. In this way the experience of blood in the mouth – typically a sign of gum disease and poor oral health – was normalised, 'I'm just used to it'. Regular bleeds could also compromise the ability to keep the mouth clean, as Finn explained:

> The worse thing is you can't floss if your gums are bleeding ... because every time I floss, it's been, every time I go to the dentist they say I have a healthy mouth and then I floss, just to be even cleaner and it just bleeds every tooth bleeds, well gum. (Finn S<40)

And sometimes the amount of blood would require additional actions.

> I just hold tissue on it and put pressure on it like an it usually stops aft a while and sometimes I'd have to inject myself and it just stops then, it's crazy like. (Niall S<40)

> Well it feels warm and you know it's there because you taste it and you can feel it warm - but then when it builds up you can feel it going down your throat and you feel like gagging and that's when you know it's a problem ... for me I remember the smell of it now and was more like big lumps of liver and jelly I was spitting out ... if you get what I mean. (Tomas M>40)

As can be seen by the examples given here, much of the bleeding expressed and experienced as mundane and ordinary by people with haemophilia would likely be considered traumatic and worrying by those without the condition. It is also worth noting that this normalised bleeding occurs predominantly in the privacy of the home, people are unlikely to have company whilst cleaning their teeth, which may affect how they respond to this leaking.

In these accounts, everyday leaking of blood from the mouth is common, resulting from everyday oral hygiene activity and largely normalised. Less routine episodes of bleeding from the mouth resulted from trauma, tongue or cheek biting, gum disease, sports injuries and following dental surgery. Associated with these bleeds were experiences of fear, panic, nausea, choking, extended periods of hospitalisation, anaemia and blood loss sufficient to impact on consciousness. For those with access to factor for home use, the mouth was singled out as qualitatively different. Other causes of less routine bleeds were largely unavoidable and unexpected, whereas bleeds following dental treatment (once diagnosed) were expected and potentially manageable. Most participants with access to factor reported prophylactic use of large amounts before allowing people to examine their mouths. In those without access to factor, dental phobia and avoidance of dental care was common.

## Reflections on the role of the mouth in haemophilia

The experiences of people with haemophilia presented here build on the key themes of this chapter. The first ties in with issues highlighted in the chapter's introduction and reflects the separation of the mouth and the body: in the routine provision of services for people with haemophilia (as illustrated through the use of specialist dental services and the absence of the body from factor self-management risk systems); through the relative lack of research on the mouth in haemophilia; and through the experience of dental care as uniquely traumatic and threatening. The second theme focuses on the way the mouth is experienced by people with haemophilia themselves as different, and as the site where internal bleeding (discredited deviance) becomes visible and visceral. These themes are tied together through the concept of the 'leaky' body.

The majority of participants in this study, regardless of the severity of their haemophilia, or their success in managing bleeding in other sites in the body, experienced bleeding through their mouth. In this way the mouth becomes the focal point of the leaky body. Many individuals with mild disease had been diagnosed following dental treatment. For these participants, their bleeding identity was tied to their mouths and their sole use of factor treatment was related to bleeding from the mouth and associated with a significant fear of all dental treatment. At the severe end, participants reported living with the daily taste of blood in their mouth and waking up with blood on their pillowcases. In all of these examples, it was not just leaking but the public visibility of that leaking that was significant, precipitating exposure of difference and tying in with Longhurst's (2000) work problematising leaky bodies in public spaces. Respondents also reported altering their food choices in public or avoiding intimacy with their partners through fear of bleeding from the mouth. This fits with Goffman's strategy of managing information to avoid becoming discredited (1968), further suggesting that, even in countries with excellent support and healthcare regimes in place for people with haemophilia, the mouth is experienced differently from other parts of the body. Bleeding from the mouth is common and impacts significantly on daily life.

In this context, the mouth is the site where the immediate, visceral reality of a condition which remains largely enclosed within the material body becomes visible. The mouth is the boundary through which the body leaks (Shildrick, 2015). This research highlights the way that the mouth reveals 'deviance' and challenges the ability to use 'body idiom' to communicate social position amongst people with haemophilia (Goffman, 1968). The feeling of distaste associated with visceral bleeding is clear in the accounts above and this visible difference can lead to felt and enacted stigma. Building on the work of McDowell (1993) and Longhurst (2000), we argue that men with haemophilia are forced to reconstruct their sense of self around the awareness that their internal body leaks into their external social world, predominantly through visible bleeding from the mouth. Thus, regular bleeding is normalised or hidden within the home where possible and activities which are likely to result in extensive visible bleeding are managed by specialists in the discreet location of the special care dental clinic, often geographically and socially distant from local community services. The findings of this study emphasise the importance of the routine inclusion of the mouth in information and management regimes for people with haemophilia, as with those with a vast range of other long-term conditions.

# References

Alpkilic Baskirt, E., Ak, G. and Zulfikar, B. (2009) 'Oral and general health-related quality of life among young patients with haemophilia', *Haemophilia*, 15, pp. 193–198.

Azhar, S., Yazdanie, N. and Muhammad, N. (2006) 'Periodontal status and IOTN interventions among young hemophiliacs', *Haemophilia*, 12, pp. 401–404.

Boyd, D. and Kinirons, M. (1997) 'Dental caries experience of children with haemophilia in Northern Ireland', *International Journal of Paediatric Dentistry*, 7, pp. 149–153.

Brewer, A. K. (2008) 'Advances in minor oral surgery in patients with congenital bleeding disorders', *Haemophilia*, 14(Suppl 3), pp. 119–121.

Colvin, B. T., Astermark, J., Fischer, K., Gringeri, A., Lassila, R., Schramm, W., Thomas, A. and Ingerslev, J. (2008). European principles of haemophilia care. Haemophilia, 14(2), pp. 361–374.

Dogan, M.C., Yazicioglu, I. and Antmen, B. (2013) Anxiety and pain during dental treatment among children with haemophilia. *International Journal of Paediatric Dentistry*, 14(4), pp. 284–288.

Elias, N. (1978). The civilizing process: The history of manners.

Franchini, M., Rossetti, G., Tagliaferri, A., Pattacini, C., Pozzoli, D., Lorenz, C., Del Dot, L., Ugolotti, G., Dell'Aringa, C. and Gandini, G. (2005). Dental procedures in adult patients with hereditary bleeding disorders: 10 years experience in three Italian Hemophilia Centers. *Haemophilia*, 11(5), pp. 504–509.

Fox, N. (2018) 'Reconceptualising Bodies', in: Scambler, G. (ed.) *Sociology as applied to health and medicine*. 7th edn. London: Palgrave.

Goffman, E. (1968) *Stigma – notes on the management of spoiled identity*. London: Penguin.

Gooday, G. and Sayer, K. (2017) 'Purchase, use and adaptation: interpreting 'patented' aids to the deaf in Victorian Britain', in: Jones, C. L. (ed.) *Rethinking modern prostheses in Anglo-American commodity cultures, 1820–1939*. Manchester: Manchester University Press, pp. 27–47.

Gregory, S. and Fenton, K. (2014) *Delivering better oral health: an evidence-based toolkit for prevention*. London: Public Health England.

Gringeri, A., Ewenstein, B. and Reininger, A. (2014) 'The burden of bleeding in haemophilia: is one bleed too many?', *Haemophilia*, 20, pp. 459–463.

Hewson, I., Makhmalbaf, P., Street, A., Mccarthy, P. and Walsh, M. (2011) 'Dental surgery with minimal factor support in the inherited bleeding disorder population at the Alfred Hospital', *Haemophilia*, 17, pp. e185–e188.

Hitchings, E. (2012) *The oral health of individuals with haemophilia: a mixed method investigation*. MCommDent: University of Otago.

Kabil , N., ElAlfy , M. S. and Metwalli , N. (2007) Evaluation of the oral health situation of a group of Egyptian haemophilic children and their re-evaluation following an oral hygiene and diet education programme. *Haemophilia*, 13(3), pp. 287–292.

Kalsi, H., Nanayakkara, L., Pasi, K. J., Bowles, L. and Hart, D. P. (2012) 'Access to primary dental care for patients with inherited bleeding disorders', *Haemophilia*, 18, pp. 510–515.

Longhurst R. (2000) *Bodies: exploring fluid boundaries*. London:Routledge.

Lupton, D. (1994) 'Consumerism, commodity culture and health promotion', *Health Promotion International*, 9(2), pp. 111–118.

McDowell, L. (1993) 'Space, place and gender relations: Part I. Feminist empiricism and the geography of social relations', *Progress in Human Geography*, 17(2), pp. 157–179.

Mathieson, C. and Stam, H. (1995) 'Renegotiating identity: cancer narratives', *Sociology of Health and Illness*, 17(3), pp. 283–306.

Nettleton, S. (1992) *Power, pain and dentistry*. London: Open University Press.

O'mahony, B., Noone, D., Giangrande, P. L. and Prihodova, L. (2013) 'Haemophilia care in Europe - a survey of 35 countries', *Haemophilia*, 19, pp. e239–e247.

Park, J., Scott, K. and Benseman, J. (1999) 'Dealing with a bleeding nuisance: a study of haemophilia care in New Zealand', *The New Zealand Medical Journal*, 112, pp. 155–158.

Ritchie, J., Lewis, J., Nichols, C. and Ormston, R. (2013) *Qualitative research practice: A guide for social science students and researchers*. London: Sage.

Shildrick, M. (2015) *Leaky bodies and boundaries: feminism, postmodernism and (bio) ethics*. London: Routledge.

Shtereva, N. (2006) 'Aging and oral health related to quality of life in geriatric patients', *Rejuvenation Research*, 9, pp. 355–357.

Sonbol, H., Pelargidou, M., Lucas, V. W., Gelbier, M. J., Mason, C. and Roberts, G. J. (2008) 'Dental health indices and caries-related microflora in children with severe haemophilia', *Haemophilia*, 7(5), pp. 468–474.

Srivastava, A., Brewer, A. K., Mauser-Bunschoten, E. P., Key, N. S., Kitchen, S., Llinas, A., Ludlam, C. A., Mahlangu, J. N., Mulder, K., et al. (2013) 'Guidelines for the management of Haemophilia', *Haemophilia*, 19(1), pp. e1–e47.

Sweet, R. (2017) 'Get the best article in the market': prostheses for women in nineteenth- century literature and commerce', in: Jones, C. L. (ed.) *Rethinking modern prostheses in Anglo-American commodity cultures, 1820– 1939.* Manchester: Manchester University Press, pp. 114–136.

World Federation of Haemophilia (2006) 'Guidelines for dental treatment of patients with inherited bleeding disorders', *Monograph 40.* Montreal: WFH.

Ziebolz, D., Stuhmer, C., Hornecker, E., Zapf, A., Mausberg, R. F. and Chenot, J. F. (2011) 'Oral health in adult patients with congenital coagulation disorders–a case control study', *Haemophilia*, 17, pp. 527–531.

# 11 'Having work done': the teeth, mouth and oral health as a body project

*Barry J. Gibson, Jennifer Kettle, and Lorna Warren*

That's a crown because the nerve had gone dead in it. And then I've got … I've just got one back tooth here, that's crowned. I've got no back teeth at all there. I've got one up here and one up there. And then the six teeth at the front, they're my own. And just these like few front teeth at the front are my own, and the rest I've got part dentures, top and bottom. But (Clears Throat) even then, whenever … my part dentures at the bottom, they just slip on and off. My top ones, that's what they were like at first and I didn't like them, because at the palate I used to feel sick and I hated wearing them. So, when I changed dentist (Clears Throat) I changed dentist because I went back to work and I was working in town, and my husband was already going to that dentist in town … so I started going there. And Mr [name] he was only a young dentist then, and we had a long talk and I explained to him how I felt about it and I've got this thing about blood and everything. And I said, 'I can't get on with these dentures that I've got'. And he said, 'Well, we can do different dentures for you'. (Wendy, 77)

Wendy's account of oral care and dental treatment is quite a common one among people from 'her generation'. A recent study of the 'significance of the mouth in older age'[1] (Gibson et al., 2019; Kettle et al., 2019; Warren et al., 2020) reported on a repository of 'mouth talk' (Warren, et al., 2020) from groups of older people about their experiences of oral care over the life course. 'Mouth talk' encapsulates how older people talk about their embodied experience of holding onto and maintaining their teeth. It reveals how some talk about themselves as a particular person with 'a particular moral approach to life … demonstrating … willingness to invest time and effort to achieve a desired goal' (Warren et al., 2020, p. 1261). In this chapter, we discuss one aspect of that goal which was to get to older age with some teeth intact through 'having work done'.

This chapter demonstrates that a close analysis of 'mouth talk' from the project 'the significance of the mouth in older age' can reveal a dimension of dentistry that has remained underanalysed in sociology and social science in dentistry. In this chapter, we point out that dentistry is a fundamentally 'embodied' enterprise. By this we mean that the experience of oral care involves active people with living bodies who undergo work as thinking feeling subjects.

DOI: 10.4324/9781003047674-14

In doing so people experience their oral care primarily through their mouths and bodies. Just as embodiment was hidden in the sociology of health and health care in general (Turner, 1984), the embodied nature of oral care is something that has remained largely 'hidden' from sociological accounts of oral health and dentistry. In this chapter, we build on an ongoing grounded theory study of 'oral health as a life course project' by exploring what it means to 'have work done' on one's mouth and teeth (Gibson et al., 2019).[2] We do so by starting with a very brief introduction to oral care as a life-course project before going on to provide a detailed analysis of participants' accounts of the work of dentists. After this, we go on to examine the 'embodied' nature of dental work before making some more general observations about the nature of dental work in relation to pre-existing approaches in the social sciences as applied to oral health and dentistry.

The chapter draws on the concept of 'body work' (Gimlin, 2007, 2002; Kang, 2003; Wolkowitz, 2002; Twigg, 2000) which is a concept that is used to describe the work people undertake on their own bodies as well as the work that is conducted on the bodies of others in the form of paid work. The sociology of body work also covers the 'emotional labour' that body work demands as well as the underlying processes that 'produce bodies' through the workplace (in terms of how the body is shaped because of one's involvement in certain types of work). Being the subject of dental care is effectively to make oneself available to dentists to be worked on and as they work they perform 'body work' or 'body labour' (Kang, 2003). This subject has been examined to reveal the social impacts and dynamics of this work for those who work on bodies. So, for example, a now famous study of the work of air stewardesses established how the constant need to manage emotions and the body by constantly smiling and appearing cheerful and calm had negative emotional and physical impacts on the bodies of air stewardesses (Hochschild, 1983). Twigg (2000) argued that body work is typically conducted at a distance by health care professionals, especially those who are of higher status. This of course does not hold for dental health care professionals all of whom come into regular contact with the mouth and teeth and whose work, up until relatively recently, has been dominated by direct work on the bodies of patients. This work has received almost no attention from social scientists and this is despite the fact that these ideas are relevant to the experience of dental care.

## Oral care as a life course project

In a previous paper we introduced the underlying theory of oral care as a life course project (Gibson et al., 2019). This theory was informed by grounded theory methodology underpinned with phenomenological reflections. Our goal was to explain how participants discussed embarking on a socially sustained, biographical project to keep their teeth into later life. Such findings are not new, after all it has been recognised for some time in social histories of dentistry that the profession emerged out of the 'personal care market' (Davis, 1980). One of the early sociologists of oral health and dentistry, Peter Davis, argued that the single primary reason respondents gave at that time for attending the dentist on a regular basis was the retention of teeth in whatever form[3] (Davis, 1987). It is now well established and within the dental literature where there are clear examples of patients doing anything to retain even their last couple of teeth (Cronin et al., 2009). The ability to participate in such a project requires meeting certain preconditions including having access to the social world of dentistry and then recognising the values, practices and common sense structures that people encounter as they do so. To study oral care as a life course project involves studying such common sense constructs. Within sociological research, these are termed 'ideal typifications' (Schutz, 1962, 1967).[4] One such ideal typification present in mouth talk is 'having work done'.

## 'Having work done'

> I'd had quite a lot of dental work because I remember when I first came to Sheffield … he absolutely blitzed my mouth and took all my fillings out and replaced them. And I've got this, I've got a bridge here and he did that and you know, I had a lot of dental work done then and it was all replacements … In fact, I had the majority of work done as a younger person then as I got sort of into my 30s (Sylvia, 72).

Sylvia represents a typical member of the 'heavy metal generation' (Ettinger, 1993) in dentistry. This group of patients were the first to encounter dentistry in the era of the high-speed handpiece. The narrative goes that dentists got the ability to work on teeth and enthusiastically engaged in 'drilling and filling'. This resulted in a generation who have wide-reaching experiences of dental treatment and who have also come to embody this era in dentistry. 'Having work done' involves there being 'objects' for the work to be done '*on*'. This includes teeth, gums, jaws and previous (sometimes failing) dental work. Having work done also involves objects to be working towards,[5] fillings, bridges, crowns and implants, amongst other things. Having work done is therefore filled with the 'intention' to have objects worked on, produced and fixed within the mouth. In this sense then the 'body work' of dentistry involves 'in-order to' (Schutz, 1989) projects that are performed directly on the body. It also may or may not arise from an important precondition, the 'dys-appearing body' (Leder, 1990).

> I can't fault the dentist at all but there's a great big gap between these two at the end and all the food goes between it. I've got those wooden toothpicks. And say you go out for a meal you're doing this with your tongue to try and get the food out all the time. So, I said to her last time, 'You know I've got all this' and I said, 'It still hurts a little bit, this tooth, underneath'. (Doris, 83)

Such 'embodied' 'dysappearances' (Leder, 1990) of oral disorders and 'dys-functions'[6] have long been the subject of oral and dental research. They comprise disruptions to the flow of everyday experience in the form of, pain, gaps in teeth with attendant problems such as difficulties speaking and food getting stuck between teeth. Whilst we have noted this before (Gibson et al., 2019; Kettle et al., 2019; Warren et al., 2020), such ideas have yet to be fully integrated into emerging sociological theorisations of oral health and dentistry. Yet such points are already well-established within dentistry as a whole, where the impact of oral conditions has formed the basis of a large body of research around the presence and 'dys-appearances' of the mouth in everyday life in the guise of work on oral health-related quality of life (Locker and Gibson, 2006; Locker and Gibson, 2005; Locker and Allen, 2007; Slade, 1997). It is also central to much of the research in restorative dentistry looking at the impact of removal of partial dentures and dental implants (Cronin et al., 2009; Trulsson et al., 2002; Grey et al., 2013).

Whilst the 'dys-appearance' of the mouth and teeth appears to set a negative tone for the work of dentists, it encapsulates the positive goal of *returning the body to its pre-reflective harmony with the world* (Schutz, 1967; Gallagher, 1995). Success is therefore judged on the basis to which this is achieved.[7] Such re-flections form a sizeable chunk of research in restorative dentistry effectively also providing a whole series of useful data on the goals of treatment and what good treatment outcomes look like (Grey et al., 2013). For example, Osman et al. (2014) interviewed a sample of 16 participants (3 females and 13 males) utilising semi-structured interviews and focused thematic analysis on their accounts of implanted partial overdentures. One of the participants stated:

> I can eat my pineapple chunks now; they don't shift all over the place. No, it's just so convenient. They're just like, probably having normal teeth back again. That's what I find with them, you eat and they don't jump up and down and get stuff stuck underneath them when you're out at a restaurant.
> (Participant 8 in Osman et al., 2014, p. 589)

Such reporting on the 'restoration' of functions such as smiling, eating and improvements in social confidence are said to lead to a renewed sense of at-tractiveness, self-esteem and confidence in everyday life (Osman et al., 2014). Dentistry's focus has traditionally been on improving functional status and so-cial confidence as markers of success. The sociology of oral care over the life course adds to this by identifying first, that dentists *and* patients are simulta-neously engaged in this 'body work', and second, that the goal of this work is the development of ongoing 'body-mouth schemas' (Merleau-Ponty, 2002; Crossley, 1995; Staudigl, 2007). The concept of body schema refers to non-conscious pre-reflective schemas that result in various bodily postures and movements that, in turn, incorporate the environment into our experience (Head, 1926; Gallagher, 1995). In oral care as a life course project 'having work done' involves at-tempting to 'restore' the pre-reflective harmony between the 'body-mouth schema' and the world. As such, then, the success of dentists is judged on the basis to which this work returns the 'body-mouth schema' back to its pre-reflective state. These findings can be integrated into a sociology of oral health and dentistry and suggests that we should renew our focus on the embodied dental subject and these 'body-mouth schemas'. In the next section, we pick this up and demonstrate that a large part of mouth talk is precisely about such 'body-mouth schemas'.

### Embodiment and dental work

> The bottom veneer on this side (participant's left), not the veneer, the cap, you know, where it's thinner at the bottom where it moulds around your teeth. Some of that cracked off. And I think this may possibly have been a result of my bite being changed when I had the veneers and things done at the top. I used to have a very big oversized ugly tooth there (top left for dentist). So that was taken down and the crown made more to match the size of the others. But of course that big tooth used to be the first point of contact when the teeth came together. So as that had moved, I think this side (right for dentist) now happened to be the first point of contact … she took the cap off to see whether it was good enough to redo it, but it wasn't so she extracted it under injection. She had to cut the tooth in half and then pull each half out. And I did go a bit faint while she was doing that. (Chuckles). It wasn't so much that she was inflicting any pain on me because I'd had the injection. I think I was just worrying about if it all broke up and she might have to go 'through the flesh'. (Kathleen, 69)

As we can see, an adjustment was made to Kathleen's teeth because of how her teeth looked and felt. Adjustments to an oversized tooth led to a change in her bite and this then had consequences for her other teeth, leading to a further investigation of an existing crown that subsequently was damaged in the treatment. A consequence of this was the eventual removal of the tooth. Like 'whack-a-mole',[8] the dentist was engaged in a constant struggle to maintain work and fix past work that was damaged from the treatment performed within Kathleen's mouth. Here, the primary focus of the dentist's intervention is 'embodied' and involves working on teeth in a three dimensional cavity – the mouth. The work itself results in adjustment to the patient's 'body-mouth schema', making the outcomes of treatment unpredictable. Such 'body-mouth schemas' constantly move and change in response to treatment and disease processes. Kathleen's primary reference point in her narrative is the embodied experience of having this work done as well as the ongoing struggle to maintain her unstable 'body-mouth schema'. Cronin et al. (2009) also provide some excellent examples of this focus:

> I went back into the dental hospital to have my gum reduced, cut down and I don't know what else he did, you'd have to talk to him, but it was more,

you know he was doing a lot of scraping, it took about half an hour or 45 min of work, so that there would be enough depth, height, you know, to have the crown attached.

(Esther, 55–64 years in Cronin et al., 2009, p. 139)

Research in restorative dentistry has indeed focused on the bodily space of the mouth and teeth. Dental work manipulates the three dimensional bite. This involves a fundamental disruption to the pre-reflective flow of everyday life – to the 'body-mouth schema'. The mouth has to be presented for treatment, held in place for the dentist to 'scrape, 'gouge' and 'cut'.

And I have to say the *first*, the very *first* part of it when he started going into the jaw bone, I actually thought I would never have done this if I knew what I was going to experience, it was horrible, a horrible feeling and all that. But you know, like everything you get over it and will I do it again? Yes, if I have to.

(Emily, 45–54 years in Cronin et al., 2009, p. 140)

In what follows, Yvonne had gone through significant amounts of dental treatment in the past. Some of her teeth continued to decline. In her narrative, she jokingly refers to herself as a failing patient. But we can also see that previous work acted as a condition for further work but also how this further work threatens to undo the previous work.

I was perfectly all right when I went on Wednesday morning for this check-up, and ever since, it's gotten worse. It's sensitive, so yeah, so I've got a toothache now. I think … well, I've been thinking that tooth is probably going to go eventually. It's been griping for about a year, off and on, slightly, but yeah, I know the signs. I think it's a root, probably. But it comes and goes and I try not to eat on it. That'll mean that'll disrupt the denture again, so here we go again, you know. I don't know why he doesn't send me to another dentist. I don't know why he doesn't beg another dentist to take this horrible patient off him. (Laughter). (Yvonne, 66)

Yvonne's 'body-mouth schema' is unstable leading to the loss of the pre-reflective harmony between her body and everyday life.

Research in dentistry has highlighted the sensitivity people can have to wearing removable partial dentures (RPDs) which can be challenging to live with (Smith, Entwistle, and Nuttall, 2005). But our data indicate that this can also be true for implant supported dentures. As Frances indicates these can also require patients to undergo significant periods of adaptation:

It was just painful. They have to sew up the gums. Horrible, with a huge needle, big fat needle, that long, you know, and thread. When you see it coming at you, (Laughter). It was really horrible. But you think you have to grin and bear it. So, I did.

[Researcher] How did they feel when they were first ... ?

Well, at first, they feel as though they don't belong to you at all. It takes ages at least a year, at least a year, for them to feel as though it's something foreign in your mouth. Even now, because I can't feel anything. It's totally dead. But that's all right.

[Researcher] Is that ever an issue with say eating or drinking anything?

I'm very careful about eating apples or anything like that because I'm so worried that something could go wrong. Because you have to go back. I think it's two years after they're in. I've had them 10 years so far, for check-ups. And they said, 'You just have to be that bit careful'. So, I never eat an apple with my front teeth. No (Frances, 79)

Frances' account demonstrates enduring a significant change in 'body-mouth schema'. This involved the excruciating horror of having her gums sewn with a large needle, albeit told with a sense of humour. Undergoing such treatment is presented as an achievement. Frances then explains how she adapted to her new 'body-mouth schema' adjusting what she was eating. The consequences of the 'body-mouth schema' therefore went beyond her mouth and teeth to affect her diet.

Dental research suggests that providing personal support or providing video or written self-help aids can enable adaptation to such new 'body-mouth schemas' (Smith, Entwistle, and Nuttall, 2005; Klages, Esch, and Wehrbein, 2005; Szentpetery et al., 2005; Wostmann et al., 2005). What is clear from this literature is that there is no underlying theory behind how such 'fit' and 'function' is developed; much of this research is service oriented, focused on satisfaction and oral health-related quality of life. Exley et al. (2009) focused on the costs of implants but did not have much to say about the underlying embodied experience of care (Exley et al., 2009). Here we show that 'having work done' involves considerable time and effort on the part of patients in making themselves subject to the work and then adapting to the consequences of the work itself. It is not just dentists' labour that is engaged in 'having work done', patients engage in considerable amounts of work too.

Successful adaptations result in a sense of achievement associated with arriving at the destiny of older age with some 'natural' teeth intact. This leads to a hypothesis that the more someone has experienced 'having work done' during their life course, the greater the sense of achievement when they get the destiny of older age with some of their 'own teeth' intact. Even when interventions failed, participants could still report success. Indeed some might pay significant amounts of money to have the ultimate piece of work done – dental implants. Frances indicated:

When they crumbled. What made me decide? It was hideously expensive. I think it cost £ 6,000 to have the three teeth done, £ 2,000 a tooth. But one of my friends rang me up and said, 'Look. I've got to insist. You must have implants'. And she said, 'It's the best thing I've ever done in my life'. She'd had them and I'm so grateful that she did say that, so very, very grateful. Because there've been nobody ... I mean, you can see they're incredibly good ... they're doctors of dentistry, not just bachelors but doctors of dentistry. I mean, they were really at the top end of the profession. And I thought they did a fantastic job on it. I don't think you'd know, would you? (Frances, 79)

In this instance, the credentials of the dentist acted as a significant factor in Frances' decision to have the implants placed. This is despite a ban on using the title Dr in the United Kingdom.[9] Clearly, there are conditions surrounding 'having work done' that relate to the knowledge of the dentist and their authority whereby dimensions of power play a significant role in the process. This has been the subject of considerable discussion in the social science of oral health and health care (Freeman, Whelton, and Gibson, 2010; Nettleton, 1992, 1989, 1994) and these data indicate that a much wider debate about the power dynamics underpinning these interactions should be of interest to a sociology of oral health and dentistry. This is especially the case when the expense of treatment is so high that there are 'vulnerabilities' associated with the situation in which patients find themselves. The case of Gladys reveals why this is so important.

I decided to have an implant in a front tooth and I thought about it for a long time and then decided I would have it done ... I had no idea when I embarked on that journey that it would be so painful, so intrusive, and so bruising. I do bruise very easily, but the bruising was unbelievable. And I was unlucky inasmuch the bone had deteriorated and I think I'd had an infection in the bone and so the bone when they were inserting the implant had to be dug out and then built up again and I think that caused considerably more problems than I might have had. So I think, you know, it wasn't just a straightforward implant. There were complications. But I certainly would hesitate greatly to ever embark on that again. And what I didn't realise until I happened to be having coffee with a friend and her tooth dropped out and she said, 'Oh dear, that's my implant. It keeps dropping out'. And I thought, 'Well, implant can't drop out'. But when I spoke to the dentist about it later, he said, 'Well, if you've got very receding gums', and I do suffer from receding gums as I think a great many older people do, but perhaps I'm worse, I don't know, that this can happen. And I had never been warned about that. And I believe that you can have to have, you know, considerable work done on implants within a number of years of them being done. And, you know, I was never warned about that, so I was really a bit cross when I found out. (Gladys, 78)

This case reveals that a central property of 'having work done' is the underlying 'vulnerabilities' associated with the intervention itself. First there is the need to undergo gouging, scraping, sucking and grinding. There are 'vulnerabilities' associated with dys-appearing body, disturbances to the 'body-mouth schema' and here we also have the 'vulnerabilities' associated with the potential to be exploited by dentists. We are not claiming that Gladys was exploited but are pointing out how the work she had done taken alongside the bad experiences of her friend have exposed her to her own 'vulnerability'. This, in turn, leads Gladys to have significant concern about her own implants. She went on to state:

> So now I'm extra careful to brush around my implant and hope that my receding gums are not receding any further. I think that's now currently my biggest worry, receding gums. (Gladys, 78)

This underlying 'vulnerability' is a key property of 'having work done'. It exposes the fundamentally embodied experience of oral disease and dental treatment. Aspects of these vulnerabilities have long been recognised as a part of the encounter with dental treatment. In dental research, this has been thematised with reference to the concepts of dental anxiety and phobia (Cibirka, Razzoog, and Lang, 1997; Klingberg and Broberg, 2007; Carrillo-Diaz et al., 2012; Keles et al., 2018). Yet this underlying vulnerability remains under-theorised in sociological accounts of oral health and dentistry. Vulnerability has been the subject of phenomenological reflection (Staudigl, 2007) where it has been examined in relation to the violations of bodily integrity. Staudigl (2007) argued that it is through 'violations' that our 'intentional openness to the world' is 'oppressed, expropriated and alienated by another person (or collective agency) whose action imposes relevancies that force the experiencing subject's exclusive attention'. He goes on to state:

> Inasmuch as this imposition implies the impossibility of withdrawing from that condition and maintaining a distance from one's non-intentional sensible immediacy – a distance wherein reflection becomes possible and henceforth meaning – this imposition causes pain, which consequently turns out to be a constitutive part of any violation.
>
> (Staudigl, 2007, p. 244)

'Having work done' can involve different types of violation: (1) spatial violation, when body space is restricted and constrained (while having work done); (2) temporal restriction, which may happen to one's living horizon so that what one thought was possible (having teeth in older age) is no longer possible; and finally (3) interpersonal violation, where individuals find themselves judged or stereotyped because of their oral and dental condition. Yet at the same time, these data provide an overwhelmingly positive picture whereby such violations can be overcome. The goal of 'having work done' is to return the 'body-mouth schema' to equilibrium. This then results in the sense of 'I can do this again' and so we get a cycle of dental work that progresses throughout life. This of course is reflected in the sense of achievement our participants had when they had kept their teeth into older age.

## Conclusion

This chapter provides a preliminary analysis of what it means to have work done in oral health and dentistry. 'Having work done' is a fundamental practice associated with oral care over the life course. The underlying construct of oral care over the life course is functionalist since it constructs the achievement of having teeth in older age to largely have resulted from participating in oral care practices. These practices are sustained by various organisational contexts in the 'social world of oral health' (Gibson et al., 2019). The underlying theory fits the accounts of older people in 'the significance of the mouth in older age study'. This chapter focuses on 'having work done' as one of the practices associated with this 'life-course project'.

'Having work done' demonstrates the importance of understanding the embodied nature of dental work and the centrality of bodily 'dys-appearances' to the everyday experience of oral health and health care for this group of people. These themes have been largely ignored by the sociology of oral health and dentistry, only recently being highlighted as part of the significance of mouth in older age study (Gibson et al., 2019; Kettle et al., 2019; Warren et al., 2020). In this chapter, we go further to demonstrate that the underlying purpose of oral care is the constant modification of 'body-mouth schemas' designed to return the body to its pre-reflective state. 'Having work done' is therefore presented as an 'in-order to' 'body-mouth' project aimed at restoring this balance through the work of the dentist and patient. Consequences of this work are that it can lead to violations of body-space, body temporality and interpersonal relationships. Yet here we find that the underlying story is overwhelmingly positive. 'Having work done' over such a sustained period of time brought with it a palpable sense of achievement. A fundamental dimension, therefore, of the underlying body-mouth project is this embodied achievement.

These analyses demonstrate that 'body work' is not just accomplished by professionals but that in dental care it clearly involves a degree of 'work' in controlling the body in order to receive 'care'. In addition, clearly the work that is being done by dentists is on the bodies of patients requires 'looking after' and this, in turn, involves the need for patients to continue the work of daily care when they are not at the dentist. What results from the body work of the dentist becomes the body work of the patient, leading to intense inter-relationships that are not particularly well covered by the concept of 'body work'. We therefore will need to move beyond such kinds of sociology to find a better 'fit' for our conceptualisation of 'what is going on' (Glaser, 1967, 1978) in such relationships. Likewise these reflections do not touch on how the politics of the dental industry can have profound impacts on these relationships (see Chapter 3 in this volume).

There are several future directions that this analysis might take. First, there is room for further study of the relationship between embodied dys-appearance and the success of dental work. Significant research has been conducted in dentistry around oral pain and the 'discomfort' of removal of partial dentures in prosthodontics (Klages, Esch, and Wehrbein, 2005; Szentpetery et al., 2005; Wostmann et al., 2005; Strassburger, Kerschbaum, and Heydecke, 2006; McGuire, Millar, and Lindsay, 2007; Fueki, Yoshida, and Igarashi, 2011). This research reflects the dominance of functionalist perspectives in oral biology, and the social and behavioural sciences in dentistry as a whole. Whilst this chapter is not the place to provide a fuller analysis of what this means, a few comments are worth making.

In the sociology of health and illness, there is a tendency to relegate functionalism to the dustbin of history; this is because there is a widespread perception that the structural functionalism of Parsons (Parsons, 1949) has had its day. This seems odd. After all, functionalism remains dominant in psychology, it clearly underpins the biopsychosocial models associated with Oral Health Related Quality of Life (OHRQoL) (Locker, 1988; MacEntee, 2006) and there remain functionalist theories in sociology that have had more success in dealing with the complexity of modern society (Luhmann, 1995). Even those approaches that start out critiquing early functionalist accounts of the emergence of the dental profession are themselves based on functionalist accounts of power (Nettleton, 1988, 1991, 1992; Brenner, 1994).

There remains little or no theory building in dentistry with which to grapple with these themes, most work is based on further review of existing approaches with little or no real examination of the underlying theoretical assumptions or 'fit' of existing accounts. Theory pieces of the kind being articulated in this chapter are only the beginning of the process of making sense of dental work. It may well be that 'biopsychosocial' functionalisms are inadequate to explain the complexity of 'what is going on' in dental work and how this intersects with the body of the patient as a thinking feeling subject, experiencing and becoming responsible for the work of the dentist which is, in turn, incorporated into patients' 'body-mouth schemas'. As a consequence, further theory building is required that fits these relationships more closely.

Following the principles of grounded theory (Gibson and Hartman, 2014), the challenge we face is the type of data that we have and the limitations of these data. Although the narratives in the study were rich, we have yet to examine the actual performance of work as it is done in the present. Other data is needed based on direct observations of what it means to have work done *in the present* rather than being derived from memory which itself can be problematic to analyse (Fuchs, 2012). There is a move in dentistry to go beyond simply relying on interview data with a range of methods being used (Horne et al., 2020). Data looking at particular treatments focused on the 3D space of the mouth and teeth along with resulting adjustments to the 'body-mouth schema' are warranted. Such work could draw on ethnographic methodologies bolstered with interviews of both the dentist and the patient. It may also be that more careful analysis of 'body-mouth schema' drawing on experimental methods and neuroscience may produce alternative interdisciplinary perspectives relevant to dental research.

## Notes

1 The original study on which this chapter is based was funded by GlaxoSmithKline. This funding has in no way affected what the authors would like to say about the data and there are no conflicts of interest in the writing of this chapter.
2 The background study along with details of the sample are provided in previous papers (see Kettle et al., 2019; Warren et al., 2020; Gibson et al., 2019).
3 The prevention of the loss of teeth at the time came a distant second.
4 We believe that the study of such constructs is entirely in keeping with the pragmatic tradition in grounded theory.
5 Corresponding to 'in-order to' motives or projects (Schutz, 1967).
6 Leder (1990) pointed out that the body is usually taken for granted as a frame for everyday life; it 'disappears' and is only brought to attention when there are disturbances in the flow of everyday consciousness through pain or disfunction. In such instances, it 'dys-appears'; this means it appears in a disturbed form.
7 Except, perhaps, with respect to aesthetics where the goal is to transform the very nature of the pre-reflective state by elevating or adjusting the appearance of the teeth and therefore the relationship between the participant and their teeth. The details of such reflections are nonetheless beyond the scope of this paper.
8 'Whack-a-mole' is a game in which toy moles appear at random and players use a mallet to attempt to hit them back into their holes. Used colloquially, the term signifies a repetitive and commonly futile task.
9 See Lala in this volume.

## References

Brenner, N. (1994) 'Foucault's new functionalism', *Theory and Society*, 23(5), pp. 679–709.
Carrillo-Diaz, M., Crego, A., Armfield, J. and Romero, M. (2012) 'Self-assessed oral health, cognitive vulnerability and dental anxiety in children: testing a mediational model', *Community Dentistry and Oral Epidemiology*, 40(1), pp. 8–16.
Cibirka, R., Razzoog, M. and Lang, B. (1997) 'Critical evaluation of patient responses to dental implant therapy', *Journal of Prosthetic Dentistry*, 78(6), pp. 574–581.
Cronin, M., Meaney, S., Jepson, N. and Allen, P. (2009) 'A qualitative study of trends in patient preferences for the management of the partially dentate state', *Gerodontology*, 26(2), 137–142.
Crossley, N. (1995) 'Merleau-Ponty, the elusive body and carnal sociology', *Body & Society*, 1(1), pp. 43–63.
Davis, P. (1980) *The social context of dentistry*. London: Croom Helm.
Davis, P. (1987) *Introduction to the sociology of dentistry: comparative perspectives*. Otago: University of Otago Press.
Ettinger, R. (1993) 'Cohort differences among aging populations: a challenge for the dental profession', *Special Care in Dentistry*, 13(1), pp. 19–26.

Exley, C., Rousseau, N., Steele, J., Finch, T., et al. (2009) 'Paying for treatments? Influences on negotiating clinical need and decision-making for dental implant treatment', *BMC Health Services Research*, 9(7).

Freeman, R., Whelton, H. and Gibson, B. (2010) 'Toothbrushing rules: power dynamics and toothbrushing in children', *Social Science and Dentistry*, 1(1), pp. 37–47.

Fuchs, T. (2012) 'The phenomenology of body memory', in: Koch, S., Fuchs, T., Summa, M., and Muller, C. (ed.) *Body Memory, Metaphor and Movement*. Amsterdam: John Benjamins Publishing Company.

Fueki, K., Yoshida, E. and Igarashi, Y. (2011) 'A structural equation model relating objective and subjective masticatory function and oral health-related quality of life in patients with removable partial dentures', *Journal of Oral Rehabilitation*, 38(2), pp. 86–94.

Gallagher, S. (1995) 'Body Schema and Intentionality', in: Bermudez, J., Marcel, A., and Eilan, N. (eds.) *The Body and the Self*. Boston, USA: MIT Press.

Gibson, B. and Hartman, J. (2014) *Rediscovering Grounded Theory*. London: Sage.

Gibson, B., Kettle, J., Robinson, P., Walls, A., et al. (2019) 'Oral care as a life course project: A qualitative grounded theory study', *Gerodontology*, 36, pp. 8–17.

Gimlin, D. (2002) *Body work: beauty and self-image in American culture*. Berkeley, CA: University of California Press.

Gimlin, D. (2007) 'What is 'body work'? A review of the literature', *Sociology Compass*, 1(1), pp. 353–370.

Glaser, B. (1978) *Theoretical sensitivity: advances in the methodology of grounded theory*. California: Sociology Press.

Glaser, B. and Strauss, A. (1967) *The Discovery of Grounded Theory*. Chicago: Aldine Publishing Company.

Grey, E., Harcourt, D., O'sullivan, D., Buchanan, H., et al. (2013) 'A qualitative study of patients' motivations and expectations for dental implants', *British Dental Journal*, 214, pp. E1–E1.

Head, H. (1926) *Aphasia and kindred disorders of speech, vol 1*. Cambridge: Cambridge University Press.

Hochschild, A. (1983) *The managed heart: the commercialization of human feeling*. Berkeley, CA: University of California Press.

Horne, P., Foster Page, L., Leichter, J., Knight, E., et al. (2020). 'Psychosocial aspects of periodontal disease diagnosis and treatment: A qualitative study', *Journal of Clinical Periodontology*, 47, pp. 941–951.

Kang, M. (2003) 'The managed hand: the commercialization of bodies and emotions in Korean immigrant-owned nail aalons', *Gender and Society*, 17(6), pp. 820–839.

Keles, S., Abacigil, F., Adana, F., Yesilfidan, D., et al. (2018) The association between dental anxiety and oral health related quality of life among individuals with mild intellectual disability', *Meandros Medical and Dental Journal*, 19, pp. 9–18.

Kettle, J., Warren, L., Robinson, P., Walls, A., et al. (2019) 'I didn't want to pass that onto my child, being afraid to go to the dentist': making sense of oral health through narratives of connectedness over the life course', *Sociology of Health and Illness*, 41(4), pp. 658–672.

Klages, U., Esch, M. and Wehrbein, H. (2005) 'Oral health impact in patients wearing removable prostheses: Relations to somatization, pain sensitivity, and body consciousness', *International Journal of Prosthodontics*, 18(2), pp. 106–111.

Klingberg, G. and Broberg, A. (2007) 'Dental fear/anxiety and dental behaviour management problems in children and adolescents: a review of prevalence and concomitant psychological factors', *International Journal of Paediatric Dentistry*, 17(6), pp. 391–406.

Leder, D. (1990) *The absent body*. London: The University of Chicago Press.

Locker, D. (1988) 'Measuring oral health: a conceptual framework', *Community Dental Health*, 5(1), pp. 3–18.

Locker, D. and Gibson B. (2006) 'The concept of positive health: a review and commentary on its application in dental research', *Community Dentistry and Oral Epidemiology*, 34(3), pp. 161–173.

Locker, D. and Allen, F. (2007) 'What do measures of 'oral health-related quality of life' measure?', *Community Dentistry and Oral Epidemiology*, 35(6), pp. 401–411.

Locker, D. and Gibson, B. (2005) 'Discrepancies between self-ratings of and satisfaction with oral health in two older adult populations', *Community Dentistry and Oral Epidemiology*, 33(4), pp. 280–288.

Luhmann, N. (1995) *Social systems*. Stanford, California: Stanford University Press,.

MacEntee, M. I. (2006) 'An existential model of oral health from evolving views on health, function and disability', *Community Dental Health*, 23, pp. 5–14.

McGuire, L. C., Millar, K. and Lindsay, S. (2007) 'A treatment trial of an information package to help patients accept new dentures', *Behaviour Research and Therapy*, 45, pp. 1941–1948.

Merleau-Ponty, M. (2002) *Phenomenology of perception*. London: Routledge & Keegan Paul.

Nettleton, S. (1988) 'Protecting a vulnerable margin - towards an analysis of how the mouth came to be separated from the body', *Sociology of Health & Illness*, 10(2), pp. 156–169.

Nettleton, S. (1989) 'Power and the location of pain and fear in dentistry and the creation of a dental subject', *Social Science and Medicine*, 29(10), pp. 1183–1190.

Nettleton, S. (1991) 'Wisdom, diligence and teeth: discursive practices and the creation of mothers', *Sociology of Health & Illness*, 13(1), pp. 98–111.

Nettleton, S. (1992) *Power, pain and dentistry*. Buckingham: Open University Press.

Nettleton, S. (1994) 'Inventing mouths: disciplinary power and dentistry', in: Jones, C. and Porter, R. (eds.) *Reassessing Foucault: Power, Medicine and the Body*. London: Routledge.

Osman, R., Morgaine, K., Duncan, W., Swain, M., et al. (2014) 'Patients' perspectives on zirconia and titanium implants with a novel distribution supporting maxillary and mandibular overdentures: a qualitative study', *Clinical Oral Implants Research*, 25, pp. 587–597.

Parsons, T. (1949) *The structure of social action*. New York: Glencoe Free Press.

Schutz, A. (1962) *Collected papers I: the problem of social reality*. London: Kluwer Academic Publishers.

Schutz, A. (1967) *The phenomenology of the social world*. Evanston, Illinois: Northwestern University Press.

Schutz, A. (1989) *The structures of the lifeworld Volume II*. Evanston, Illinois: Northwestern University Press.

Slade, G. (1997) 'Measuring oral health and quality of life', in: Slade, G. (ed.) *Measuring oral health and quality of life*. North Carolina: Department of Dental Ecology.

Smith, P., Entwistle, V. and Nuttall, N. (2005) 'Patients' experiences with partial dentures: a qualitative study', *Gerodontology*, 22(4), pp. 187–192.

Staudigl, M. (2007) 'Towards a phenomenological theory of violence: reflections following Merleau-Ponty and Schütz', *Human Studies*, 30, pp. 233–253.

Strassburger, C., Kerschbaum, T. and Heydecke, G. (2006) 'Influence of implant and conventional prostheses on satisfaction and quality of life: A literature review. Part 2: Qualitative analysis and evaluation of the studies', *International Journal of Prosthodontics*, 19, pp. 339–348.

Szentpetery, A., John, M., Slade, G. and Setz, J. (2005) 'Problems reported by patients before and after prosthodontic treatment', *International Journal of Prosthodontics*, 18, pp. 124–131.

Trulsson, U., Engstrand, P., Berggren, U., Nannmark, U., et al. (2002) 'Edentulousness and oral rehabilitation: experiences from the patients' perspective', *European Journal of Oral Sciences*, 110, pp. 417–424.

Turner, B. S. (1984) *The body and society*. London: Basil Blackwell Publisher.

Twigg, J. (2000) 'Carework as a form of bodywork', *Ageing and Society*, 20(4), pp. 389–411.

Warren, L., Kettle, J., Gibson, B., Robinson, P., et al. (2020) 'I've got lots of gaps, but I want to hang on to the ones that I have': The ageing body, oral health and stories of the mouth', *Ageing and Society*, 40(6), pp. 1244–1266.

Wolkowitz, C. (2002) 'The social relations of body work', *Work, Employment and Society*, 16(3), pp. 495–508.

Wostmann, B., Budtz-Jorgensen, E., Jepson, N., Mushimoto, E., et al. (2005) 'Indications for removable partial dentures: A literature review', *International Journal of Prosthodontics*, 18, pp. 139–145.

# Part IV

# State, surveillance, and social justice

# 12 'Enlightened employers of labour?':[1] oral health in the British factory, 1890–1930

*Claire L. Jones*

## Introduction

In the current business world, the oral health of a company's workforce can have a significant impact on productivity. By the late 1980s, about 12 million work days were reportedly lost to dental causes in Britain (Feaver, 1988, p. 41). In Canada in 2013, over 40 million hours per year were reportedly lost due to dental problems and treatment, corresponding to productivity losses of over one billion dollars (Hayes et al., 2013, p. 1). It is therefore in the interests of both employers and employees for companies to provide some form of dental health welfare and indeed, many large companies do so under private medical insurance. But the inclusion of dental health in the occupational welfare provided by British businesses is a relatively recent phenomenon, as is the idea that good oral health is vital to maintain company productivity. Britain's large industrial cotton manufacturers were among the first employers to provide medical care for their workers from the late eighteenth century making them the first industrial paternalists. Yet, it was only from the late nineteenth century that large manufacturers began to recognise the mouth as important bodily organ separate from the rest of the body and began to provide their factory workers with oral health care. These manufacturers, alongside the state and the dental profession, became increasingly concerned that poor oral health was one of the leading reasons for absence from work, a growing number of sick days and was responsible for decreasing productivity. Indeed, tooth decay was so widespread in the late nineteenth century workplace and beyond that it was labelled 'the people's disease' (e.g., Terman, 1913, p. 11. See also Strong's chapter in this volume). Accordingly, manufacturers across different industries increasingly employed dentists to inspect workers' mouths, promote oral hygiene and provide dental treatment. And yet, despite its importance, historians have largely overlooked the development of oral health care as a part of occupational health and industrial welfarism. The growing literature on the history of occupational health mentions oral health only briefly, if at all (Bartrip, 2002; Harrison, 1996; Long, 2011; Long and Marland, 2009; Russell, 1991; Weindling, 1985).

Instead, histories of industrial dental welfare have tended to be subsumed into more narrowly defined histories of the dental profession, often written by dental

DOI: 10.4324/9781003047674-16

professionals themselves. In aligning industrial dentistry with professional, medical and technological developments within dentistry, these histories generally provide a teleology; they accept at face value the testimony of contemporary dental practitioners who argued that industrial dentistry was adopted by 'enlightened employers of labour' (Anon, 1922c, p. 926) for the wholesale good of workers, the nation and its citizens and was a development that filled the gap in universal dental provision until the foundation of the National Health Service in 1948 (e.g., Gelbier, 1999; Feaver, 1988). The adoption of this progressive perspective is unsurprising, given the fact that most available evidence in the form of professional journals, correspondence and company reports all present an enlightened vision of saving the teeth of Britain's workforce. But by incorporating employee voices into the narrative, we learn that dental welfarism had a much wider and multi-sided set of significances.

In analysing industrial dental welfarism in the late nineteenth and early twentieth centuries in its broader context of public and occupational health, this chapter demonstrates how its introduction was squarely in the interests of dental practitioners and factory bosses. Indeed, its introduction was far from inevitable and was not solely a response to a perceived need by the enlightened. As we will see, regardless of any benefit to individual workers, industrial dental welfare was not only a tool used to enhance company productivity but also aimed to make the workforce politically compliant, thus mirroring concomitant state attempts to survey and regulate the public's health. Much of this oral health provision then centred on power relations and represented employer attempts to control the industrial worker's mouth. Drawing on Foucault's concepts of governmentality and biopower, historians and sociologists have long discussed power relations of this kind as forming a central part of public health with its emphasis on prevention (Armstrong, 1983; Lupton, 1995). Moreover, as sociologists have long argued, the mouth, as the boundary between the internal and external body, is a body part that is uniquely placed to become regulated and controlled (Nettleton, 1992. See also Chapter 10 and 11 in this volume). As employers, dentists and the state began to argue, the industrial worker's mouth was the gateway to the rest of the body and a barometer of general bodily health; its control had far reaching implications for not only the overall health of the population but of the body politic. However, as we will also see, such control was not always achieved. The processes of control were messier than has typically been acknowledged and some employees resisted attempts at control of their mouths. Employee opinion is, of course, notoriously difficult to uncover; the records of such are rarely extant. Nonetheless, some insight into worker reception of dental welfare provision will be gleaned through neglected sources, some of which demonstrate that employees rejected dental welfarism at worst and were apathetic about it at best.[2] In order to facilitate a comparative analysis, this chapter will chronologically outline the development of dental welfare by drawing on prominent early examples within three different British industries – match-making, confectionery and biscuit-making.

## Phossy jaw in the match factory, c. 1890–1912

As various acts of legislation began to place oral health and hygiene increasingly under state and medical control in the late nineteenth century, the question of oral health in the factory first came to prominence in Britain's 25 match factories. Under the Public Health Act of 1875 and the Factory and Workshops Acts of 1878, 1883, 1891 and 1895, medical officers of health and sanitary and factory inspectors began to survey the oral health of Britain's 4,300 match factory workers, prompted by the presence of phosphorous necrosis (or 'phossy jaw' as it became commonly known). Since the 1830s, match making had involved dipping wooden splints into white or yellow phosphorous; the chemical reaction it fostered when matches were struck produced the yellow flame, but phosphorous was also highly poisonous. Workers, particularly those who dipped matches over sustained periods of time in poorly ventilated work rooms, suffered from painful inflammation, putrid abscesses on the face, mouth and gums and disintegration of the jaw; some died as a result. Treatment involved tooth and bone extraction. Poor oral health was widespread in the match factories; workers were described as being 'of the poorest and most down-trodden appearance' and dental caries in particular were thought to predispose individuals to the condition (Squire, 1927, p. 55). Much state, medical and employer emphasis then rested on preventing caries through mouth surveillance and the promotion of self-regulation of the mouth through oral hygiene.

While the reported number of cases each year remained relatively low by the 1890s (estimated at about 1 per cent of the workforce), phossy jaw's identification as an industrial disease with horrific symptoms made it a powerful weapon in the political struggles around working conditions, welfare and state regulation (Harrison, 1996, p. 68). The match factory worker's mouth was at the centre of these struggles. Public and state attention mostly focused on Bryant and May, Britain's largest match maker with its factory in London's East End. The company's poor reputation as an employer with non-existent welfare provision had been highlighted by the infamous Match Girl Strike of 1888, during which women employees walked out of its factory in protest at low wages and the firm's system of fines.[3] Sensational stories of phossy jaw at the factory in the local and national press further blemished the company's reputation. The *Star*, in particular, not only revealed the firm's poor working conditions but also exposed its cover-up and underreporting of cases, resulting in a widespread feeling of injustice that the firm's owners were profiting from the sweated labour of their workers (Emsley, 2000, p. 106). Bryant and May also threatened employees with non-payment if they dared to report phossy jaw cases (Harrison, 1996, p. 68). The Salvation Army was so concerned about conditions in British match making that it established its own factory in 1891 to produce 'safety' matches made from the non-poisonous red phosphorous, although the continued popularity of 'strike anywhere' matches with white or yellow phosphorous meant that the venture was commercially unsuccessful and was taken over by Bryant and May in 1901. New legislation in 1892 and 1896 required match factories to provide adequate ventilation, washing facilities and report cases of phossy jaw to the factory inspectorate, although the cover-up of cases continued (Satre, 1982). At its own expense, Bryant and May employed a dentist, C. Laurence Gill, to regularly examine and treat workers' teeth. By the end of 1898, over 450 of the firm's 1,300 workforce had been inspected and 104 received dental treatment and were subsequently certified as having sound mouths (Thorpe, Oliver and Cunningham, 1899, p. 86).

Similarly, The Diamond Match Company, Bryant and May's biggest rival and Britain's second-largest match producer, feared the adverse publicity from phossy jaw and stated that it was 'so great a source of continuous anxiety that the directors resolved that they must definitely and absolutely prevent the disease or give up the industry' (Thorpe, Oliver and Cunningham, 1899, p. 145). As an American company, it drew on oral health measures already established in the United States. Westerton, the Company's dentist, examined and treated the mouths of factory workers, while the Company required workers to have the appropriate dental work carried out at their own expense. The firm paid the worker's wages for the period of time they were incapacitated from dental treatment and provided artificial teeth where necessary. The Company also urged its employees to thoroughly cleanse the mouth, teeth and gums after meals, using a tooth brush with borax and Castile soap-powder every morning and evening in their homes. Tooth brushes and tooth powder were supplied free (Thorpe, Oliver and Cunningham, 1899, p. 17).

By the time the Home Office began its inquiry into the use of phosphorous and its health impact on the match making workforce in 1898, both the Diamond Match Company and Bryant and May could demonstrate their provision of dental welfare. With input from leading dental public health advocate George Cunningham, the 1899 *Report* from the inquiry highlighted the excellent facilities 'voluntarily' introduced by the firms and called the companies pioneers (Thorpe, Oliver and Cunningham, 1899, pp. 18, 86). The *Report* also offered fourteen recommendations to Britain's other 23 match factories, including the employment of a resident dentist, the employment of workers with sound teeth, the installation of hot and cold-water basins and soap, and a regime of systematic gargling with an antiseptic mouthwash, as well as introducing measures to ensure worker compliance, such as erecting instructive notices around the factory. Many of these recommendations were turned into rules in revised Factory Acts.

But while dental welfare became common to British match factories by the turn of the twentieth century, it did not transform the industry nor the overall oral health of the workforce and thus was not a successful exercise in worker coercion. Small firms remained unconvinced that the financial outlay for dental welfare was economically beneficial and were unhappy with the state meddling in their private affairs; they resented the factory dentist and saw him, his office and equipment as a financial burden and suffered reduced earnings from the reduction in working hours when individuals were being examined and treated, and thus only provided the bare minimum required by law (Anon, 1899).

Similarly, not all dentists were convinced of the benefits of promoting oral hygiene in the factory; dentists often saw workers as the impediment to their own good oral health. Westerton, of The Diamond Match Company, stated that giving toothbrushes to workers had proven to be no good whatsoever because the teeth of these workers from the working-class districts of Liverpool were in such a bad state to begin with (Thorpe, Oliver and Cunningham, 1899, p. 148). Gill estimated that only 5 per cent of the Bryant and May factory had sound teeth, reflective of the poor oral health of the population of the East End more widely (and also of army recruits for World War One, as demonstrated by Strong in Chapter 9 in this volume). Cunningham stated, 'To my mind, the only matter for wonder is not that they [match factory workers] suffer from necrosis, but that so many of them escape' (Thorpe, Oliver and Cunningham, 1899, p. 208). Older women employees were particularly susceptible to poor oral health, partly because they were less likely than men and younger workers to admit to it for fear of having all of their teeth removed (Thorpe, Oliver and Cunningham, 1899, p. 86).

Moreover, there is little evidence to suggest that individual workers appreciated the introduction of dental welfare. Visits to factory dentists, while high in number, were compulsory and do little to highlight worker enthusiasm. The 1899 *Report* recognised that compulsory dentistry 'was not likely to be welcome by all the persons employed' and found that the majority of the hundred strong workforce at Albright & Wilson's phosphorous factory in Oldbury, Birmingham, objected to oral examinations and refused to clean their teeth (as well as their hands), resulting in the company's abandonment of compulsory preventive measures (p. 134). Women workers at Bryant and May would not 'submit to the extraction of their teeth' and potential female employees were deterred from applying for available factory positions as word spread through the East End of the factory's introduction of a compulsory dental examination on admittance, making it difficult for the firm to have a full workforce (Thorpe, Oliver and Cunningham, 1899, pp. 86, 182). Some Bryant and May workers suffered from phossy jaw after having teeth removed by practitioners outside the factory before returning to work, which went against company rules to not return to work after tooth extraction until the wound had healed, given the increased susceptibility to necrosis. Periodic dental inspection also prompted some Glasgow factory workers to take strike action, the very action firms wished to avoid (Bartrip, 2002, p. 211).

Bryant and May and The Diamond Match Company amalgamated in 1901. In the subsequent decades, the enlarged firm obtained a reputation as a prominent welfarist employer and argued that its provision of dental welfare, alongside other forms of welfare, had helped to increase productivity and workers' use of freely distributed toothbrushes and toothpaste had led to a reduction in sickness days (Marshall, 1912, p. 6). But its introduction of dental welfare was not primarily motivated by benevolent intentions; it was the adverse publicity of having an employee suffer or die from phossy jaw and the threat of further industrial unrest that had prompted it and thus represented a method of worker coercion (Fitzgerald, 1989, p. 52). Demonstrating the limitations of dental welfare in the match making industry, oral hygiene practices were actively resisted by some workers. It was the decline in the commercial popularity of the 'strike-anywhere' match, the state's prohibition of white phosphorous from 1910, as well as growing automation in production, that had a larger impact on the decline of phossy jaw and overall improvement in the oral health of match factory workers.

## Enhancing worker efficiency and the benevolent paternalism of confectioners, c. 1904–1925

As the phossy jaw scandal was on the wane, a number of large confectioners employing thousands of workers established dental clinics and associated oral hygiene programmes for their employees. While Rowntree and Company Ltd of York established its clinic in 1904, the clinic established by Cadbury's of Birmingham in 1905 was the most comprehensive and became a model clinic for other firms. Company dentists W. Courtney Lyne and from 1908, T. P. Wolston Watt subjected the firm's 5,000 employees to a systematic programme of teeth and mouth examination and treatment (if necessary), which soon became compulsory and a condition of employment (Gelbier, 1999, p. 15). The firm's dental staff continued to grow in the 1920s and 1930s (Figure 12.1). To encourage workers' self-regulation of the mouth, the dentists displayed 'care of the teeth' charts in lavatories and other prominent places around the manufactory, provided toothbrushes and toothpaste at a discounted rate and wrote regular articles and reports on oral hygiene within the bi-monthly *Bournville Works Magazine*. By 1910, Watt claimed that nearly 9,000 teeth had been removed and over 3,000 were filled (Watt, 1910, p. 311).

What prompted the confectioners to provide dental welfare for their employees? Like those of match factory workers, the teeth of confectionery factory workers were generally poor, possibly due to the decaying effect of the high level of sugar dust in the air. And yet, the teeth of confectionary workers were reportedly no worse than workers in other industries or in the wider community (Lyne, 1907). Moreover, unlike match making, confectionery was not a dangerous trade and the industry did not have phossy jaw to contend with; neither did legislation coerce their adoption of such measures. Instead, dental welfare formed part of confectioners' expanding welfare programmes, which included medical care, pensions, sick pay, education, recreational facilities and perhaps most famously, accommodation in the form of model villages at Cadbury's Bournville and Rowntree's New Earswick. Aided by the firms' marketing, the public at the time and historians subsequently accepted that confectioners were motivated by the benevolent paternalism of their Quaker faith (Kennedy, 2000; Wagner, 1987). Yet, while confectioners were benevolent, they were also convinced that workers would be more productive if they had good oral health. Watt, Cadbury's dentist, claimed that no one could work 'satisfactorily with raging toothache' and as an advocate of the theory of focal sepsis, argued that

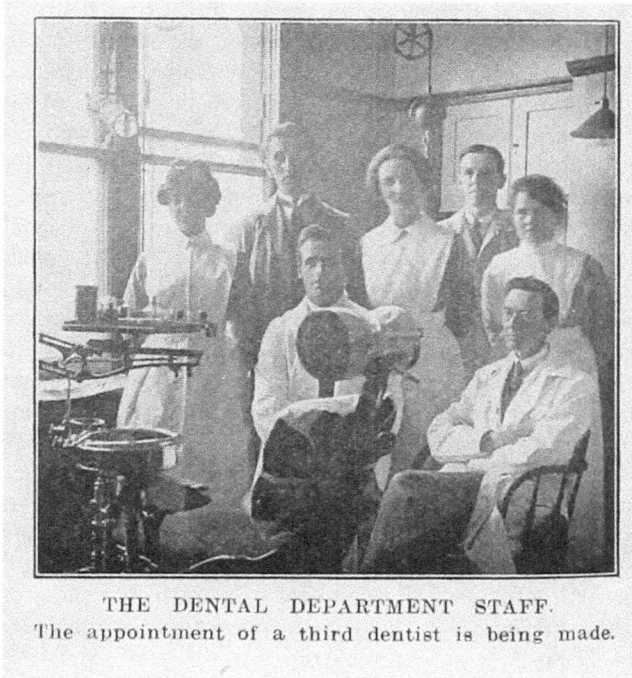

THE DENTAL DEPARTMENT STAFF.
The appointment of a third dentist is being made.

*Figure 12.1* The Dental Department Staff at Cadbury's.

Source: Cadbury Archive, Mondelēz International.

tackling oral sepsis prevented other forms of illness among the workforce (Watt, 1910; for more on focal sepsis, see Chapters 6 and 8 in this volume). Cadbury's doctor confirmed that he had witnessed an improvement in digestive troubles among workers after combatting tooth decay because poisonous micro-organisms from the mouth had been prevented from affecting the stomach; he stated that the effect on morale was positive because the worker felt that the employer was doing something for their benefit and thus productivity increased. Similarly, the doctor at Rowntree's was so convinced of the benefits of tackling poor oral health that he implored the firm: 'If you can't afford to employ both a dentist and a doctor, I advise you to get rid of me and provide a dentist for so much of the illness is due to faulty teeth that I really think his services are more necessary than mine' (Feaver, 1988, p. 41). The doctor nonetheless remained employed alongside the dentist.

Enhancing worker efficiency at the factories of the confectioners was also entwined with the state's new quest for national efficiency through greater intervention in the health of its citizens. Prompted in part by the poor oral health of army recruits for the Boer War (1899–1902) and as outlined in

Chapters 5, 6 and 9 in this volume, the Liberal government introduced a state-led programme of national regeneration through the introduction of wide-ranging welfare legislation from 1906. While all manual workers could claim free visits to general medical practitioners under the National Insurance Act of 1911, oral health was not specifically covered. Confectioners' industrial dental clinics therefore aimed to provide workers and sometimes their dependents with the dental care they believed they needed (Gelbier, 1999, p. 1). State and employer welfare provision was also an attempt at worker appeasement by limiting the appeal of more radical left-wing solutions to social problems which, according to Kevin Dowd (2001), was largely successful. Unlike at Bryant and May, several decades earlier where the match making workforce were heavily unionised, welfare provision in the confectionery factory had the effect of advancing the cause of political moderation (and Liberalism in particular) and encouraged a belief in an economic structure that industrial society operated for the mutual, almost equal, benefit of employers and employees. Indeed, it was no coincidence that both the Cadbury's and the Rowntree's were heavily involved in local and national politics. While B. Seebohm Rowntree's 1901 *Poverty: A Study of Town Life*, based on his investigation into poverty in York, inspired some of the government's reforms around unemployment and education, George Cadbury refused several times the offer of becoming a Liberal MP and instead promoted the cause of 'New Liberalism' to the working classes through his ownership of the *Daily Star* newspaper (Dowd, 2001, p. 59).

The key to both Cadbury's and the state's aims of regeneration and worker compliance was the child.[4] While the state emphasised the importance of child-rearing and education, Cadbury's oral health programme targeted workers under 16 years old. Edward Cadbury laid out the firm's scheme in his 1912 publication, *Experiments in Industrial Organisation*. He argued that treating child workers' teeth formed 'the basis of the whole dental organisation in the Works' and outlined that as a condition of employment, parents were required to authorise the dentist 'to do whatever he considered necessary for the benefit of the boys' and girls' teeth' and their treatment would be continuous until boys were 21 and indefinitely for girls (Cadbury, 1912, p. 104). Each child worker was given a tooth brush and a tin of tooth powder, which the dentists ensured were properly used, together with a leaflet on 'The Care of the Teeth'. On admission to the Works, each child worker was further introduced to the importance of oral hygiene for preventing tooth decay through a series of lectures on the structure and care of the teeth, which were illustrated by black board, drawings or lantern slides. Watt described such lectures as 'useful propaganda' and even claimed that industrial clinics were an important part of a company 'cure for a great deal of labour troubles' (Watt, 1923, pp. 2, 7).

Cadbury's oral hygiene promotion to children also expanded into local schools, which, as Nettleton (1992) has argued, were ideal observatories for routine dental surveillance and the exercise of dental power (p. 32). The firm donated a toothbrush and a tin of tooth powder to every child at the four elementary schools from which the majority of its employees came. In 1910, 97 per cent of these children were reportedly suffering from carious teeth (Watt, 1910). In turn, school teachers, who 'heartily co-operate', used these gifts in regular 'toothbrush drills' and requested more from the firm when required (Cadbury, 1912, p. 105). The promotion of oral hygiene expanded further into Birmingham's School Medical Service, established in 1907 as another Liberal government reform. Elizabeth Taylor Cadbury (1858–1951), wife of George Cadbury, was integral to championing the health of the local child stating in 1907 that 'almost all the problems of physical, mental and moral degeneracy originate with the child'. Cadbury took a special interest in child oral health by establishing and running Birmingham's school dental treatment scheme between 1911 and 1924. Helen V. Smith (2012) suggests that Cadbury's particular interest in improving the dental health of school children was based on her own childhood experience of dental problems, as well as those of her children. During her adolescence and again in adulthood, Cadbury suffered from severe dental problems, requiring an emergency extraction and a protracted series of dental surgeon visits. She also faced difficulties locating reliable dental practitioners to provide treatment for her children (p. 170). By 1914, the scheme had provided dental treatment for over 10,600 children in Birmingham elementary schools (Smith, 2012, p. 195). The dentists at the Cadbury's works watched the City's programme closely, and by 1921, Watt suggested that the fact that the number of child workers within the firm that required treatment had decreased over the past few decades was proof of its efficacy (Watt, 1921, p. 218). The firm's influence in dental matters in the city continued with the establishment of Bournville Dental Hospital in 1925, which was funded by company management, Quaker donations, run by the factory dentists and aimed to attend to the oral health of employees and their dependents (Reinarz, 2009, p. 142–3).

By the 1920s, the Bournville Dental Clinic was hailed as a great success by Cadbury management and the firm's dentists. It became a model for the British Dental Association on how employers could promote worker efficiency though an industrial dental clinic and was also an inspiration to manufacturers in other industries (Anon, 1920, 1922a). In 1921, Watt claimed that the 2,000 patients attending the Cadbury's clinic per year for toothache were back to work within an hour and by the 1930s, claimed that the clinic's programme contributed to the workforce's adoption of regular teeth cleaning (Watt, 1921, p. 218, 1937, pp. 52–3). The firm could claim the success of its oral health programme because it was compulsory. Dental surveillance over the workforce, and beyond into the local community, was therefore largely achieved. But while company records provide a wholly positive view of worker reception to company dental provision, some workers did resist such intervention. Watt confirmed that many employees, particularly young girls, initially avoided the clinic because rumours of the pain inflicted on patients circulated the manufactory. Moreover, many of the male workers that claimed to brush their teeth by the end of 1905 only did so 'about once a month and that day was usually Sunday' (Cadbury, 1912, p. 109). Company records thus are not necessarily revealing of the extent to which oral hygiene was adopted by workers. Nonetheless, workers seemed to accept interventions into their oral health, as well as other aspects of their life, more readily than those in Britain's match factories several decades earlier. Cadbury's dentists were keen to emphasise that 1,500 workers visited the Clinic of their own accord by 1910 (Watt, 1910). In addition, its provision of welfare meant that the firm seemingly succeeded in mitigating against labour unrest. The confectioners' motivation for establishing a dental welfare programme then may have been benevolent but should not be detached from the wider state aims of enhancing national efficiency.

## Industrial welfare professionalised, socialism and the biscuit maker, c. 1918–1930

The dental clinic of Peek Frean, the biscuit manufactory based in Bermondsey, London, that employed 2,000 workers, had much in common with those of the confectioners. It was established in the first decade of the twentieth century in order to provide oral examinations, treatments and programmes of prevention to the firm's workers and their dependents. It was also founded with the explicit aim of enhancing worker health and happiness and thus company efficiency and despite workers going on strike in 1911, management were convinced of its success (De La Mare, 2008). A. S. Cole, the firm's manager responsible for dental and medical welfare, stated that 'health is largely dependent on the prevention of the ailments which have as their origin defects of the teeth'. Similarly, the child was a key focus of Peek Frean's clinic and its work (Gelbier, 1999, pp. 16–7). Cole attributed a growing interest among the young workers in the health of their teeth to the work of the school dentist before they entered employment; thus, the clinic of the Peek Frean factory functioned as an extension of the dental power of schools. Yet, while the clinics of the confectioners continued to play an important role in interwar politics and industrial relations, it was the clinic of Peek Frean that had a noticeable impact both in the professionalisation of industrial welfare nationally and in the transformation of local public health during the period of reconstruction after World War One. Peek Frean contributed to these shifts in two key ways.

First, as vice-president of the Institute of Industrial Welfare Workers Incorporated (IIWWI) during the 1920s, Cole played a key role in the professionalisation of industrial welfare and in the extension of dental health surveillance in the factory (Anon, 1925; Figure 12.2).

The interwar period witnessed a flourishing of institutes, societies and publications promoting industrial welfare as employers both sought to pool together methods to improve working conditions after the devastation of the war and to assert their authority in order to prevent labour disputes. Trade union membership, which had stood at 2.5 million in 1910, grew to 6.5 million in 1918 and reached 8.5 million by 1920. Moreover, factories were now too large for

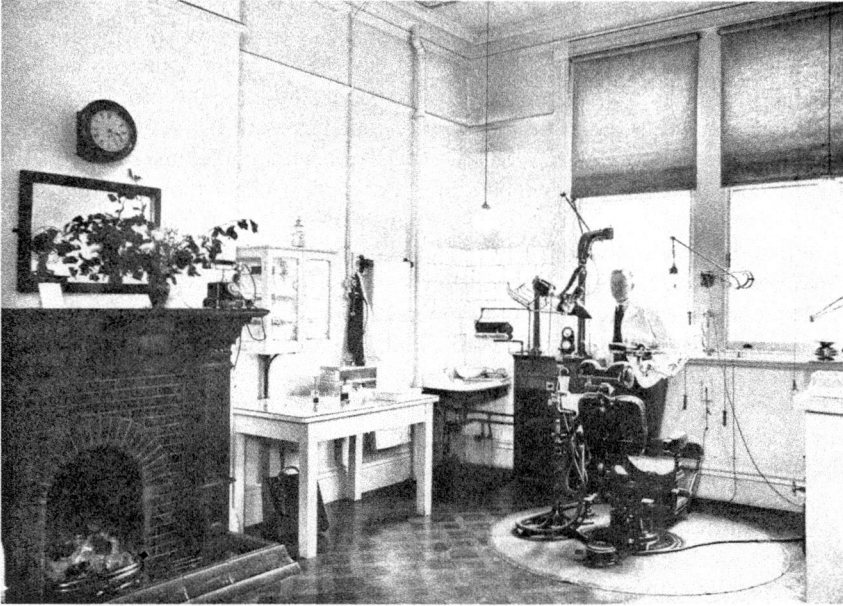

*Figure 12.2* Factory dental department, c. 1920.
Source: Wellcome Collection. Attribution 4.0 International (CC BY 4.0).

employers to know all of their workers so paternalism was difficult; many firms attempted to create and maintain a 'family spirit' through welfare. The IIWWI was small in comparison to the Industrial Welfare Society, the first national body concerned with workers' welfare under the directorship of Seebohm Rowntree and with over 700 members representing firms from all sectors of industry, but its scope was different. The Institute represented the supervisors responsible for managing company welfare, rather than being representative of the larger company as was the case with the Society (Woollacott, 1994, p. 45). Cole could therefore practically demonstrate to other members of the Institute and its local branches how the Peek Frean dental clinic produced firm efficiencies and resulted in worker compliance. Simultaneously, industrial dentistry was finding a home at the British Dental Association (BDA). Through the Association's Committee on Industrial Dental Service, the increasing number of factory dentists were keen to demonstrate the value of industrial dentistry to employers that felt financially constrained and did so through the publication of a report in 1922 (Anon, 1922c). Robert Lindsay, Dental Secretary of the BDA, argued that employers that did adopt such schemes 'got their reward in the better dental health of their work people, which resulted in more regular attendance and better work', while claiming that employers who failed to adopt such services were failing the nation: 'unless they do wake up to it, we, as a nation, shall find ourselves worse handicapped than ever in the race for industrial supremacy' (Gelbier, 1999, p. 28).

At a national level then, industrial dentistry was extending its gaze through professionalisation but at a local level, Peek Frean's dental schemes formed part of a broader public health campaign in Bermondsey. The campaign, the first of its kind conducted by a Sanitary Authority aimed at instilling personal hygiene habits into the local population of 120,000 people who worked in the Borough's various local factories, formed part of a political struggle between the local Labour Borough Council and the Tory government for the provision of universal health services (Lebas, 1995, p. 43). Under the reforming influence of Dr Alfred Salter (1873–1945), Bermondsey Labour councillor, MP and Christian socialist, and his wife Ada, the first woman Labour Mayor in Britain, Dr R. King Brown, local medical officer of health, and Grantley Smith, municipal dental surgeon, were the driving forces behind the campaign. Brown and Smith argued that 'bad teeth' (caries and pyorrhea) was the most common source of 'malignant germs' among the local population and the cause of many cases of ill health (Great Britain, 1924, pp. 37–8). Although Peek Frean was an important local employer, the majority of the population of Bermondsey were not eligible for the firm's dental welfare. Thus, in the absence of national provision for oral health, Smith argued that the only way to tackle the widespread problem of poor oral health was to combine industrial and public health efforts, thus strengthening the dental gaze across the public and private spheres.

The campaign consisted of programmes of lectures, advertisements and films on care of the teeth (Figure 12.3). Between 1923 and 1948, the Council's Public Health Department made approximately 30 films, which included footage of workers of the Peek Freans factory. An electric sign, illuminated at night and working from 7 am until 11 pm, showing 12 pictures of 'the evil effects following neglect of the teeth' was erected near to the Borough's dental clinic, which aimed to fill a gap in dental provision by treating those not provided for by Peek Frean (Anon, 1922b, 1924; Great Britain, 1924, p. 37). A second Borough dental clinic opened in 1927. Three open-air demonstrations on the teeth, delivered by Smith and held at different places in the Borough, addressed between 700 and 800 people (Great Britain, 1924, p. 39). By 1928, Brown circulated magazines to residents of the borough with information on the dental clinics (Great Britain, 1928, p. 61). By 1930, the Borough opened a Health Centre, one of the first in London to combine a dental clinic, with a tuberculosis solarium, a foot clinic, and ante-natal and child-welfare clinics (Jones, 2011).

The campaign was considered a success by campaigners. Brown claimed that the interest of the 700–800 people who attended the lectures was 'unquestionable', while the publication of the magazine was reportedly due to demand for more information and the success of the illuminated signs inspired other boroughs to erect similar (Great Britain, 1924, p. 39; 1928, p. 61). The campaign grew throughout the interwar period and as explained in a text book co-written by Donald Connan, Brown's successor, it became a model to other health authorities and used to extend local authority public health provision

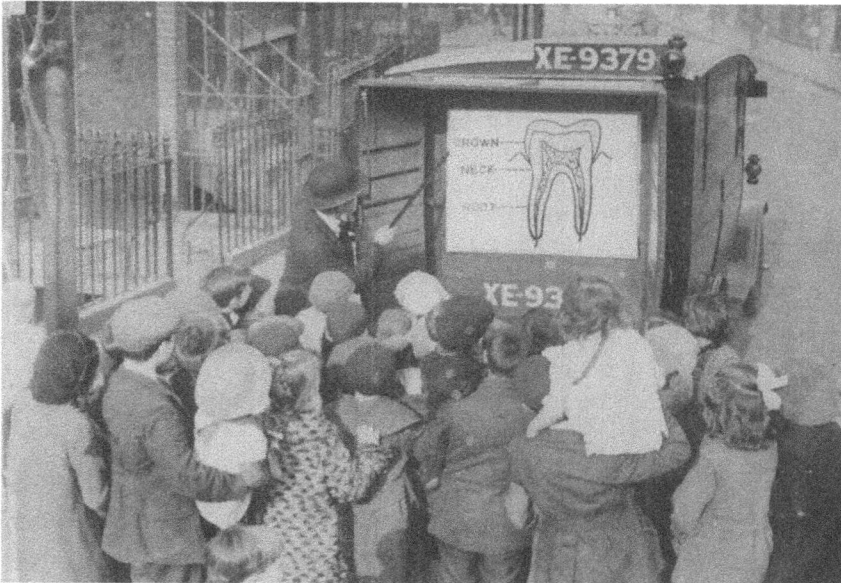

*Figure 12.3* Cinemotor van in Bermondsey showing a slide of the structure of teeth.

Source: Southwark Archives photograph, reference PB 945, with permission.

until universal provision under the National Health Service in 1948 (Connan and Bush, 1927). But of course, it was in practitioners' professional interest to highlight the campaign's success. While the local authority apparently enjoyed consistent grassroots support, there is little evidence from the population of Bermondsey that they embraced the campaign's messages about how to care for their own teeth, let alone enjoyed improved oral health. Indeed, Brown even suggested that most local people still failed to visit the local clinics and Smith stated that many were suspicious and even openly hostile towards well-meaning oral health advice. Moreover, with poor housing conditions, Salter argued that 'it was utterly impossible for them to maintain bodily cleanliness' (Brockway, 1951, p. 12. See also Ward, 2019). The campaign therefore was more of an imposition on the local population and like the provision of dental welfare by the match factories and confectioners, dental care was not something they demanded or necessarily valued. The Bermondsey public health campaign and Peek Frean's part in it nonetheless demonstrates how company dental welfare formed part of state surveillance into the mouths of local workers and vice versa with the aim of nurturing healthy and productive workers and citizens in an increasingly socialist metropolis. Both local authority and company dental welfare expanded as the Labour party took increasing control over London boroughs in the interwar period and London County Council by 1934.

## Conclusion

Oral health is a much-maligned topic in the wider historical scholarship of occupational and public health. Yet, as this chapter has demonstrated, it formed an important focus of the welfare provided by employers in at least three manufacturing industries in late-nineteenth and early-twentieth-century Britain. The provision of industrial dentistry took similar forms in match-making, confectionery and biscuit-making: dental surveillance by professionals and the promotion of self-regulation of the mouth through oral hygiene. And while each industry was prompted into providing this welfare for different reasons, it is clear that they all provided a way to regulate the industrial worker's mouth and by extension, the wider population. Through this regulation, employers aimed to improve productivity, but also to create a compliant workforce, which was enhanced by the professionalisation of industrial welfare and industrial dentistry. Regulation was most obviously aimed at the child. Both the confectioners and Peek Frean saw the key to improving workers' oral health was to instil oral hygiene practices into children both before and after employment not only to prevent dental caries but also to produce a compliant workforce. Such measures were a key feature beyond the factory too, as the state attempted to regenerate the population in the form of measures, such as the School Medical Service at the national level and public health campaigns of the Labour party at the local level. However, the extent to which these firms succeeded in regulating the mouths of their workers is more mixed. While making visits to the company dentist compulsory for workers ensured oral health surveillance some degree of success, oral hygiene practices were rejected by some workers, particularly those who had not already been exposed to such practices by school dentists. Indeed, toothbrushing did not become a common practice among workers, as among the British population more broadly, until at least the 1940s and became so for a number of reasons that are beyond the scope of this chapter. Nonetheless, this chapter has demonstrated that the beginnings of dental welfare and the aims of companies like Bryant and May, Cadburys and Peek Frean to control the worker's body cannot be divorced from the wider state frameworks of disciplinary knowledge and power.

Clearly, much more research needs to be conducted on the history of dental welfare by British employers, not only in other factory settings during the period under study here but also in divergent work places that engaged those other than the industrial worker, such the growing number of white-collar firms and in retail. Indeed, important mid-twentieth century retailers like Marks and Spencer became providers of dental welfare to its middle-class employees before universal NHS provision (Gelbier, 1999, p. 24–5). Industries were also clearly gendered. Moreover, further work needs to be carried out on worker responses to such measures. Yet, in the absence of such research, this chapter has suggested that employers played a more central role in the state's overall aim of shaping the health of workers and citizens, thus blurring the boundary between private and public provision. Indeed, it can no longer be taken for granted that workers wholesale accepted employer (or indeed state) provision of dental welfare, even though it was promoted as being in their best interest.

## Acknowledgements

Thanks to Helen Strong for her excellent research assistance.

## Notes

1 Anon, 1922c, p. 926.
2 For the provision of other worker facilities, see Hayes, 2002.
3 Labour historians have long regarded the Match Girls Strike as heralding the rise of militant trade unionism. For example, Briggs and Saville, 1971; Fitzgerald, 1989; Raw, 2009.
4 Historians have long emphasised the state's prioritisation of child health in the early twentieth century. For example, Gijswijt-Hofstra and Marland, 2003; Steedman, 1990.

## References

Anon (1899) 'Teeth in the match factory. The 'phossy jaw' inquiry', *Daily News*, 16529, 17 March. pp. 5.
Anon (1920) 'Industrial dental clinics', *Bournville Works Magazine*. July, Xviii, pp. 184.
Anon (1922a) 'Industrial dental clinics', *British Dental Journal*, 43, pp. 917.
Anon (1922b) 'Health of the Borough', *Southwark and Bermondsey Recorder*. 20 October. At: University of Reading, Peek Frean Archive, MS1216, box 7/2.
Anon (1922c) 'Report of the National Dental Service Committee on Industrial Dental Service', *British Dental Journal*, 43, pp. 925–930.
Anon (1924) 'Health propaganda – Bermondsey's campaign – a lead to the country', *The Daily Telegraph*. 20 September. At: University of Reading, Peek Frean Archive, MS1216 8/2, book 4.
Anon (1925) 'Welfare work – beneficial effect on industry', *Glasgow Herald*. 22 January. At: University of Reading, Peek Frean Archive. MS1216, 8/3, book 5.
Armstrong, D. (1983) *Political anatomy of the body: medical knowledge in Britain in the twentieth century*. Cambridge: Cambridge University Press.
Bartrip, P. W. J. (2002) *The Home Office and the dangerous trades: regulating occupational disease in Victorian and Edwardian Britain*. Amsterdam and New York: Rodopi.
Briggs, A. and Saville, J. (eds.) (1971) *Essays in labour history, 1886-1923*. London: Springer.
Brockway, F. (1951) *The Bermondsey story: the life of Alfred Salter*. London: Allen and Unwin.
Cadbury, E. (1912) *Experiments in industrial organisation*. Longmans: Green & Co.
Connan, D. M. and Bush, H. W. (1927) *Better than cure: a handbook on public health propaganda*. London: Noel Douglas.
De La Mare, U. (2008) 'Necessity and rage: the factory women's strikes in Bermondsey, 1911', *History Workshop Journal*, 66, pp. 62–80.
Dowd, K. W. (2001) *The social and political activity of the Cadbury family: a study in manipulative capitalism*. Ph.D. thesis, Swansea University.

Emsley, J. (2000) *The shocking history of phosphorus: a biography of the devil's element*. London: Pan Books.

Feaver, G. P. (1988) 'Occupational dentistry: a review of 100 years of dental care in the workplace', *Journal of the Society of Occupational Medicine*, 38, pp. 41–43.

Fitzgerald, R. (1989) 'Employers' labour strategies, industrial welfare, and the response to new Unionism at Bryant and May, 1888–1930', *Business History*, 31(2), pp. 48–65.

Gelbier, S. (1999) *Development of industrial dental services in the United Kingdom*. London: Lindsay Society for the History of Dentistry.

Gijswijt-Hofstra, M. and Marland H. (2003) *Cultures of child health in Britain and the Netherlands in the twentieth century*. Amsterdam and New York: Rodopi.

Great Britain. (1924) *Report on the sanitary condition of the borough of Bermondsey for the year 1924*. London: HMSO.

Great Britain. (1928) *Report on the sanitary condition of the borough of Bermondsey for the year 1928*. London: HMSO.

Harrison, B. (1996) *Not only the "dangerous trades": women's work and health in Britain 1880–1914*. London: Taylor and Francis.

Hayes, A., Azarpazhooh, A., Dempster, L., Ravaghi, V., Quiñonez, C. (2013) 'Time loss due to dental problems and treatment in the Canadian population: analysis of a nationwide cross-sectional survey', *BMC Oral Health*, 13, pp. 1–11.

Hayes, N. (2002) 'Did manual workers want industrial welfare? Canteens, latrines and masculinity on British building sites, 1918-1970', *Journal of Social History*, 35(3), pp. 637–658.

Jones, E. (2011) 'Nothing too good for the people: local Labour and London's interwar health centre movement', *Social History of Medicine*, 25(1), pp. 84–102.

Kennedy, C. (2000) *Family, fortune and philanthropy: Cadbury, Sainsbury and John Lewis*. London: Hutchinson.

Lebas, E. (1995) 'When every street became a cinema'. The film work of Bermondsey borough council's public health department, 1923–1953', *History Workshop Journal*, 39(1), pp. 42–66.

Long, V. (2011) *The rise and fall of the healthy factory: the politics of industrial health in Britain, 1914–1960*. Basingstoke: Palgrave.

Long, V. and Marland, H. (2009) 'From danger and motherhood to health and beauty: health advice for the factory girl in early twentieth-century Britain', *Twentieth-Century British History*, 20(4), pp. 454–481.

Lupton, D. (1995) *The imperative of health: public health and the regulated body*. London: Sage.

Lyne, C. W. (1907) 'Toothache and its prevention by the dentist', *Bournville Works Magazine*, April, V, pp. 178.

Marshall, J. S. (1912) *Mouth hygiene and mouth sepsis*. Philadelphia, London: J.B. Lippincott Company.

Murray, R. (1992) 'Peter Holland: a pioneer of occupational medicine', *British Journal of Industrial Medicine*, 49, pp. 377–386.

Nettleton, S. (1992) *Power, pain and dentistry*. Buckingham: Open University Press.

Raw, L. (2009) *Strike a light: the Bryant and May match women and their place in labour history*. London: Continuum.

Reinarz, J. (2009) *Health care in Birmingham: the Birmingham teaching hospitals, 1779–1939*. Woodbridge: Boydell Press.

Russell, A. (1991) *The growth of occupational welfare in Britain*. Aldershot: Avebury.

Satre, L. J. (1982) 'After the Match Girls' strike: Bryant and May in the 1890s', *Victorian Studies*, 26(1), pp. 7–31.

Smith, H. V. (2012) *Elizabeth Taylor Cadbury (1858–1951): religion, maternalism and social reform in Birmingham, 1888–1914*. Ph.D thesis, University of Birmingham.

Squire, R. (1927) *Thirty years in the public service. An industrial retrospect*. London: Nisbet.

Steedman, C. (1990) *Margaret McMillan. Childhood, culture and class in Britain*. London: Virago.

Terman, L. M. (1913) *The hygiene of the school child*. London: Harrap.

Thorpe, T. E., Oliver, T. and Cunningham, G. (1899) *Reports to the secretary of state for the Home Department on the use of phosphorus in the manufacture of lucifer matches*. London: HMSO.

Wagner, G. (1987) *The chocolate conscience*. London: Chatto and Windus.

Ward, P. (2019) *The clean body: a modern history*. London: McGill-Queen's University Press.

Watt, T. P. W. (1910) 'Dental department', *Bournville Works Magazine*. August, viii, pp. 311.

Watt, T. P. W. (1921) 'What the works dental department does', *Bournville Works Magazine*. September, Xix, pp. 218.

Watt, T. P. W. (1923) 'Some observations on an industrial dental clinic', *Reprinted from the Dental Surgeon*, 10(988), pp. 2–8.

Watt, T. P. W. (1937) 'Dental department', *Bournville Works Magazine*. February, ret xxxv, pp. 52–53.

Weindling, P. ed. (1985) *The social history of occupational health*. London: Croom Helm.

Woollacott, A. (1994) 'Maternalism, professionalism and industrial welfare supervisors in World War I Britain', *Women's History Review*, 3(1), pp. 29–56.

# 13 The state of tooth decay: dental knowledge, medical policy and fluoridation in Sweden, 1952–1962

*Jonatan Samuelsson*

In the decades following the 1939 establishment of Folktandvården – the Swedish Dental Service (henceforth SDS) – the issue of tooth decay moved to the centre of attention in Swedish public health. The SDS set out to provide free dental care to children up to the age of fifteen. Lack of funds, a persistent shortage of dentists and rampant tooth decay made this a daunting task. Following a slight decline in tooth decay due to World War Two sugar rations, caries rates started rising again towards the end of the 1940s. In 1950, untreated caries was present in just under 30 per cent of the teeth of Swedish seven-year-olds (Aronsson, Ordell and Aldin, 2009, p. 6). In Norrköping, a medium-sized working-class industrial town in the south eastern Swedish county of Östergötland, the chief medical officer (Förste stadsläkare, henceforth CMO) became inspired by North American attempts at combating tooth decay by means of Community Water Fluoridation (henceforth CWF), that is, adding caries-inhibiting fluorides to municipal drinking water supplies. Developed in the United States in the 1940s and 1950s, CWF was and is aiming to provide protection against tooth decay through the water tap of every home. Compared to other means of fluoride application, such as toothpastes, mouth washes or foodstuffs, CWF was often seen as preferable for being cheap, continuous and without the need to educate the population and correct its behaviour.

## Science and society: the origins and contexts of fluoridation

The connection between fluoride and caries protection began to attract attention in the United States in the 1930s. American dentists observed that people living in places with naturally high levels of fluoride in the water supply suffered less tooth decay. The first attempt at CWF was launched in 1945 in the town of Grand Rapids, Michigan. Several studies soon followed in the United States and elsewhere. The procedure commonly adopted was to fluoridate the water supply of a town, and then monitor children's caries rates and dental care needs, using a nearby unfluoridated town as a control. Most such studies soon began reporting positive results. In 1951, it was made an official policy of the US Public Health Service, and it became widely implemented throughout the following decades.

DOI: 10.4324/9781003047674-17

In many ways, CWF became the 'magic bullet' of dentistry: it was researched and promoted by the dental community as the final remedy to dental caries, putting the dental profession in a position of influence and respect vis-a-vis local and national governments (Picard, 2009).

CWF was controversial from its very inception. Among other things, opponents tended to argue that the practice was not as effective as it was claimed to be, that there were health hazards involved, and that it constituted unjustified forced medication. Protests sometimes led to referendums and bans on CWF. Studying CWF controversies, scholars have stressed the close alignment of anti- or pro-fluoridation sentiments with social, ethical and political positions and worldviews (Cf. Martin, 1991; Reilly, 2001; Carstairs and Elder, 2008; Whipple, 2010). Being so closely associated with the towering public health problem that was tooth decay in the early 1900s, the epidemiological science of CWF is particularly apt for studying what science studies scholar Sheila Jasanoff calls 'co-production'. In the edited volume *States of Knowledge*, Jasanoff (2006a) and others develop the concept of co-production to denote 'the proposition that the ways in which we know and represent the world (both nature and society) are inseparable from the ways in which we choose to live in it' (Jasanoff, 2006b, p. 2). The concept highlights the ways in which science and the social will often appear as one and the same, as they are created and moulded in tandem. The Norrköping Fluoridation Trials provide a striking example of this. They were a scientific experiment as much as they were a public health measure: the goal was to ease the pressure of caries on the town budget while simultaneously creating new knowledge about fluorides.

In time, the march of CWF across the United States slowed down, as the practice became connected to emerging issues of environmental health. As chemicals in food and environmental health hazards moved into the American mind in the 1960s, people started understanding CWF in new ways (Carstairs, 2015b). Challenging scientific reductionism and notions of naturalness, modern environmentalism, argues historian Frank Zelko (2019, p.520), 'would have made CWF a much harder sell in the 1970s than was the case at mid-century'. At the same time, the early anti-fluoridation movements of the United States, Canada, and Britain have been cast as a kind of forerunners, foreshadowing the environmental movement's holistic ontology and critique of technocratic reign (Carstairs and Elder, 2008; O'Hara, 2017; Zelko, 2019). Arguments about personal freedom and the right of the individual to choose whether or not to ingest certain substances have also been instrumental in rallying anti-fluoridation support in the United States, Canada and Britain (Martin, 1991; Reilly, 2001; Carstairs and Elder, 2008; Picard, 2009; Whipple, 2010; O'Hara, 2017). Alyssa Picard (2009) argues that prominent national issues in the United States in the 1960s, such as anti-communism and racial segregation, highlighted the question of 'the proper relationship between government authority and political liberty ... in ways that helped create a climate for a particularly bitter proxy fight over fluoride' (p. 127). CWF in Sweden evoked similar issues, but in a social and political context much different from the American one.

## Public health and the Swedish welfare state

Public health sits at a juncture of interests and identities such as state, corporate, professional, citizen, class, gender and race. Oral health is no exception. Historically as well as in the present, co-ordinated efforts to improve public oral health has been shown to further dentistry's professional interests (Lindblom, 2004, Picard, 2009), as well as those of corporations (Jones, this volume), middle-class white masculinity (Adams, 2000), and unequal dental care markets (Raskin, this volume). Although all of these dimensions play into the events of this chapter, my focus is on the intersections of state authority and interests with those of individual citizens. Berggren and Trägårdh (2006; see also Trägårdh, 1997) have proposed the notion of statist individualism to describe the way Swedish politics during the twentieth century have been geared towards securing, by means of a strong state and fine-grained social insurance and welfare systems, maximum autonomy for the individual vis-a-vis family and other mainly local communities. This has been a system in which the Swedish state has been prone to relatively far-reaching and intrusive bureaucratic interventions, expecting citizens to conform to rather narrowly conceived life courses to gain access to social benefits.

In line with this, public health (in Swedish Folkhälsa, people's health) became a core project, verging on an obsession, of the emerging Swedish welfare state – characteristically dubbed Folkhemmet, the people's home – during the hectic social reform years of the 1930s (Johannisson, 1991). Through the influence of European social hygiene, citizens' behavioural patterns became conceptualised as agents of health, paving the way for state intervention and central planning of several aspects of citizens' private lives (Johannisson, 1991). At this moment, when novel disease concepts were 'linking medical and social control together in a confusing network', repressive measures 'such as separation, confinement and sterilization seemed to be legitimized' (Johannisson, 1994, p. 177). The overall ideology was the belief in scientific rationality and its potential to order, make sense of and ultimately alter both the social and biological foundations of the state. Although persistent, the statist individualist contract has undergone changes during the twentieth century. Late modern statist individualism hinges more on the right to make informed individual choices when it comes to social benefits (Berggren and Trägårdh, 2006). Though mainly occurring during the 1970s and 1980s, this change began in the 1960s, and it had important effects on the historical trajectories of CWF science and policy in Sweden. Rather than channelling resistance to a possible expansion of state authority, CWF debate in Sweden occurred at a time when a traditionally expansive state was starting to do away with nation- and state-centred rationales for public health interventions in favour of individual-centred ones. Moreover, the issue of CWF in Sweden was intimately linked to the ongoing Norrköping Fluoridation Trials, making it particularly suitable for the incorporation of STS and CWF literature into a narrative that emphasises how science, states and citizens are made and remade in relation to one another.

This chapter examines the Norrköping Fluoridation Trials, where part of the town's water supply was fluoridated between 1952 and 1962. Through an analysis of the fluoridation collection at the Norrköping city archive, published reports and governmental publications, I follow the trials from inception to termination via two national expert committees and into the Swedish national parliament, where a law permitting CWF was created as a direct result of the fluoridation in Norrköping. The law was repealed after ten years, having never been used to fluoridate a Swedish city or town. This chapter aims to answer two main questions: How was the relationship between science and policy imagined and utilised in the reports and debates surrounding the Norrköping Fluoridation Trials? How had, by the early 1960s, health policy and the state-individual relationship changed to make CWF appear undesirable?

The remainder of the chapter begins by recounting the initiation of the trials, particularly addressing their public health and scientific underpinnings respectively. The next empirical section is centred on the two expert committees and their links to the Norrköping trials. From there, I turn to the cessation of the trials and the making of the law, before ending with a concluding section.

## Fluoridation begins in Norrköping

Fluoridation began in February 1952. By then, Allan Melander (1897–1958) had been the town's CMO for almost five years. After earning his medical licentiate degree in his native Stockholm, he went on to work as a practicing physician in a number of Swedish communities, as well as embarking on a study trip across Europe, before settling in Norrköping and his new job in 1947. Melander's correspondence hints at a daunting workload, not least stemming from dental care.

The SDS reform of 1939 has been understood as the culmination of the professionalisation of Swedish dentistry (Lindblom, 2004). With it, oral health was incorporated into the ongoing public health obsession, making it part of the making of the modern Swedish welfare state. Through the SDS, dental care for children was to be provided for free by the regional administrative units known as Landsting. Implementation was slow and laborious, as the aforementioned high caries prevalence, shortage of dentists and lack of funds made for a challenging mix of obstacles to be overcome by politicians and civil servants across the nation. At that time, Norrköping, along with five other municipalities, was not yet part of a Landsting, and so had to implement the reform by themselves.

In the United States, CWF was debated not only in ethical and political terms but also from a scientific perspective. Opponents of fluoridation argued that comparisons between communities could not adequately control for other differences, such as water and soil content or demographic and socio-economic factors. They also made the point that since local dentists were aware of the ongoing fluoridation, their judgement in registering and documenting children's caries rates could not be considered objective (Martin, 1991; Freeze & Lehr, 2009). The randomised controlled double-blind study, though novel and not yet named the gold standard, was already being considered a key benchmark for medical research (Jones and Podolsky, 2015).

Allan Melander set out to solve both these issues. When the human-sized fluoride dispenser at the Norrköping waterworks was switched on, only about a third of the town's inhabitants began pouring fluoridated water from their taps. This was because Norrköping's piping system was divided into two separate systems, drawing from the same well but serving different parts of town. These were called the 'high zone' and the 'low zone', and it was the latter which was fluoridated during the trials (Figure 13.1). This ability to divide the population into two groups – whose 'social, geographical and climatic circumstances' (Melander, 1953, p. 39) were deemed all but identical – allowed for the creation of comparable test and control groups. This was crucial in positioning the Norrköping study in relation to the growing international research field.

Double-blindness would be ensured by withholding information from both dentists and citizens about the fluoridation process. The setup was simple: Melander and his team would collect records from school dental practices, as well as conduct a total of three organised examinations of randomly selected children from each group. Then the data would be compiled and analysed, comparing the children who had been drinking fluoridated water and those who had not. Though not entirely kept a secret, knowledge of what was going on essentially remained within a small group of officials, scientists and dentists, who were all in favour of the study and its methods (Figure 13.2).

In sum, the fight for oral health had been accumulating attention in Sweden in the 1930s and 1940s. It was also proving extremely challenging. International experiences were similar, and knowledge about fluorides and CWF was growing in the United States. The Norrköping Fluoridation Trials combined these contexts, promising oral health benefits as well as scientific insights and prestige. The trials were made possible in no small part by Melander's ties to both these worlds. Not only was he a career-driven public health official but he was also a science enthusiast, well-versed in the American CWF literature and well-connected in the Swedish odontological community. Melander's success in bringing the trials to the attention of prominent Swedish scientists proved crucial in the ensuing process of rendering CWF viable as a public health measure.

## Crafting consensus: the fluoride committees

As allies to the Norrköping project became engaged in evaluating CWF as a caries-fighting tool at the national level, the unity of science and society came increasingly into focus. The National Board of Health

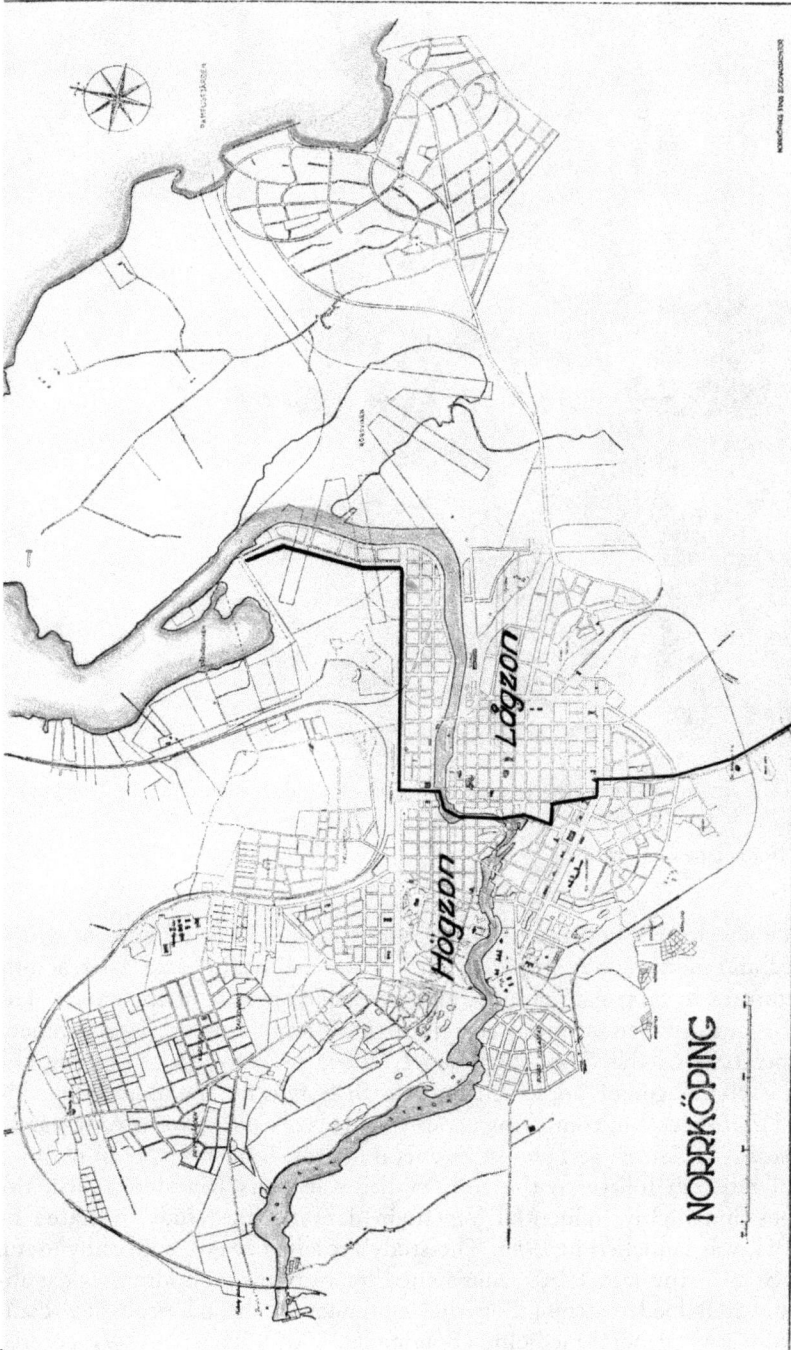

*Figure 13.1* Map showing the two zones being served by separate water piping systems.

Source: Norrköping City Archives.

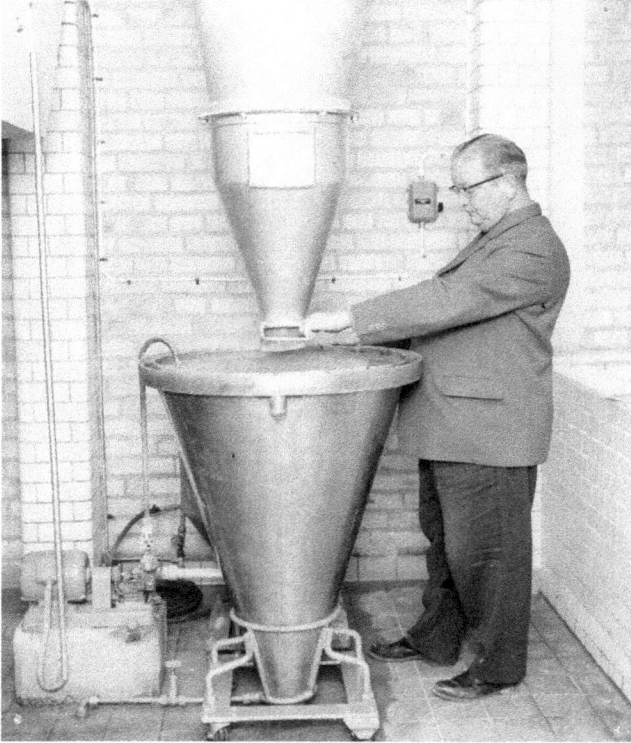

*Figure 13.2* Engineer Harry Åkerlund operating the fluoride dispenser at the Norrköping City Waterworks.

Source: Norrköping City Archives.

(Medicinalstyrelsen, henceforth NBH) had, through its many bureaus which directed and monitored multiple aspects of Swedish health care, far-reaching opportunities to propagate political and scientific agendas of their own. The NBH's Bureau of Dentistry was created in 1939 to oversee the establishment and operation of the SDS (Bommenel, 2006, pp. 68–70). Alongside the practical challenges of implementing the SDS reform, the Bureau quickly realised that success in combating caries would also require extensive research. Against this backdrop, and amidst a general interest from the state in reviving medical research following the toils of the war years (Sweden 1946), the infamous and highly influential Vipeholm dental caries study, initiated by the NBH, was launched in 1945. The study's results became politically useful as the SDS in the late 1950s campaigned for restricting children's sugar intake, and it helped to strengthen the legitimacy of the odontological community vis-a-vis general medicine (Bommenel, 2006). Thus, as CWF entered the Swedish political agenda, odontologists were in high regard among Sweden's policymakers.

In 1952, the NBH appointed an expert committee to review the use of fluoride in combatting caries. Members of the committee included Arvid Syrrist (1905–1997), associate professor of pedodontics at Malmö Dental School, and histologist Bengt Gustafsson (1916–1986), then head of the board's dental research station at Vipeholm. Syrrist had helped Melander plan the trials, while Gustafsson would begin to aid in the registering and processing of data from Norrköping only a couple of months after the meeting at the NBH. The committee worked for about a year, finalising its report in December. The report ("Fluor som medel …" 1954) clearly promotes a CWF agenda, echoing the commitment to Norrköping from some of its authors. It downplays ethical considerations and scientific uncertainties, and although its concluding call for research closely mirrors the Norrköping setup – as the report was being finalised, Gustafsson (1953) wrote cheerily to Melander: 'As you can see, the Norrköping plan is in great accordance with this final statement from the committee!' – the ongoing fluoridation is never mentioned in the report. The committee proposed that CWF be made legal under the supervision of, and obligation to seek permission from, the NBH.

Another fluoride committee was appointed in 1957. Although not as unanimous as the first one, they drew the same basic conclusions and made similar recommendations (Sellman, Ericsson and Strålfors, 1958). Neither of the two committee proposals were immediately implemented. Instead, both reports were starkly criticised by members the NBH's scientific council. Gösta Westin (1895–1969), professor of cariology and headmaster at the Stockholm dental school, was a frequently consulted expert in dental policy. Reviewing the first fluoride committee, he concluded by recommending against the committee's proposals (Westin, 1954). As he reviewed the second report, his basic evaluation was the same, yet this time he recommended the NBH to move forward with the policy proposed in the second report. Why? Because time was running out: tooth decay kept rising, verging on the uncontrollable. As a scientist, Westin could not endorse the report, which he characterised as a politicised and useless product, but as a cariologist committed to combating tooth decay he saw no other alternatives, as 'the pros and gains … outweigh the cons and flaws' (Westin, 1958, p. 409). It was Westin's change of heart that tilted the scale for the NBH, prompting them in April 1958 to make a written recommendation endorsing CWF to the government.

Historian Catherine Carstairs (2015a) has pointed out that it was the carefully crafted image of consensus, rather than actual scientific consensus, that tilted the scales in favour of CWF in post-war America. Similarly, Frank Zelko (2019, p. 537) writes: 'The fact that CWF is practiced in only a small number of countries strongly indicates that its adoption is only partly dependent on scientific consensus'. The two Swedish fluoride committees highlight this simultaneously scientific and political nature of CWF. Evidence was interpreted, downplayed or emphasised in line with what was going on in Norrköping as well as what was hoped for the future. Both committees purported to judge science and policy separately, but in reality, the two were always entangled.

## Lex Norrköping: Fluoridation halts and the Water Fluoridation Act is created

In early 1958, following an illness which had kept him in bed for the better part of a year, Allan Melander passed away. His job and the fluoridation trials were thus taken over by his deputy Sven Ljungberg. By this time, Ljungberg had already been acting in Melander's stead for most of 1957. From his sickbed, Melander was able to compile and publish the first set of results from the trials. Two articles, written in German, appeared in the Swedish dental journal *Odontologisk Revy* in 1957 (Melander, 1957a; 1957b). Results were positive, documenting a significant reduction of tooth decay in the fluoridated area. No general health data had been gathered and compared between the groups, even though such investigations had previously been identified as crucial by Melander as well as by the NBH's experts. Melander did seek help from colleagues in conducting such check-ups on several occasions, but it seems never to have been put into practice.

Publication came off the back of a few months of markedly increased communication regarding the trials. Not least other towns, both Swedish and international, corresponded with Melander from the latter half of 1956 and onwards, activities which only increased following the publication. With secrecy thus having given way to publicity, public debate and protest inevitably ensued. Protesters often cited international critiques of CWF, and their arguments generally mirrored those of the American and British anti-fluoridation movements of the time, positing it as a potentially harmful instance of forced mass medication and an unacceptable impingement by the state in individuals' lives (Martin, 1991; Reilly, 2001; Freeze and Lehr, 2009; Whipple, 2010). The most prominent Swedish anti-fluoridation organisation, Hälsofrämjandet, was also remarkably similar to its Anglo-Saxon counterparts. Founded in 1945 as Förbundet Allnordisk Folkhälsa by Finno-Swedish health philosopher Are Waerland, Hälsofrämjandet embraced the organicist, anti-statist and dietary views which historian Amy Whipple (2010) has associated with the British anti-fluoridation movement during the same period (Eklöf, 2005; Petrov, 2012; Kunkeler, 2019) (Figures 13.3 and 13.4). During the 1960s and 1970s, CWF would become one of Hälsofrämjandet's main targets. The organisation wrote letters of complaint to the Norrköping city board of health and the County Administrative Board of Östergötland, as well as a thoroughly critical response to the NBH's 1958 policy recommendation to the government.

In late 1961, the Norrköping Fluoridation Trials were addressed by the Supreme Administrative Court (Regeringsrätten), following a complaint by Hälsofrämjandet. The court concluded that the adding of fluorides was in no way intended to ensure the water's serviceability as drinking water, that

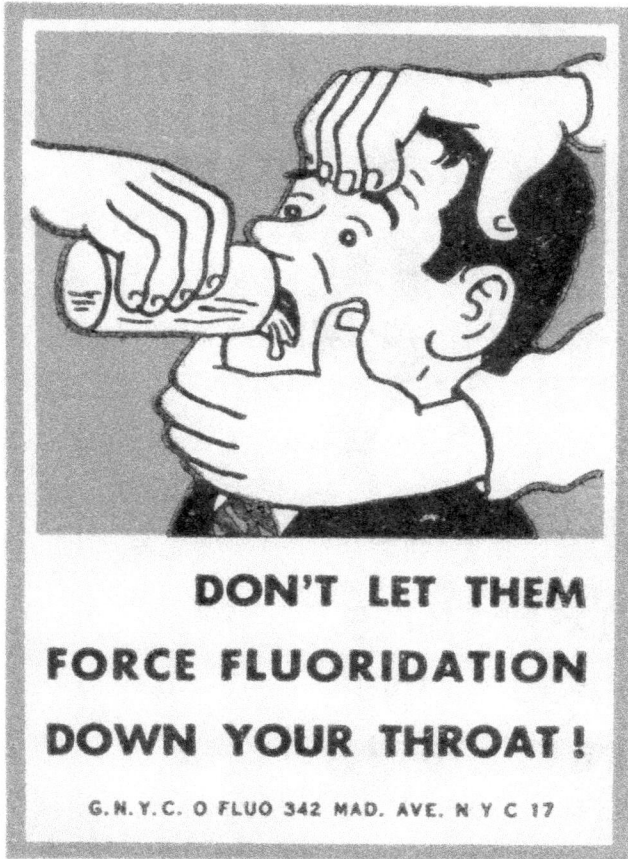

*Figure 13.3* American antifluoridation sticker.
Source: Norrköping City Archives.

long-term health risks could not be ruled out, and that those wishing to avoid consuming fluoridated water were unable to do so (Domstolsverket, 1961). Thus, the court judged the ongoing fluoridation to be illegal[1] and ordered it to cease, which it did on 1 February 1962.

Norrköping responded swiftly to these developments. The city Board of Health wrote directly to the minister of internal affairs requesting to be exempt from the law hindering CWF. There had been no significant change in overall scientific knowledge or consensus, but when the issue shifted from national CWF to the possible continuation of the Norrköping study, the tables turned in terms of the government's willingness to endorse CWF. While most consulting bodies had been reluctant to support the NBH's earlier proposals, most of the same respondents now endorsed the exemption request. However, simply

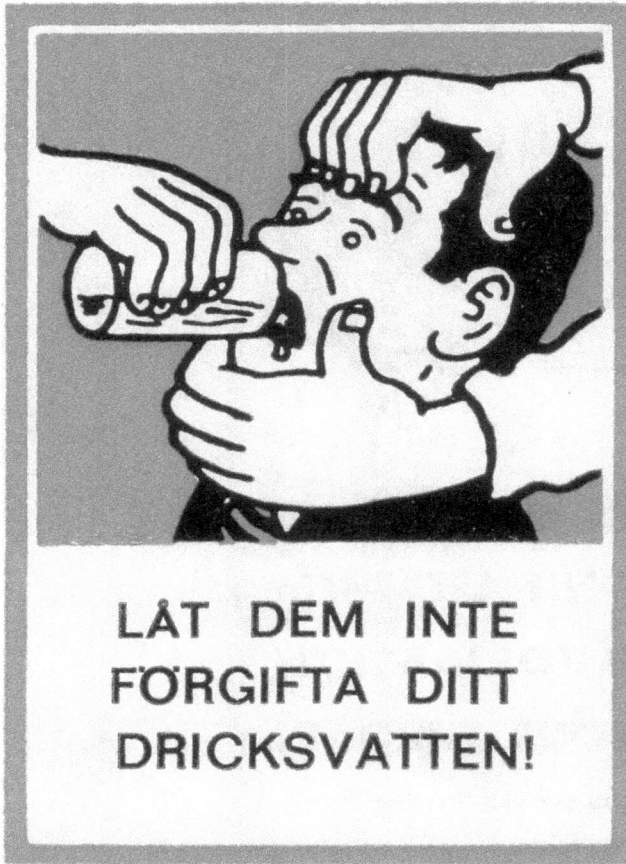

*Figure 13.4* Swedish antifluoridation sticker.

Source: Norrköping City Archives.

granting an exemption was not feasible, given the nature and reach of the overstepping of personal integrity implied: such infringements would, in principle, have to apply to all citizens.

The bill proposing the Water Fluoridation Act (henceforth WFA) was largely argued by both reference to and direct copying of the NBH's committee reports and other statements on the matter (SFS 1962, p. 588). When minister of internal affairs Rune B. Johansson put the bill to parliament, he made clear that even though the law had to be general in principle, its aim was to facilitate the continuation of the Norrköping Fluoridation Trials: in the first chamber of parliament, he referred to Norrköping's exemption request as 'the petition which forms the basis of the bill' (Sweden. Sveriges riksdag 1962a, p. 25). The bill stipulated that CWF would be made legal, subject to permission from and supervision by the government (specifically through the NBH). Johansson told both chambers of parliament that only Norrköping would be granted such permission for at least the first five years, before the safety of the procedure had been more firmly ascertained (Sweden. Sveriges riksdag 1962a; 1962b).

The bill passed by 221 votes to 96, with 23 abstaining, following long and intense debates in both chambers. Unsurprisingly, technical aspects were downplayed in favour of a values-and-principles oriented discussion which mainly focused on CWF as an act of forced medication and the legitimate grounds for the state to impinge on the individual's autonomy and freedom of choice. For the proponents, tasking the state with remedying tooth decay would have to entail favouring the all-encompassing solution over individual choice. In principle, the opposition subscribed to the same view but argued the need for a sense of proportionality and wariness of abuse of power (Sweden. Sveriges riksdag 1962a; 1962b).

The fact that the parliamentary debate primarily revolved around values rather than facts does not imply that science was not present. To the contrary, both sides of the debate drew upon science to support their arguments. While opposers of CWF highlighted scientific uncertainty with regard to potential risks, proponents downplayed them, denied them or framed them in Popperian terms: harm from fluoridation could well be scientifically ascertained, but given ever so many studies and ever so much data, it could never – just like the potential risks of any human activity – be wholly dismissed.

In March 1963, two months after the WFA had come into effect, the Norrköping board of health applied with the NBH for permission to resume fluoridation of the low zone. Due to a prolonged process at the NBH of defining rules and guidelines and processing applications, the permission and the necessary preparations were not in place until 1968. By then, six years had passed since the trials had been terminated, and Ljungberg deemed it scientifically pointless to resume the study. He also did not want to risk a backlash for other, increasingly successful, fluoride applications by re-igniting the anti-fluoridation movement (Ljungberg, 1968).

In 1971, following an intense campaign spearheaded by Hälsofrämjandet, and what has been described by one indignant dentist (Petterson, 1972) as a filibustering coup, parliament voted to repeal the WFA (Sweden. Sveriges riksdag 1971). By then, CWF had yet to be commenced in the handful of cities which had obtained permission to fluoridate during the 1960s. Despite the combination of epidemic caries and an extensive publicly funded oral health programme, Norrköping remains to this day the only Swedish municipality ever to fluoridate its water supply. Between 1977 and 1981, the parliamentary Flouride Commission revisited CWF, deeming the practice both effective and money-saving (Sweden. Socialdepartementet, 1980). Due however to the now familiar civil rights and personal freedom issues as well as some environmental uncertainties, the committee opted not to propose a renewed Water Fluoridation Act (Sweden. Socialdepartementet, 1981). In sum, CWF once came on the verge of becoming a part of Sweden's already-far-reaching, at times even re-pressive, public health and social engineering project. Yet in the end, it never did. This fact can be only partly explained by falling caries rates and im-plementation of other means of fighting tooth decay.

While caries rates did not drop sharply until the 1970s, all but plummeting in the 1980s and 1990s, they began dropping slowly already in the 1960s. In 1957, the results from Vipeholm underpinned a campaign promoting modesty in the consumption of sweets: a campaign which introduced Swedes to the enduring concept of Lördagsgodis, Saturday Sweets. Also crucial was the introduction in the early 1960s of nation-wide fluoride rinsing in elementary schools as well as the introduction of the first fluoridated toothpastes. Less caries meant less ur-gency in fighting it. However, although on the decline, caries was still highly prevalent throughout the 1960s. A law already put into effect would have been a readily available tool in bringing it down. Yet it was never used. The final fate of CWF in Sweden has to be explained using other contexts, highlighting how the state-individual contract was renegotiated and how public health policies shifted from a societal rationale to an individual one, where the state informs and guides rather than prescribes and decides.

In the late twentieth century, the statist individualist contract changed, be-coming more market- and individual-choice-oriented (Berggren and Trägårdh, 2006). Individual responsibility towards society or the common good was pushed back in favour of responsibility towards the self and there was increasing de-mands for influence and personal choice regarding societal services. Although most striking during the 1980s and 1990s, this change began with the authority-questioning and individualism of the radical 1960s, which, in turn, has roots in the 1950s (Östberg, 2018; see also Ekström von Essen, 2003; Agar, 2008). Health care policy and organisation, at the same time, developed along similar lines. Historian Mattias Tydén (2000, p. 71) describes the 1950s as a crucial breaking point in Swedish sterilisation practices, where 'a dominating force was replaced by a dominating voluntariness, [and] sterilisation for the good of society was replaced by sterilisation for the good of the individual'. In 1958, liberal exemption clauses were introduced into the mandatory smallpox inoculation programme, rendering it practically – albeit not strictly – voluntary (Sweden. Sveriges riksdag 1958). In 1960, the SDS was reformed along similar lines (Bommenel, 2006, ch. 8). All in all, the national health care system began its reorientation – which was to be fully embraced by the end of the century – towards conceptualising the patient as a consumer rather than as a citizen (Nordgren, 2003).[2]

## Conclusion

Scientific uncertainty sat rhetorically at the heart of the parliamentary CWF debate. The arguments of both sides revealed their shared view of science and its relation to policy. To their minds, science was a servant to policy, to be called upon when facts which are deemed relevant for the issue at hand seem uncertain or are unknown. However, the ways in which CWF figured in the debate and in the story I have told in this chapter, as both as an abstract entity and as the very tangible Norrköping trials, highlight instead how science and policy were co-produced. In the parliamentary debate, the trials became a way out of two simultaneous dilemmas: their continuation could potentially disperse some of the uncertainties surrounding health risks, while also embodying a promising solution to the problem of tooth decay gone rampant. Considering a concrete case in the legal context of general CWF made possible a crucial oscillation between the tangible and the abstract, as well as between the issue's scientific and political poles. The ongoing research in Norrköping was considered valuable for gaining knowledge, as a potent weapon in combating caries, and for strengthening Swedish science's international reputation. This triad of scientific and political aims had to be co-imagined for CWF to appear as a promising avenue for political action.

Rather than successfully moving the issue into either the scientific or the political domain, both the issue and the domains themselves had to be moulded to fit together. The crucial balancing act was making the science behind CWF appear solid, while at the same time calling for more: to continue the Norrköping Fluoridation Trials, and to ensure strict medical surveillance of CWF's subjects. At the political end, general CWF had to come across as desirable and at the same time not as the actual goal, which was instead to enable the trials to go on. In the end, the conjoining of Norrköping and general CWF turned a yes vote in parliament into two yes votes: yes, CWF is good and yes, we need more research before using it. Though hinged simultaneously on the solidity of the existing science, the desirability of CWF and the need for caution and more science (preferably of the kind that had already been done, in the United States and in Norrköping), the decision was never entirely dependent on any of them. The science, politics and promises of fluoridation were co-produced.

The story of the Norrköping Fluoridation Trials and the WFA thus provide a telling example of the broader societal changes taking place. In the early 1950s, such grand-scheme, one-size-fits-all social measures seemed palatable. By the turn of the 1960s, they were not quite as appetising, and certainly going out of style. The state was en route to becoming less of a dominating patriarch and more of a guiding enabler. As previous research has convincingly argued, the initial embrace and subsequent resistance and caution elicited by CWF aligns with the historical trajectories of the environmental movements and the critique of expert society. Moreover, the history of CWF projects many of the widely adopted sentiments of those movements further back in time than the 1960s in which they are normally placed.

The case of the Norrköping fluoridation and CWF in Sweden confirms this picture, adding an avenue for further historicising the individual rights-component of the CWF debate. The close alignment of CWF debates and contemporary political issues addressing conflicts between state authority and individual rights has previously been demonstrated. The Swedish case invites further pursuit along this line of inquiry, unearthing ideas about individual rights and liberties in relation to state power in the field of public health, where a critique of the paternalistic and far-reaching state apparatus was formulated earlier than might have been generally assumed. This paves the way for future research, where international comparisons might help us further understand the different trajectories of CWF around the world, as well as those of late modern individualism and the science-state nexus. Positing CWF as a crucial phenomenon in redrawing the boundaries at the intersection of citizens, states, and science enhances understanding of contemporary fluoridation debates and the values at stake.

## Notes

1 It is worth noting that the court's ruling was essentially a review of the legal competence of local Boards of Health or Public Waterworks to conduct CWF, rather than an assessment of the safety of the procedure or of the science involved. Much like O'Hara (2017) has pointed out regarding a similar British court ruling in 1983, the court's decision was nevertheless used as an argument for the non-safety of CWF later on.

2 In Sweden, the figures of the consumer and that of the citizen have been far from opposite or exclusive. To the contrary, a long-running, state-organised consumer guidance programme has been in place, underpinned by the notion that citizens acting as well-informed consumers would function as a kind of check on the economy, weeding out ineffective industries and raising the overall standard of production and welfare (Alexius and Löwenberg, 2018). However, for the purposes of this chapter and in the context of the Swedish health care system, the distinction between the citizen as one who is entitled to services simply by virtue of being part of the nation and the consumer as one who is entitled to making well-informed personal choices by virtue of being a taxpayer is both useful and historically valid.

## References

Adams, T. L. (2000) *A dentist and a gentleman: gender and the rise of dentistry in Ontario.* Toronto: University of Toronto Press.

Agar, J. (2008) 'What happened in the sixties?', *British Journal for the History of Science,* 41(4), pp. 567–601.

Alexius, S., and Löwenberg, L. (2018) 'Shaping the consumer: A century of consumer guidance', in: Brunsson, N. and Jutterström, M. (eds.) *Organizing and reorganizing markets.* Oxford: Oxford University Press, 2018.

Aronsson, K., Ordell, S. and Aldin, C. (2009) *Tandhälsans utveckling i sverige och ostergötland under 1900-talet. Några Fakta.* [Development of oral health in Sweden and Ostrogothia in the 20th century. Some facts.] Rapport 2009:4. Linköping: Folkhälsovetenskapligt centrum.

Berggren, H. and Trägårdh, L. (2006) *Är svensken människa? Gemenskap och oberoende i det moderna Sverige.* [Are Swedes human? Community and independence in modern-day Sweden.]. Stockholm: Norstedts.

Bommenel, E. (2006) *Sockerförsöket: Kariesexperimenten 1943-1960 på Vipeholms sjukhus för sinneslöa.* [The sugar trials: The 1943—1960 caries experiments at the Vipeholm hospital for the mentally ill.] Ph.D. thesis, Linköping University. Lund: Arkiv förlag.

Carstairs, C. (2015a) 'Debating water fluoridation before Dr. Strangelove', *American Journal of Public Health*, 105(1), pp. 1559–1569.

Carstairs, C. (2015b) 'The environmental critique of water fluoridation', *Scientia Canadensis*, 38(1), pp. 1–21.

Carstairs, C. and Elder, R. (2008) 'Expertise, health, and popular opinion: Debating water fluoridation, 1945–80', *Canadian Historical Review*, 89(3), pp. 345–371.

Domstolsverket [The Swedish National Courts Administration] (1961) 'Fråga om fluoridering av vattenledningsvatten'. [Issue concerning fluoridation of drinking water.], in: *Regeringsrättens årsbok*. Stockholm: Fritzes. pp. 143–151.

Eklöf, M. (2005) 'Vegetarisk (rå)kost och det reformerade livet: Maximilian Bircher-Benner och de svenska hälsokoströrelserna'. [Vegetarian (raw)food and reformed life: Maximilian Bircher-Brenner and the Swedish health food movement.], *Lychnos: Annual of the Swedish History of Science Society*, 70(1), pp. 245–272.

Ekström von Essen, U. (2003) *Folkhemmets kommun: socialdemokratiska idéer om lokalsamhället 1939—1952*. [The commune of the People's Home: Social democratic ideas about local community 1939—1952.] Ph.D. thesis, Stockholm University. Stockholm: Atlas.

Esping-Andersen, G. (1992) 'The making of a social democratic welfare state', in: Misgeld, K., Molin, K., and Åmark, K. (eds.) *Creating social democracy: a century of the Social Democratic Labor Party in Sweden*. English transl. and rev. ed. University Park: Pennsylvania State University Press. pp. 35–66.

Fluor som medel mot tandröta. Utredning verkställd av expertkommitté genom medicinalstyrelsens försorg. (1954) [Fluoride against tooth decay. Investigation conducted by an expert committee under the auspices of the Royal Board of Health.]. *Svensk tandläkare-tidskrift*, 47(1), pp. 1–28.

Freeze, R. and Lehr, J. H. (2009) *The fluoride wars: how a modest public health measure became America's longest running political melodrama*. Hoboken, NJ: John Wiley & Sons.

Gustafsson, B. (December 22, 1953) *Letter to Allan Melander*. Norrköping: Norrköping City Archives, Board of Health (hereafter: NCA:BH), F4:1.

Jasanoff, S. ed. (2006a) *States of knowledge: the co-production of science and social order*. 1st paperback ed. International Library of Sociology. New York: Routledge.

Jasanoff, S. ed. (2006b) 'The idiom of co-production', in: Jasanoff, S. (ed.) *States of Knowledge*, pp. 1–12. New York : Routledge.

Jones, D. S. and Podolsky, S. H. (2015) 'The history and fate of the gold standard', *The Lancet*, 386(9977), pp. 1502–1503.

Johannisson, K. (1991) 'Folkhälsa. Det svenska projektet från 1900 till 2:a världskriget'. [The people's health. The Swedish endeavour from 1900 until World War 2.], *Lychnos: Annual of the Swedish History of Science Society*, 56(1), pp. 139–195.

Johannisson, K. (1994) 'The people's health: public health policies in Sweden', in: Porter, D. (ed.) *The history of public health and the modern state*. Clio medica 26. Amsterdam: Rodopi, pp. 165–182.

Kunkeler, N. (2019) 'Sven Olov Lindholm and the literary inspirations of Swedish fascism', *Scandinavian Journal of History*, 44(1), pp. 77–102.

Lindblom, C. (2004) *I väntan på tandvård: hur tandrötan blev politik*. [Awaiting dental care: How tooth decay became politics.] Ph.D. thesis, Linköping University. Stockholm: Carlssons.

Ljungberg, S. (December 13, 1968) *Letter to The Norrköping City Board of Health*. Norrköping: NCA:BH, F4:8.

Martin, B. (1991) *Scientific knowledge in controversy: the social dynamics of the fluoridation debate*. SUNY series in science, technology, and society. Albany: State University of New York Press.

Medicinalstyrelsen [Royal Board of Health, the; RBH] (1958) 'Skrivelse till Kungl. Maj:t ang. användning av fluorider i kariesförebyggande syfte'. [Letter to the Royal Majesty on the use of fluorides to prevent caries.], *Svensk tandläkare-tidskrift*, 51(6), pp. 426–429.

Melander, A. (November 19, 1952) *Letter to Arvid B. Maunsbach*. Norrköping: NCA:BH, F7:1.

Melander, A. (1953) 'Kort redogörelse för försöken med fluoridering av dricksvatten i Norrköping'. [Short report on the drinking water fluoridation trials in Norrköping.], in *Årsberättelse för 1952*. Norrköping: Hälsovårdsnämnden, pp. 36–45.

Melander, A. (July 4, 1955a) *Letter to Gaston Backman*. Norrköping: NCA:BH, F4:1.

Melander, A. (November 30, 1955b). *Letter to the Kiruna City board of health*. Norrköping: NCA:BH, F4:1.

Melander, A. (1957a) 'Kurzer Bericht über den Versuch der Fluoriderung des Trinkwassers in Norrköping, Schweden'. [Short report on water fluoridation in Norrköping, Sweden.], *Odontologisk Revy*, 8(1), pp. 57–72.

Melander, A. (1957b) 'Ergänzungsericht über den Versuch der Fluoriderung des Trinkwassers in Norrköping, Schweden'. [Progress report on water fluoridation in Norrköping, Sweden.], *Odontologisk Revy*, 8(4), pp. 474–479.

Nordgren, L. (2003) *Från patient till kund: Intåget av marknadstänkande i sjukvården och förskjutningen av patientens position*. [From patient to customer: The introduction of market thinking in health care and the repositioning of the patient.] Ph.D. thesis, Lund University.

O'Hara, G. (2017) *The politics of water in post-war Britain*. London: Palgrave Macmillan.

Östberg K. (2018) *1968 — När allting var i rörelse*. [1968 — when everything was in motion.]. Johanneshov: Bokförläggarna Röda Rummet.

Petrov, K. (2012) 'Från blodbesudlat kolonialsocker till livsviktigt blodsocker: Svensk-europeiska teman i sockrets globala kulturhistoria'. [From blood-stained colonial sugar to essential blood sugar: Swedish-European themes in the cultural history of sugar.], *RIG: Kulturhistorisk tidskrift*, 95(3), pp. 129–154.

Petterson, E. O. (1972) 'Abolition of the right of local Swedish authorities to fluoridate drinking water', *Journal of Public Health Dentistry*, 32(4), pp. 243–247.

Picard, A. (2009) *Making the American mouth. Dentists and public health in the twentieth century*. New Brunswick: Rutgers University Press.

Porter, D. (1994) 'Introduction', in: Porter, D. (ed.) *The history of public health and the modern state*. Clio medica, 26. Amsterdam: Rodopi, pp. 1–44.

Reilly, G. (2001) *'This poisoning of our drinking water': the American fluoridation controversy in historical context, 1950–1990*. Ph.D. thesis, George Washington University.

Sellman, S., Ericsson, Y. and Strålfors, A. (1958) 'Kariesprofylax genom fluor'. [Caries prophylaxis by means of fluoride.], *Svensk tandläkare-tidskrift*, 51(6), pp. 303–379.

Sweden. Ecklsesiastikdepartementet. De medicinska högskolornas organisationskommitté [Organizational committe of medical colleges, the.] (1946) *Organisatoriska åtgärder till främjande av medicinsk forskning*. [Organizational measures promoting medical research.] SOU 76 [Parliamentary investigation report no. 76].

Sweden. Sveriges riksdag [Swedish Parliament] (1958) *Förslag till lag om ympning av smittkoppor* [Smallpox Inoculation Bill], Prop:111. Stockholm: Riksdagen.

Sweden. Sveriges riksdag [Swedish Parliament]. (1962a) *Första kammarens protokoll* [Debates of the first chamber of parliament], 21 November, 1962, No. 32. Stockholm: Riksdagen, pp. 21–57.

Sweden. Sveriges riksdag [Swedish Parliament]. (1962b)*Andra kammarens protokoll* [Debates of the second chamber of parliament], 21 November, 1962, No. 33. Stockholm: Riksdagen, pp. 112–154.

Sweden. Sveriges riksdag [Swedish Parliament]. (1962c) *Lag om tillsättning av fluor till vattenledningsvatten* [Water Fluoridation Act], SFS 1962:588. Stockholm: Riksdagen.

Sweden. Sveriges riksdag [Swedish Parliament]. (1971) *Lagen om upphävande av lagen (1962:588) om tillsättning av fluor till vattenledningsvatten* [Water Fluoridation Repeal Act], SFS 1971:859. Stockholm: Riksdagen.

Sweden. Socialdepartementet. (1980) Fluorberedningen [Fluoride commission, the.]. *Lönar det sig att tillsätta fluor i dricksvattnet? En samhällsekonomisk utvärdering för perioden 1981–2025. Rapport till Fluorberedningen.* [Is adding fluoride to drinking water worth it? A socio-economic evaluation for the period 1981–2025. Report to the Fluoride Commission.] SOU 13 [Parliamentary investigation report no. 13].

Sweden. Socialdepartementet. (1981). Fluorberedningen [Fluoride commission, the.]. *Fluor i kariesförebyggande syfte.* [Fluorides in caries prevention.] SOU 32 [Parliamentary investigation report no. 32].

Trägårdh, L. (1997) 'Statist individualism: on the culturality of the Nordic welfare state', in: Sørensen, Ø. and Stråth, B. (eds.) *The cultural construction of Norden.* Oslo: Scandinavian University Press, pp. 253–285.

Tydén, M. (2000) *Från politik till praktik: de svenska steriliseringslagarna 1935-1975. Rapport till 1997 års steriliseringsutredning.* [From politics to practice: Swedish sterilization laws 1935–1975. Report to the 1997 sterilization committee.] SOU 2000:22 [Parliamentary investigation report no. 22, 2000]. Stockholm: Fritzes.

Vattenfluoridering: Symposium. [Water fluoridation: Symposium.] (1955). *Svensk tandläkare-tidskrift,* 48(4), pp. 430–434.

Westin, G. (1954) *Letter to the RBH [typed copy].* Norrköping: NCA:BH, F4:1.

Westin, G. (March 19, 1958). *Letter to the RBH [typed copy].* Norrköping: NCA:BH, F4:6.

Whipple, A. C. (2010) 'Into every home, into every body': organicism and anti-statism in the British anti-fluoridation movement, 1952–1960, *Twentieth Century British History,* 21(3), pp. 330–349.

Zelko, F. (2019) 'Optimizing nature: invoking the "natural" in the struggle over water fluoridation', *History of Science,* 57(4), pp. 518–539.

# 14 The cultural politics of dental humanitarianism

*Sarah E. Raskin*

## Introduction

Multiple intersecting sociopolitical trends underlie US residents' unmet oral health care needs in the early twenty-first century: advanced decay and periodontal disease that could have been halted and possibly reversed with early and dependable preventive care, pain relief, extractions, aged appliances, modest restorations as well as full sets of properly fitted dentures, and their associated physical and psychosocial suffering. Since the late 1990s, federal austerity measures have obliterated state-level budgets for dental public health provisions and community dental services. Dental Medicaid optimization has been stymied by reimbursement rates that lagged inflation, floundering acceptance among private practitioners, and the exclusion of meaningful adult dental benefits in most states. Organised dentistry has obstructed proposals to regularise its social obligations vis-a-vis dental coverage in national health insurance reform, substantive workforce recruitment to underserved communities, universal patient acceptance, or the licensure of multi-disciplinary semi-autonomous dental team members, in particular mid-level providers (Edelstein, 2009; Lee and Divaris, 2014; Balasubramanian et al., 2019; Moeller and Quiñonez, 2020; Otto, 2017). At the same time, dental charitable volunteerism has arisen in the United States as a, if not *the*, predominant manifestation of dental social responsibility, as evinced in the number of events organised, provided hours donated, patients treated, and services and value of care delivered. The disjuncture between the systemic failures demonstrated by the persistence of patients' unmet needs and professional and public enthusiasm for dental charitable volunteerism—an impermanent approach by definition—merits critical consideration.

Charitable dental volunteerism in the United States comprises three main types. The American Dental Association–branded annual Give Kids a Smile Day and its ongoing donated dental services programmes 'match' private practitioners through their state membership organizations to deliver free short-term care to patients from specific categories: low-income children and elders, and people living with disabilities. In these two types of charitable care—one, a continuous trickle for qualifying individuals, and the other a single day event each year—episodic care is delivered in providers' offices. There is no

DOI: 10.4324/9781003047674-18

expectation of providers enrolling matched patient for ongoing services beyond the temporary volunteer milieu.

The third major type of dental volunteerism in the United States is the temporary dental charity event, where tens or even a few hundred dental providers deliver services en masse to thousands of patients who wait out the line—sometimes by overnighting in their vehicles—often alongside medical, ophthalmological, and veterinary services. Events in this model trace to at least 1985, when the non-profit organisation Remote Area Medical (or, RAM as it is popularly known) included dentistry among comprehensive health care services that it began bringing to domestic medically underserved communities in the style of short-term experiences in global health (STEGHs). Short-term dental volunteerism has proliferated since 2000 with the founding of the brand Missions of Mercy (or, MOM) by the Virginia Dental Association Foundation; Thirty-two state dental associations now produce at least two MOMs per year as does the American Dental Association annually, in formal partnership with the city hosting its annual convention. They have also become the most publicly known events, due in part to prolific national and global media coverage.

In contrast to the contraction of substantive resources and reforms to address unmet dental needs in a systematic and sustained way, short-term dental volunteer events, which generally last from one-and-a-half to five days, proliferated from 2000–2019. They also fomented significant new commitments: portfolios from dental philanthropists and line items in state budgets, a niche sub-industry in event administration and specialised equipment rentals, advocacy to permit short-term cross-state licensure permissions, advertising opportunities for volunteers and donors, and community-based dental education (CBDE) opportunities for students. Their popularisation is succinctly demonstrated by two encounters I had at either end of a decade of ethnographic research in the dental safety net in Virginia, including at short-term dental volunteer events. In 2011, at the flagship MOM in the rural Appalachian town of Wise Virginia, I met an attendee who had travelled from Haiti to obtain dental care after hearing about the annual event on a Francophone radio programme two years prior. A decade later, at a state coalition meeting on workforce resilience amid COVID reopening, a fellow task force member passionately advocated scaling up MOMs in excess of prior years and regardless of community health, arguing that events needed to expand because *providers* missed volunteering at them. While short-term dental volunteer events' popularity among attendees is understood to reflect patients' desperation to have their unmet needs treated amidst the United States' exclusionary private dental system and asystematic and inadequate public system, the widespread enthusiasm for these events among providers across twenty years indicates their ubiquity in *professional* culture, including the socialisation of new professionals, as well.

Domestic short-term dental volunteerism has thrived despite critiques of the impoverished ethics of 'band-aid solutions' to address unmet dental needs (Holden, 2020; Mouradian, 2006), recognition by their own organisers of their inadequate impact on population-level oral health disparities (Arefi et al., 2020; Edelstein et al., 2020; Raskin, 2015), and calls for global dentistry to strengthen sustained justice commitments (Dharamsi et al., 2007; Freeman et al., 2020; Holden and Quiñonez, 2020; Moeller and Quiñonez, 2020; Patthoff, 2007; Treadwell and Northridge, 2007).[1] It has also perpetuated individualising and stigmatising notions of patients' responsibility for disease risk, calcified the relegation of state obligations of care to the privatised marketplace, and privileged individual provider heroism over the systemic reform necessary to successfully advance oral health equity (Health and Story 2021; Rivkin-Fish, 2011; Otto 2017). Short-term volunteerism justifies and even concretises the discordance between dentists' claims of moral inclusivity and denial of duty to care for under-resourced people, as described by Yu and colleagues in this volume (see Chapter 2). It has also provided an outlet to formalise the profession's evangelism, exemplified by a dentist-penned invocation adopted by the American Dental Association in 1991, which begins: 'Thank you, O Lord, for the privilege of being a dentist, For letting me serve as your instrument in ministering to the sick and afflicted' (Kalil 2020; for an example see Meyer and Meyer 2020).[2]

In other words, the moral economy of normative temporary dental volunteerism prioritises (presumptively homogeneous) providers' value(s) over patients; fosters patients' dependence on periodic and irregular treatment opportunities while continuing to exclude them from predictable access to care, particularly for prevention and early-stage disease; and subjugates structural reform to a market based status quo.[3] Thus, volunteerism as organised dentistry's primary modality of social obligation disassociates patients' oral suffering from the relations of power through which that suffering is produced (see also Lala et al., 2021). Taking at face value the stated aims of these projects—to deliver care to underserved patients—we must ask *how* and, moreover, *why* has this shift occurred? Critical humanitarian perspectives gives us important insights.

## Envisioning critical dental humanitarianism

Humanitarianism is the foundational belief in the value of human life. It is commonly operationalised as the relief of suffering, in which state- and non-state actors provide material, legal, and other resources to victims of war, natural disasters, and other emergencies, often but not exclusively in transnational contexts. While oral suffering has not been at the forefront of humanitarianism, its role in overall health and the centrality of medical concerns in humanitarianism merits its inclusion in reflections on humanitarianism in the early twenty-first century, as does the ways that short-term dental charity events are modelled after global medical humanitarianism, in particular religious missions. In particular, temporary dental volunteer events exhibit key characteristics that have been objects of critical analysis.

Historically, humanitarianism was grounded in both secular and religious institutions' sense of obligation to respond to victims' claims of sociopolitical rights. Critical humanitarian scholar Didier Fassin describes humanitarianism as the 'introduction of moral sentiments into human affairs' (Fassin, 2013), or the application of justice-based rationalism to emotional concerns like relieving strangers' suffering. During the twentieth century, emergencies that imperilled groups of people diversified, multiplied, and in many cases extended to longer-term and even semi-permanent needs. Concurrently, the array of humanitarian responses—public, private, volunteer-driven, profit-making—pluralised and formalised, as did governmental and non-governmental institutions' under-standings of their legal and ethical obligations to respond to individuals' claims to relief, commonly on the grounds of sociopolitical rights (Fassin, 2012). Initial universalising frameworks of humanitarianism were replaced by administrative, moral, and affective logics through which individuals *qua* institutions evaluated victims' requests for legitimacy, merit, and deservingness. This shift from justice-driven objective universalism to emotionally driven subjective gatekeeping unveiled and magnified power imbalances 'between the one giving aid and the one receiving it' (Fassin, 2012, p. 193) at both higher structural levels such as bureaucratic policy and at more intimate interpersonal levels of human in-teraction. It also extended underlying systems of power inequities, such as commoditised human services under late capitalism (Baillie Smith and Laurie, 2011; Rivkin-Fish, 2011), and underlying contexts, such as the journalistic objectification of stigmatised health behaviours and conditions (Adams, 2017; Rozario, 2003).

In light of these insights from critical humanitarianism, dental social re-sponsibility in the United States merits specific consideration. On one hand, oral health care in the US has *always* existed outside of state obligations, even as medical coverage became a public entitlement for specific populations and as public dental benefits depend on private practitioners' acceptance. On the other hand, the well-agreed uniqueness of having physical and psychosocial suffering due to unmet dental needs is starkly juxtaposed against the empirical, demon-strating these unmet needs' grounding in the profession's veneration of periodic volunteerism and obstructionism of systemic reform. In this chapter, I analyse temporary dental volunteer events through Fassin's understanding of humani-tarianism's moral economy as being grounded in the everyday determinations that occur in the power-imbalanced space between claimants and providers, such as clinical decisions made in situ, and macro-level decisions made at in-stitutional levels, for example, the institutionalization within professional training programmes of temporary dental volunteerism as social responsibility.

## Affective relations and moral decisions at the dental charity fair

To consider how temporary dental volunteer events exemplify the humani-tarian reason described by Fassin, it is helpful to first understand how they operate. Planning among partners including local host organizations, dental professionals, and auxiliary groups (e.g., a local health department), begins a year prior, often at a post-event review of the immediately concluded clinic.

Organisers recruit volunteer clinicians to staff the event, which might range from dozens of nearby providers who serve for one day to hundreds of multidisciplinary dental team members including oral surgeons and endodontists who drive fifteen hours or more and spend multiple nights in local hotels, as well as large teams of faculty and students from dentals schools across the state, as well as local dentists to provide short-term emergency follow-up care if needed, particularly for surgical procedures. They also secure non-clinical volunteers and staff (e.g. security), permits (e.g. traffic), rentals (e.g. portable dental chairs, portable x-ray), dental supplies, in-kind donations, advertising, media coverage, a space of 6,500 feet minimum (e.g. education sector gymnasium, civic centre, airport hangar and county fairgrounds), and hospitality provisions, including on-site food for volunteers, negotiated fee hotel room blocks, and a higher-end event where organisers, donors, and esteemed guests such as elected officials socialise. They also fundraise to cover costs of approximately $50,000 per event day, or per approximately 500 patients (Virginia Health Care Foundation, 2013); and write protocols including credentialing, the handling of pathogens, and prescription procedures.

Following walk-throughs at various intervals in the months and weeks preceding the event, on-site set up typically begins two days before the first patient is registered and medically screened for services. A core team of experienced volunteers and any paid staff (e.g. from the state dental association) finalise layout and patient flow; erect portable dental equipment and stations (e.g. patient waiting area, instrument sterilization, data collection, media); secure clean water, electricity, and biowaste resources; and innumerable other tasks. In the late afternoon of the day prior to the event's early morning start of multi-day events, more volunteers arrive for orientation. Amplified upbeat music turns the event space's sombre, focused, and sometimes frantic morning tone to joyful and goal-oriented after lunch. The event director gives a rousing speech. Wide-smiled long-time volunteers reunite in the adjacent parking lot, amidst equipment trailers branded with the names of private practices or affiliate organizations. They rib each other good-naturedly: Who brought the most assistants and hygienists from their private practice? Which dentist will skip dinner to persist with the last complex case? Some clinicians adjust or customise their assigned portable operatories. The majority of volunteers depart the space to eat supper, rest, and return by 6:00 am. Meanwhile, a line of patients has been continuously growing at the entrance, sometimes from three days before the event; would-be patients commonly sleep in their vehicles in hopes of arriving to the event early enough to qualify for a first-come, first-served ticket or, at some events, pre-registration beginning approximately twelve hours prior to the official start.

Each event day follows a predictable cycle. The earliest front-end volunteers arrive by 4:30 am to begin communicating with and granting event entrance to patients in groups of approximately twenty at a time. Patients complete electronic registration and medical and dental triage, then wait in an area categorised by procedure type until they are called for services: cleanings, extractions, or restorations. Once services are complete, patients may recover within a dedicated space then check out; depending on the setting, they may peruse a health education area if they feel well enough. From the moment volunteers arrive until the event's close each day, myriad improvisations also occur within the highly orchestrated event. At outdoor events, for example, severe weather may temporarily halt services. Other times they reflect generally scheduled interruptions such as an opening invocation from a local religious leader or the arrival of a state legislator, governor, or other esteemed guest, whose expectations of small talk and photos with patients and volunteers must be considered amongst other dynamics such as patient flow and safety protocols.

While many changes respond to extrinsic factors, others reflect the micro-decisions through which humanitarian logics occur. A fearful patient may change their mind about a procedure once they get into the dental chair; the dental team will have to decide how long to spend calming and coaxing them, knowing that a line of ready-and-willing patients sits in folding chairs within view, waiting their turn. Inevitably each year, after the front-end volunteers have regretfully turned away patients who arrived after all tickets were dis-tributed, a slow trickle of late-arriving patients makes its way in, as operatories are freed up faster than anticipated and dental teams decide they have the endurance to volunteer for one more hour. These cases are often negotiated through leadership, who assess capacity based on the late-arriving patient's needs: Simple needs such as cleanings, simple extractions, and crown repairs may be intaked quite easily. More complex cases such as root canals require more negotiation, and assessment of the dental team's stamina.

Patients' self-comportment often bears on these decisions, especially as multi-day events advance towards their conclusion. Returning patients who have pre-viously experienced long waits and decide, instead, to try arriving once the event is underway often met with gentle scolding and less enthusiasm, on the part of the leadership team, to negotiate extended time with volunteers than are patients whose tardinesss was beyond their control due to vehicle troubles, inability to miss work, or childcare challenges. Immediately evident dental emergencies such as abscesses also compel late entry, while missed appointments to receive dentures—verboten given their rarity—elicit far less sympathy and only occa-sionally a revision in service delivery. These hidden practices are no less core to temporary dental volunteer events than the patient-side factors more commonly described by the prolific media coverage of dental charity fairs. Not uncommonly, such coverage relies on tropes through which poor people are objectified, and thereby poverty distanced from recognition as a *choice* of governance, and through which the scripted articulations of uneven power between patients and providers are brought to life (Adams, 2017; Rivkin-Fish, 2011).

Coursing through these micro-decisions is the fragility of the effects of the moral decisions and affective relationships that occur therein. Take, for example, this vignette from my fieldwork in July 2011:

> I recognized Jeff from two days before, when he asked to enter the
> fairground before the event had begun, to wash his face and refill his

canteen. He carried a large canvas backpack. Jeff sought surgical extraction of three impacted wisdom teeth that had been diagnosed two years earlier. He couldn't afford the procedure and had been self-managing his pain with topical headache powder and white willow branch, avoiding infection by rinsing with warm salt water, and planning his trip to the annual charitable event. Living without a vehicle in this rural location that lacked adequate public transportation, Jeff took a public van from his hometown to within 20 miles of the fairground then walked the rest of the way, sleeping outdoors as he went. As the line moved forward, he expressed his nervousness not at the procedure, but at the hours afterward. In budgeting for the trip, Jeff hadn't calculated for the public van not running on Sundays. He feared a delayed return that would result in him missing work, but also agonized over the decision between two different ways to care for himself in the 36 hours following surgery: pay for one night in a local motel and limit his food expenditures as planned, or sleep outdoors an extra night and absorb an extra day of food expenses. I saw Jeff in recovery a few hours later, his mouth bursting with blood-tinged white gauze and his facial expression concerned with the decision. The event director also noticed his state and came over to inquire. Determining 'We can do better than that', the event director returned to the intake line to ask if anyone was from Jeff's hometown and had room for one more in their vehicle. About fifty people down the line, a man who sought three small fillings and a crown repair raised his hand. 'Congratulations', the event director said, palming him $40 for gas, 'You are now number one in line for services'.

The commonness of such interactions betrays providers and patients' familiarity with rarity of universal dental access and, therefore, the events' high stakes. This results in a shared drive to enrol just one more patient, or deliver one more service to a patient needing multiple services before the close of day. In their pursuit to treat as many unmet patients' needs as possible, dental providers and administrators reflect the heroic side of the power asymmetries described by Fassin's concept of humanitarian reason: bypassing the 'first come, first served' rule of order, contributing funds, supporting patient recovery even if it means arranging transportation, or, in some cases, delivering services as long as possible, even after fellow volunteers have taken scheduled breaks to eat, rest, and enjoy time with colleagues. The potentiality of such 'above-and-beyond' services always privileges providers' capacity above the claims to the right of health care of the patient, who must patiently and often in a pain-filled state await word of whether they will be seen.

The irrefutably qualifying moral and emotional appeal of a man who walked twenty miles and slept outside to receive services signalled to volunteers his stark sacrifice above and beyond the everyday suffering of having unmet dental needs, and prompted action on their part. Similarly, I have observed (and numerous journalists have documented) many other experiences in which the clinical encounter in temporary dental volunteer events is understood by providers and patients alike to interweave *both* of their tenacity as an indicator of moral righteousness, occasionally through a mercurial lens of good luck or, more often, spiritual delivery. At the same time, the determination of services ultimately rests with the provider-volunteer. Foremost among these examples are the distinctions in provider responses to the limited number of patients randomly selected to receive customised dentures the following year in the 'denture lottery'.

For those patients who have attended the event for multiple sequential years to obtain disease management and simple procedures, and tried repeatedly to 'win' the denture lottery, volunteer responses are, not unusually, deeply emotional. Those patients, providers have told me, make their arduous and completely optional volunteer commitment 'worth it'. For these providers, the personal reward of rejuvenating a 'deserving' patient's smile stokes their return to volunteer in subsequent years, thus serving for higher-level gatekeeping on subsequent event success. By contrast, providers have shared with me their ambivalence when lucky patients win the denture lottery at first entry or early in their tenure at these events; while these providers deliver the promised service of denture preparation, it is at times with a stated expectation that those patients won't attend subsequent appointments for fitting, adjusting, and so forth, and that the opportunity has therefore been 'wasted'. Similarly, providers have expressed to me their dampened enthusiasm for volunteering and unwillingness to exceed the standard course of services for patients who they suspect of misusing opioids, who they evaluate to have poor home hygiene, who they believe to be lying about their low-income qualification, or who they perceive as being entitled, for example, expressing disappointment about the limited types of treatments available as the day advances and the concluding hour approaches.

Such interactions obviate the seeming humanitarian universalism—clinicians' relief of strangers' unmet dental needs and their associated physical and psychosocial suffering—engendered in temporary dental volunteer events. They can also have material effect if they reduce service delivery or increase gatekeeping. When considered within the context of dental professional training in the United States, we can also see how they perpetuate a dental social responsibility that exemplifies humanitarian reason.

## Socialising affective morality through dental professional training

In 2019, the annual July MOM in Wise, Virginia, moved indoors for the first time in its twenty-year history. This physical relocation from large tents erected on the county fairgrounds into a local university's multiuse facility gave me a new vantage point to observe social interactions in a more concentrated manner than in prior years. Among other fieldnotes, I wrote this reflective observation:

> After helping some fellow non-clinical volunteers do some set-up and planning about patient flow from pre-registration to registration, I took a

moment to peer over the civic centre's mezzanine to the pre-event action on the main floor. Around thirty volunteers set up the physical space in a clear chain of command, originating with the event director, then to experienced logistics volunteers, then to volunteers present for the sheer physical power of carrying materials … Throughout their hustle, I could see the volunteers pausing to welcome in someone who just arrived, introducing new volunteers—many of them students from my university's dental school, recognizable in branded scrubs or t-shirts—to the established practitioners who would supervise them on the floor. Not infrequently, I overheard a good-humoured burst in the style of 'six degrees of separation'—'Oh, you post-bacced with Dr. L? Great dentist!'—often followed by an exchange of contact information. These social interactions, previously elusive in the serpentine paths of the tents on the outdoor fairgrounds and sometimes literally dampened in the July humidity, seemed to take on a new buoyancy within this high-ceilinged, open view, climate-controlled space. While the Saturday night volunteer appreciation cook-out remained the most formalised networking opportunity, it occurred to me how the new physical space also fostered new social opportunities throughout the three-day event. (Wise, Virginia; 11 July 2019)

As a long-term volunteer at the Wise MOM, I was accustomed to encountering students, who comprise a sizeable labour force at temporary dental volunteer events nationwide. Long-term volunteers joke that as they advance in age, they need the younger, heartier 'next generation' to do the literal heavy lifting of equipment, pallets of chairs, and boxes of materials. Pre-clinical students often invigorate increasingly impatient children each late afternoon, when they draw on their youthful stamina to facilitate silly games in the waiting areas. Conversely, students who find their limited skillset superfluous or the tasks or patient gratitude 'not judged to be worth the time' (Rivkin-Fish, 2011, p. 184) may socialise for an extended time in the volunteer refreshment area or rove the event's exterior. Thus, student volunteerism at temporary dental events exceeds pedagogical and clinical skill development. Through student volunteerism, future dental providers are also socialised as 'ethical clinician-citizens' (Rivkin-Fish, 2011, p. 187), and therefore to specific sociopolitical logics about not only how they can choose to enact their moral and professional responsibilities but also why underserved patients need them to.

Student volunteerism at temporary dental events reflects institutionalised curricular changes that, in the 1990s-era United States, began replacing dental public health and community dentistry specialty training as public practice options were reduced or eliminated and the dental safety net was being privatised (Bailit, 2017; Edelstein et al., 2020). Community-based dental education (CBDE),[4] sometimes described as service-learning, formalised the professional dentistry value of 'service-mindedness' in 2009 and became an elective coursework accreditation requirement in 2015 following nearly two decades of discussion about training programmes' responsibility to address oral health disparities (Centore, 2017; Mathieson et al., 2013). CBDE delivers substantial volumes of care to patients with unmet dental needs; one dental school estimates providing over $5 million in free or reduced fee care to over 14,000 patients annually (Mays & Maguire, 2018).[5]

CBDE-enrolled students deliver supervised care to historically excluded patient populations in 'real-world' settings, then reflect on and interpret their experiences (Hood, 2009; Mays, 2016; Simon et al., 2018).[6] Although coursework addresses social determinants of health and health policy (Mays, 2016), the philosophy and content of training can overlook critical analyses of the systems of power that underlie dental disparities such as how structural racism underlies the inequitable distribution and gatekeeping of oral health services (Bastos et al., 2020; Elaine Muirhead et al., 2020; Lala et al., 2021; Leadbeatter 2020; Lévesque et al., 2017; Moeller and Quiñonez, 2020). Moreover, with the rare exception of dentals schools organised around pathways to careers in community settings, CBDE has not yet demonstrably produced the sustained community-based efforts indicated in its mission to 'serve the oral health needs of society not only by educating oral health care providers, but also by being collaborators in solutions to problems of access to care' (ADEA, 2009; Edelstein, 2020; Gordon et al., 2019; Mays et al., 2019; McQuistan et al., 2014).[7] For example, while clinicians in one state who participated in CBDE report a higher sense of service-mindedness and delivery of charitable care in their office, the annual value of the free or reduced care provided per dentist was comparable to those who didn't participate in CBDE ($11,000 vs. $13,000) (McQuistan et al., 2014).

Even among CBDE students who report improvements in their understanding of the role and functioning of dental safety net policy and practice, intent to work in those settings remains flat (Simon et al., 2018). Although students report that their new understanding of social justice gleaned from CBDE fosters a commitment to addressing oral health disparities (Behar-Horenstein et al., 2015; Sager and Blue, 2019, see also Smith and Mays, 2019), student interest in, empathy towards and sense of social obligation to select patient groups—in particular those who were low-income, Medicaid-insured, rural-residing and non-English speaking—measurably *declines* following CBDE experiences, even among the half of CBDE students whose service commitment exceeds four weeks (Evans, 2019; Major et al., 2016; Mays et al., 2019; Sherman and Cramer, 2005). At least one-third of CBDE students complete their service in short-term intensive placements such as international and domestic temporary dental events that occur, often annually, in locations or among populations where disparities in both oral health outcomes and care persist (Mays, 2016). These now-popular placements are considered prestigious, and in many schools foment competition. Students vie not only for limited spots overall but also for, when eligible to deliver clinical services, unofficial mentorship via placements with potential future employers and, when pre-clinical, assignment to preferential tasks; occasionally, a student who has volunteered for multiple years will be rewarded with a team lead role. Given the intense focus in the environment on delivering the maximum number of services to patients, and thus the demand on providers' time, students often experience substantial autonomy when they are not completing discrete tasks resulting in, as described earlier, students deciding if and when to return to tasks of what they consider low status or limited value. Thus, through CBDE students are socialised into logics that valorise, incentivise, and even gamify through competition the inherently temporary milieu of the volunteer event. Patient needs are supplanted to students' own motivations of participation, whether charitable, competitive, disinterested, or sceptical. Indeed, as the evidence bears out, many students who participate in CBDE learn to 'apply the assumptions built into the moral economy of commodified health care to make sense of the health disparities they observe' (Rivkin-Fish, 2011, p. 187) rather than to understand the structural conditions that underlie oral health disparities in the United States. Accordingly, dental education's value foregrounds social obligation as complementary to rather than constitutive of a career and as of benefit to the future provider apart from, and in some ways superior to, the patient. This is prestige pedagogy, in which students can fulfil service-learning requirements while also networking for future employment.

## Conclusion

The rise and institutionalization of temporary dental care in the United States in the first two decades of the twenty-first century has inhered moral logics in which both established and future providers reproduce the very sociopolitical conditions that have necessitated their creation: optional participation among providers; gatekeeping of services that bypasses claims of universalism; the valorization of elites' charity; and hierarchical decision-making that privileges providers' perspectives over patients. As oral health disparities persist, and as new attention in the field turns to examining power to advancing dentistry's social responsibility *to all* in training, practice, and policy, including viewing dental volunteerism in light of the recent COVID-19 pandemic and racial justice uprising (Bastos et al., 2020; Freeman et al., 2020; Holden and Quiñonez, 2020; Jamieson et al., 2020; Lala et al., 2021; Moeller and Quiñonez, 2020; Quiñonez and Vujicic, 2020), dental humanitarianism merits closer attention, critical analysis, and substantive changes lest it continue to eclipse sustained public health, community, and otherwise universalising dentistry.

## Notes

1 International dental mission trips, whether religiously affiliated or secular, are also a concern for global dental social responsibility. While deserving of critical analysis, they are beyond the scope of this chapter.
2 The ADA House of Delegates rescinded the invocation in 2020, in favour of 'a personal moment of reflection or silent prayer' in order to recognise religious diversity as part of a broader focus on inclusivity (Versaci 2020).

3 While these dynamics are also undoubtedly present through Give Kids a Smile and donated dental services, those types of charitable care are beyond the scope of this chapter.
4 The literature reflects different perspectives on the similarities and distinctions between service-learning and community-based dental education. Generally, service-learning is understood to benefit students' educational development and address underserved communities' needs, often in shorter-term efforts that also offer students 'cross-cultural' experiences both domestically and internationally. Community-based dental education is understood to also often benefit community clinics by providing semi-continuous staffing coverage and revenue streams of billable services.
5 Revenue has also been an important part of the case for schools to adopt CBDE. See, for example, Bailit, 2017.
6 Three US dental schools have explicit missions focused on community dental education. The limited literature suggests that they are more successful than other dental schools in placing students in career trajectories that centre service, for example as FTE dentists at community health centres.
7 The dental student debt burden in the United States is also a structural impediment to practice in dental public health and community-based clinics.

# References

Adams, M. (2017) This annual free Clinic has become 'ground zero' for parachute journalists writing about healthcare in Appalachia', *One hundred days in appalachia* [online]. 25 July 2017. [Viewed 8 September 2021]. Available from: https://www. 100daysinappalachia.com/2017/07/annual-free-clinic-become-ground-zero-parachute-journalists-writing-healthcare-appalachia/

ADEA. (2009) 'ADEA statement on professionalism in dental education [online]'. [Viewed 8 September 2021]. Available from: https://www.adea.org/Pages/Professionalism.aspx

Arefi, P., Cardoso, E. and Azarpazhooh, A. (2020) 'Reexamining dental outreach programs: A model for local empowerment and sustainable development', *Journal of the American Dental Association* [online], 151(5), pp. 340–348. [Viewed 8 September 2021]. Available from: doi: 10.1016/j.adaj.2020.01.023

Bailit, H. L. (2017) 'Are dental schools part of the safety net?', *Journal of Dental Education* [online], 81(8), pp. eS88–eS96. [Viewed 8 September 2021]. Available from: doi: 10.21815/JDE.017.012

Baillie Smith, M. and Laurie, N. (2011) 'International volunteering and development: Global citizenship and neoliberal professionalisation today', *Transactions of the Institute of British Geographers* [online], 36(4), pp. 545–559. [Viewed 8 September 2021]. Available from: doi: 10.1111/j.1475-5661.2011.00436.x

Balasubramanian, M., Brennan, D. S., Short, S. D. and Gallagher, J. E. (2019) 'A strife of interests: a qualitative study on the challenges facing oral health workforce policy and planning', *Health Policy* [online], 123(11), pp. 1068–1075. [Viewed 8 September 2021]. Available from: doi: 10.1016/j.healthpol.2019.07.010

Bastos, J. L., Constante, H. M., Celeste, R. K., Haag, D. G. and Jamieson, L. M. (2020) 'Advancing racial equity in oral health (research): more of the same is not enough', *European Journal of Oral Sciences* [online], 128(6), pp. 1–8. [Viewed 8 September 2021]. Available from: doi: 10.1111/eos.12737

Behar-Horenstein, L. S., Feng, X., Roberts, K. W., Gibbs, M., Catalanotto, F. A. and Hudson-Vassell, C. M. (2015) 'Developing dental students' awareness of health care disparities and desire to serve vulnerable populations through service-learning',

*Journal of Dental Education* [online], 79(10), pp. 1189–1200. [Viewed 8 September 2021]. Available from: doi: 10.1002/j.0022-0337.2015.79.10.tb06012.x

Centore, L. (2017) 'Trends in behavioral sciences education in dental schools, 1926 to 2016', *Journal of Dental Education* [online], 81(8), pp. eS66–eS73. [Viewed 8 September 2021]. Available from: doi: 10.21815/jde.017.009

Dharamsi, S., Pratt, D. D. and MacEntee, M. I. (2007) 'How dentists account for social responsibility: economic imperatives and professional obligations', *Journal of Dental Education* [online], 71(12), 1583–1592. [Viewed 8 Septiber 2021]. Available from: doi: 10.1002/j.0022-0337.2007.71.12.tb04435.x

Edelstein, B. L. (2009) 'Putting teeth in CHIP: 1997–2009 retrospective of Congressional Action on children's oral health', *Academic Pediatrics* [online], 9(6), pp. 467–475. [Viewed 8 September 2021]. Available from: doi: 10.1016/j.acap.2009.09.002

Edelstein, B. L. (2020) 'Pediatric dental care and oral health: past successes and current challenges', *Academic Pediatrics* [online], 20(7), pp. 885–888. [Viewed 8 September 2021]. Available from: doi: 10.1016/j.acap.2020.06.139

Edelstein, B. L., Perkins, J. and Vargas, C. M. (2020) *The role of law and policy in increasing the use of the oral health care system and services.* Washington DC: Office of Disease Prevention and Health Promotion. [Viewed 8 September 2021]. Available from: https://www.healthypeople.gov/sites/default/files/OH_report_2020-07-13_508_0.pdf

Elaine Muirhead, V., Milner, A., Freeman, R., Doughty, J. and Macdonald, M. E. (2020) 'What is intersectionality and why is it important in oral health research?', *Community Dentistry and Oral Epidemiology* [online], 48(6), pp. 464–470. [Viewed 8 September 2021]. Available from: doi: 10.1111/cdoe.12573

Evans, C. A. (2019) 'Preparing future dentists to address oral health inequities: the continuing need', *Journal of Dental Education* [online], 83(11), pp. 1251–1252. [Viewed 8 September 2021]. Available from: doi: 10.21815/jde.019.128

Fassin, D. (2012) *Humanitarian reason: a moral history of the present.* Berkley: University of California Press. [Viewed 8 September 2021]. Available from: https://hdl-handle-net.proxy.library.vcu.edu/2027/heb.33897

Fassin, D. (2013) 'The predicament of humanitarianism', *Qui Parle: Critical Humanities and Social Sciences* [online], 22(1), pp. 33–48. [Viewed 8 September 2021]. Available from: doi: 10.5250/quiparle.22.1.0033

Freeman, R., Doughty, J., Macdonald, M. E. and Muirhead, V.M. (2020) 'Inclusion oral health: advancing a theoretical framework for policy, research and practice', *Community Dentistry and Oral Epidemiology* [online], 48(1), pp. 1–6. [Viewed 8 September 2021]. Available from: doi: 10.1111/cdoe.12500

Gordon, S., Warren, A. C. and Wright, W. G. (2019) 'Influence of community-based dental education on practice choice: preliminary data from East Carolina University', *Journal of Dental Education* [online], 83(9), pp. 1000–1011. [Viewed 8 September 2021]. Available from: doi: 10.21815/jde.019.101

Holden, A. C. L. (2020) 'Exploring the evolution of a dental code of ethics: A critical discourse analysis', *BMC Medical Ethics* [online], 21(1), pp. 1–7. [Viewed 8 September 2021]. Available from: doi: 10.1186/s12910-020-00485-3

Holden, A. C. L. and Quiñonez, C. (2020) 'The role of the dental professional association in the 21st Century', *International Dental Journal* [online], 70(4), pp. 239–244. [Viewed 8 September 2021]. Available from: doi: 10.1111/idj.12563

Hood, J. G. (2009) 'Service-learning in dental education: meeting needs and challenges', *Journal of Dental Education* [online], 73(4), pp. 454–463. [Viewed 8 September 2021]. Available from: doi: 10.1002/j.0022-0337.2009.73.4.tb04716.x

Jamieson, L., Gibson, B. and Thomson, W. M. (2020) 'Oral health inequalities and the corporate determinants of health: a commentary', *International Journal of Environmental Research and Public Health* [online], 17(18), pp. 6529. [Viewed 8 September 2021]. Available from: doi: 10.3390/ijerph17186529

Lala, R., Gibson, B. J. and Jamieson, L. M. (2021) 'The relevance of power in dentistry'. *JDR Clinical and Translational Research* [online]. [Viewed 8 September 2021]. Available from: doi: 10.1177/2380084421998619

Leadbeatter, D. and Holden, A. C. L. (2020) 'How are the social determinants of health being taught in dental education?', *Journal of Dental Education* [online], 85(4), pp. 1–16. [Viewed 8 September 2021]. Available from: doi: 10.1002/jdd.12487

Lee, J. Y., and Divaris, K. (2014) 'The ethical imperative of Addressing Oral Health Disparities', *Journal of Dental Research* [online], 93(3), pp. 224–230. [Viewed 8 September 2021]. Available from: doi: 10.1177/0022034513511821

Lévesque, M., Levine, A. and Bedos, C. (2017) 'Humanizing oral health care through continuing education on social determinants of health: evaluative case study of a Canadian Private Dental Clinic', *Journal of Health Care for the Poor and Underserved* [online], 27(3), pp. 971–992. [Viewed 8 September 2021]. Available from: doi: 10.1353/hpu.2016.0139

Major, N., McQuistan, M. R. and Qian, F. (2016) 'Changes in dental students' attitudes about treating underserved populations: a longitudinal study', *Journal of Dental Education* [online], 80(5), pp. 517–525. [Viewed 8 September 2021]. Available from: doi: 10.1002/j.0022-0337.2016.80.5.tb06111.x

Mathieson, K. M., Gross-Panico, M. L., Cottam, W. W. and Woldt, J. L. (2013) 'Critical incidents, successes, and challenges of community-based dental education', *Journal of Dental Education* [online], 77(4), pp. 427–437. [Viewed 8 September 2021]. Available from: doi: 10.1002/j.0022-0337.2013.77.4.tb05488.x

Mays, K. A. (2016) 'Community-based dental education models: an analysis of current practices at U.S. dental schools', *Journal of Dental Education* [online], 80(10), pp. 1188–1195. [Viewed 8 September 2021]. Available from: doi: 10.1002/j.0022-033 7.2016.80.10.tb06201.x

Mays, K. A., and Maguire, M. (2018) 'Care provided by students in community-based dental education: helping meet oral health needs in underserved communities', *Journal of Dental Education* [online], 82(1), pp. 20–28. [Viewed 8 September 2021]. Available from: doi: 10.21815/jde.018.003

Mays, K. A., Scheffert, D. R., Maguire, M., Lunos, S., Johnson, R., Jackson, L. and Riggs, S. (2019) 'Dental students' intent to practice in rural communities before and after community-based rotations in a rural area', *Journal of Dental Education* [online], 83(11), pp. 1296–1303. [Viewed 8 September 2021]. Available from: doi: 10.21815/jde.019.142

McQuistan, M. R., Mohamad, A. and Kuthy, R. A. (2014) 'Association between dentists' participation in charitable care and community-based dental education', *Journal of Dental Education* [online]. 78(1), pp. 110–118. [Viewed 8 September 2021]. Available from: doi: 10.1002/j.0022-0337.2014.78.1.tb05662.x

Moeller, J. and Quiñonez, C. R. (2020) 'Dentistry's social contract is at risk', *Journal of the American Dental Association* [online], 151(5), pp. 334–339. [Viewed 8 September 2021]. Available from: doi: 10.1016/j.adaj.2020.01.022

Mouradian, W. E. (2006) 'Band-Aid solutions to the dental access crisis: conceptually flawed-A response to Dr. David H. Smith', *Journal of Dental Education* [online], 70(11), pp. 1174–1179. [Viewed 8 September 2021]. Available from: doi: 10.1002/j.0022-033 7.2006.70.11.tb04194.x

Otto, M. (2017) Teeth: The story of beauty, inequality, and the struggle for oral health in America. The New Press.

Patthoff, D. E. (2007) 'The need for dental ethicists and the promise of universal patient acceptance: response to Richard Masella's "renewing professionalism in dental education', *Journal of Dental Education* [online], 71(2), pp. 222–226. [Viewed 8 September 2021]. Available from: doi: 10.1002/j.0022-0337.2007.71.2.tb04269.x

Quiñonez, C. and Vujicic, M. (2020) 'COVID-19 has clarified 2 foundational policy questions in dentistry', *JDR Clinical and Translational Research* [online], 5(4), 297–299. [Viewed 8 September 2021]. Available from: doi: 10.1177/2380084420941777

Raskin, S. (2015) *Decayed, missing, and filled: Subjectivity and the dental safety net in central Appalachia*. Ph.D. thesis, The University of Arizona. [Viewed 8 September 2021]. Available from: https://media.proquest.com/media/pq/classic/doc/3834553901/fmt/ai/rep/NPDF?_s=XDG7osc9QAJhXDXY3uMCoeNO8EU%3D

Rivkin-Fish, M. (2011) 'Learning the moral economy of commodified health care: "community education," failed consumers, and the shaping of ethical clinician-citizens', *Culture, Medicine and Psychiatry* [online], 35(2), pp. 183–208. [Viewed 8 September 2021]. Available from: doi: 10.1007/s11013-011-9208-0

Rozario, K. (2003) 'Delicious horrors': mass culture, the Red Cross, and the appeal of modern American humanitarianism', *American Quarterly*, 55(3), pp. 417–455. [Viewed 8 September 2021]. Available from: https://www.jstor.org/stable/30041983

Sager, J. J., and Blue, C. M. (2019) 'Reflective learning outcomes of community-based experiences: a qualitative study', *Journal of Dental Education* [online], 83(5), 530–535. [Viewed 8 September 2021]. Available from: doi: 10.21815/jde.019.061

Sherman, J. J. and Cramer, A. (2005) 'Measurement of changes in empathy during dental school', *Journal of Dental Education* [online], 69(3), pp. 338–345. [Viewed 8 September 2021]. Available from: doi: 10.1002/j.0022-0337.2005.69.3.tb03920.x

Simon, L., Shroff, D., Barrow, J. and Park, S. E. (2018) 'A reflection curriculum for longitudinal community-based clinical experiences: impact on student perceptions of the safety net', *Journal of Dental Education* [online], 82(1), 12–19. [Viewed 8 September 2021]. Available from: doi: 10.21815/jde.018.004

Smith, P. D. and Mays, K. A. (2019) 'Dental students' non-clinical learning during community-based experiences: a survey of U.S. dental schools', *Journal of Dental Education* [online], 83(11), pp. 1289–1295. [Viewed 8 September 2021]. Available from: doi: 10.21815/jde.019.130

Treadwell, H. M. and Northridge, M. E. (2007) 'Oral health is the measure of a just society', *Journal of Health Care for the Poor and Underserved* [online], 18(1), 12–20. [Viewed 8 September 2021]. Available from: doi: 10.1353/hpu.2007.0021

Virginia Health Care Foundation. (2013) *Models that made it: Mission of Mercy*. Viewed 8 September 2021]. Available from: http://www.vhcf.org/wp-content/uploads/2010/09/MOM-Guidebook-FINAL.pdf

# Index

Note: Page numbers in *italic* indicate figures and in **bold** indicate tables, and page numbers followed by 'n' refer to notes.

For Product Safety Concerns and Information please contact our EU
representative  GPSR@taylorandfrancis.com
Taylor & Francis Verlag GmbH, Kaufingerstraße 24, 80331 München, Germany

www.ingramcontent.com/pod-product-compliance
Lightning Source LLC
Chambersburg PA
CBHW060248220326
41598CB00027B/4024